CONCEPTS AND THEORIES
IN CARCINOGENESIS

CONCEPTS AND THEORIES IN CARCINOGENESIS

Proceedings of the 4th Annual Symposium of the European Organization for Cooperation in Cancer Prevention Studies (ECP) Brugge, Belgium, June 11–13, 1986

Editors:

Alain P. Maskens
Medical Co-ordinator, ECP, Brussels, Belgium

Peter Ebbesen
The Institute of Cancer Research, The Danish Cancer Society, Aarhus, Denmark

A. Burny
Department of Molecular Biology, University of Brussels, Rhode-St-Genese, Belgium

 1987

EXCERPTA MEDICA, Amsterdam - New York - Oxford

International Congress Series No. 732
ISBN 0 444 80869 8

Published by:
Elsevier Science Publishers B.V. (Biomedical Division)
P.O. Box 211
1000 AE Amsterdam
The Netherlands

Sole distributors for the USA and Canada:
Elsevier Science Publishing Company Inc.
52 Vanderbilt Avenue
New York, NY 10017
USA

Library of Congress Cataloging in Publication Data:

```
European Organization for Cooperation in Cancer
    Prevention Studies.  Symposium (4th : 1986 :
    Bruges, Belgium)
    Concepts and theories in carcinogenesis.

    (International congress series ; no. 732)
    Includes index.
    1. Carcinogenesis--Congresses.  I. Maskens,
Alain P.  II. Ebbesen, Peter.  III. Burny, A.
IV. Title.  V. Series.  [DNLM: 1. Neoplasms--
etiology--congresses.  W3 EX89 no.732 /
QZ 202 E89 1986c]
RC268.5.E96  1986      616.99'4071      86-32993
ISBN 0-444-80869-8 (U.S.)
```

Printed in The Netherlands

Foreword

ECP (European Organization for Cooperation in Cancer Prevention Studies) was established in 1981 with the object of fostering the development of preventive studies on a European basis, since the activities of EORTC (European Organization for Research on Treatment of Cancer) were restricted to research on cancer treatment.

In order to achieve this aim, various working groups - to deal with specific cancers or aspects of cancer aetiology, and to explore the opportunities for advances on a cooperative European basis - were established. It was also decided to hold annual symposia to draw general attention to a field in which there seemed to be many opportunities for progress in matters of prevention.

At present, eight working groups are active in fields such as cancer of the respiratory tract, cancer of the breast, colorectal cancer, diet and cancer, sexual factors and cancer, viruses and cancer, AIDS and cancer, and, finally, public information in the field of cancer prevention. Annual symposia have been devoted to themes of high priority for cancer prevention: 'Tobacco and Cancer' (1983), 'Hormones and Sexual Factors in Human Cancer Aetiology' (1984), and 'Diet and Human Carcinogenesis' (1985).

This volume contains the proceedings of the 1986 symposium, held in Bruges, Belgium, June 11–13, on 'Concepts and Theories in Carcinogenesis'. The aim this time was to review our current knowledge on more theoretical or experimental aspects of carcinogenesis, as a basis for the design of new approaches in preventive oncology. Owing to the high level of the contributions, participants were exposed to an outstanding, up-to-date overview on the many aspects of this field, from molecular level to the cell, tissue, organism and finally at the environmental level. It also became apparent that conceptual and even terminological differences clearly exist between the various 'subfields'; differences which however, could be partially reduced or were, at least, better identified during the discussions, or during the workshop which followed the symposium. The symposium was also enriched by an especially valuable poster session, the abstracts of which have been published in a special issue of 'Cancer Letters' (Vol. 30, suppl. June 1986).

We are indebted to the speakers for their contributions during the symposium and the workshop, and for their prompt submission of manuscripts. The help of Professor J. Pontèn from Uppsala and Drs H. Barbason from Liège and A. Hall from London in the Program Committee was also much appreciated.

We are grateful to the sponsors of this symposium, especially the World Health Organization and the Association Contre le Cancer (Belgium). ECP also acknowledges with gratitude the support provided by the Fonds National de la Recherche Scientifique (Brussels), the City of Bruges, the Province of West-Flander, the Fonds Anne-Lise pour la Lutte contre le Cancer (Brussels), and the members of the ECP Foundation Belgium.

Our appreciation also goes to Mrs. C. Cattoir for the excellent organization of the Symposium, and to Ms. C. Gueur and Mr. Ph. Maes for their help in preparing the scientific aspects of the symposium as well as these proceedings.

The 1987 ECP symposium will be on preventive strategies of cancers related to immune-deficiency syndromes. It will be held in Brussels, on May 8–10.

Alain Maskens
Arsène Burny
Peter Ebbesen

Contents

The tissue level: Multistep carcinogenesis

Internal and external environment

Index of authors

INTRODUCTORY LECTURE

© 1987 Elsevier Science Publishers B.V. (Biomedical Division)
Concepts and theories in carcinogenesis. A.P. Maskens et al. eds.

NORMAL VS NEOPLASTIC TISSUE BEHAVIOR : WHAT DIFFERENCES ARE ESSENTIAL ?

J. PONTEN

University of Uppsala, Department of Pathology, University Hospital, S-75185 Uppsala, Sweden

The remarkable dynamic equilibrium which exists within multicellular organisms presents one of the most vexing unresolved problems in biology. The programs, controls and environmental guidelines and clues which cells will have to follow in order to preserve optimal population size and interactions during fetal development and adult life under constantly varying external and internal conditions are only vaguely understood. Neoplasia can be conceived of as the most important departure from this homeostasis, which must be evolutionary ancient and a prerequisite for endowing multicellular life with competitive strength compared to the unicellular life-style.

Much ingenuity has been invested in defining one single ("pathognomonic") feature of neoplastic cells which would absolutely distinguish them from their normal counterparts. All such claims have, however, never stood up to experimental tests and we still cannot define neoplasia in any unambigous and insightful manner. But for descriptive purposes I will use the following operational list (table 1). It summarizes the essential ways in which neoplastic cell populations depart in their behavior from normal tissues. It is phrased in terms of "transformations" to emphasize the irreversibility. In contrast to hyperplasia, which is polyclonal, neoplasia always seems to be monoclonal.

A. LACK OF PROPER PROLIFERATION CONTROL (UNRESTRAINED GROWTH TRANSFORMATION)

In all organs the number of cells is kept roughly constant by different complicated schemes. The mechanisms for this important regulation are still poorly understood, but a picture begins to emerge where an intricate "microendocrine" network operates in solid tissues via secretion of polypeptides which adjust proliferation and its close companion - differentiation according to physiologic needs.

The network is decisively modified by the responsiveness of the cells themselves. Some cells do not have receptors for the secreted growth factors and are therefore inaccessible to their action. Even when provided with adequate numbers of receptors cells in dense mutual contact will not - at least in vitro - respond with proliferation even under heavy bombardment by growth factors, "contact inhibition". They stay "switched off" until they regain responsiveness, for instance after traumatic cell loss.

This general scheme is modified in hematopoietic tissues. Some growth factors act over long distances. Responsiveness of cells is largely governed by receptors which are turned on or off depending on the stage of differentiation of the target cells.

Unrestrained growth transformation is the basis for the capacity of malignant (and benign) tumors to increase in mass even though there is no demand for more cells of that particular kind. The dynamic ways by which this will unfold varies from tissue to tissue, for instance depending on whether it - in its normal state - is "constantly regenerating" (e.g. bone marrow, epidermis) or "resting" (e.g. liver, connective tissue, glia). The respective contribution to unrestrained growth transformation by excessive production of growth factors, abnormal responsiveness to growth stimuli by cells, failure to become "switched off" even at high local cell density and unknown factors remains enigmatic.

Unrestrained growth is a population phenomenon where the relative contribution by excessive multiplication or prolonged life span will vary from case to case. It can be assessed in vitro in cells growing on a solid support as a failure to suppress DNA synthesis at progressively increasing local cell density - "lack of density inhibition of mitosis".

B. CHANGED, INTERCELLULAR "SOCIAL" BEHAVIOR (IRREGULAR MIGRATION
   TRANSFORMATION)

Cells are normally equipped with well developed senses of local orientation. Epithelium is for instance separated from stroma by a barrier - the basal membrane. Displaced epidermis is reported not to survive as if specific contact with the upper dermis is required for growth. Evidence begins to accumulate that cell surface molecules (glycoproteins and - lipids ?) mediate this type of recognition.

Irregular migration transformation alters these finely tuned intercellular relations. In carcinoma in situ, cells within the epithelial layer become more randomly arranged than normally, signalling deficient regulation of mobility. When invasion supervenes carcinoma cells have acquired the additional capacity to thrive also beyond the basal membrane and occupy new territories.

Mesenchymal cells from solid tissues, which normally are not geographically constrained by any basement membranes show their irregular transformation for instance by a capacity to penetrate into vessels.

Lymphocytes which normally wander between cells, move in and out of vessels and thrive at certain preferred sites will show their irregular migration transformation by departure from this highly developed behavior for instance by a failure to enter the blood stream and follow normal ones for their "homing".

The manifestations of irregular migration transformation will differ depending on the properties of the cells in the non-transformed state. The common denominator is a permanent departure from normal locomotory and homing behavior. It can be assessed in vitro as lack of contact inhibition of membrane movement resulting in overlapping 'criss - cross' growth.

It is generally believed that irregular migration transformation explains not only the capacity for local invasion by malignant tumors but also their metastazing ability.

C. ESCAPE FROM CELLULAR SENESCENCE (INFINITE GROWTH TRANSFORMATION; IMMORTALIZATION)

Populations of normal somatic cells, with the possible but unproven exception of certain stem-cells, only seem to have two options if forced to multiply excessively a) gradual loss proliferative capacity leading to total reproductive sterility. This so called cellular senescence occurs after a predetermined number of divisions characteristic for different organs and species or b) acquire capacity for infinite growth which, with some exceptions, is coupled to growth as a malignant tumor. Apparently, malignant tumor cell populations have this ability of increase in net cell number for an indefinite period of time. The mechanism behind infinite growth transformation remains elusive, but its dynamics may again differ between malignancies originating in constantly regenerating "stem-cell" tissues such as bone-marrow or epidermis and stationary "non-stem cell" tissues such as liver, glia or connective tissue.

Infinite growth transformation, which should be regarded as a population phenomenon is present when creation of new cells by mitosis over extended time exceeds the rate of cell death. It explains why malignant tumors but not normal tissue can be indefinitely transferred in vivo or in vitro.

D. GENOMIC ALTERATIONS (GENETIC DIVERSITY TRANSFORMATION)

Each kind of normal cells is homogenous in the sense that only a predetermined set of genes characteristic of the respective kind is expressed. This is the basis for harmonic development and differentiation.

Normal embryonic development occurs via sequential commitment of clones of cells to increasingly specialized tasks. The mechanism is largely unknown but it involves the permanent deactivation of large blocks of specific genes which cannot any more be transcribed. Whith the exception of the creation of B- and T-lymphocyte clones, which requires orderly gene rearrangements, no alteration of the genomic linear nucleotide sequence accompanies normal development and differentiation.

A malignant clone will not follow this pattern. It may activate otherwise silent genes and more importantly may express genes in a discordant fashion with reexpression of fetal antigens and paraneoplastic symptoms as possible consequences. Indirect evidence suggests that recombination of preexisting genes also may occur with formation of proteins never seen in normal cells.

With few possible but unproven exceptions malignancies have genetic alterations. They vary within a wide range. Most squamous cell carcinomas and adenocarcinomas have gross abnormalities with large increase in number of chromosomes which also show multiple rearrangements. Other malignancies mainly of hematopoietic or endocrine origin may not show measurable changes in DNA content or chromosome alterations with routine techniques. Banding methods and detailed structural DNA anlyses have, however, disclosed subtle alterations also in malignant cells previously considered karyotypically normal. This has strongly reinforced the old 'somatic cell mutation hypothesis' for cancer. It seems very reasonable to assume that the irreversible malignant phenotype which seems to be invariably passed on to each daughter cell of a malignant population is caused and maintained by permanent genotypic change.

Genetic changes ranging from chromosomes abnormalities to point mutations are, of course, also a prominent feature in many non-neoplastic somatic cells. A peculiar feature of genomic disturbances in malignant, in contrast to normal cells, may be their progressive nature. In serially propagated cancer cell populations new genotypes will evolve. In vivo malignancies which originally are diploid (chronic leukemias in man for example) often end up with aneuploidy as so called blast crises.

Modern methods have permitted extensive analysis of malignant cells. They have shown a multitude of structural and functional changes in virtually every metabolic pathway. Cancer cells are thus more profoundly disturbed than previously thought. The total pattern of these disturbances differs from case to case so that each one seems to have its own unique set of departures from normal. No single aberration or set of abnormalities has been found which distinguishes neoplastic from normal cells. This would explain the unpredictable behaviour of individual malignancies with respect to growth rate, development of metastases, systemic effects, response to therapy etc.

Most malignancies display considerable intercellular variability with respect e.g. to expression of antigens, chromosomes constitution and ultrastructure. These features almost certain by form the basis for two key microscopic criteria of malignancy - atypia (=profound structural disturbance) and pleomorphism (=intercellular variability). The reason for this remarkable relaxation of strict control of the genotype and permission of creation of new viable phenotypes remains unknown. It may well differ in degree between various malignancies. In man most common carcinomas are extremely heterogenous, whereas lymphomas, leukemias, a proportion of mammary cancers especially the tubular carcinomas, well differentiated thyroid carcinomas and certain neuroendocrine tumours such as carcinoids are predominantly diploid and presumably considerably less heterogenous in their genomes.

The existing heterogeneity can be thought of as soil for Darwinian selection of increasingly fit cells. It would explain development of drug resistance because of selection of unresponsive cell variants. It would also explain progression from in situ to invasive carcinoma. It predicts that many if not all malignant tumours are mosaics of different clones in spite of the fact that they all are progeny of one primarily fully transformed cell according to the generally accepted theory of monoclonal origin of malignant tumors.

INDEPENDENCE OF THE FOUR COMPONENTS OF THE MALIGNANT TETRAD

Two items are necessary to clarify before elaborating on this central question. The <u>relative stability</u> of cells from different species and <u>benign</u> versus - <u>malignant</u> neoplasia.

Abundant observations in vitro have made it clear that vast differences exist between normal tissues with respect of their "spontaneous" tendency to undergo a malignant change. One extreme is represented by the mouse where all cells capable of at least some degree of multiplication in vitro have a definite probability of forming established lines, which become tumorigenic. The other end of the spectrum is represented by human and avian cells which apparently never undergo malignant transformation spontaneously in vitro. That this is a species - rather than organ - dependent difference is demonstrated by the fact that mesenchymal, epithelial and hematopoietic cells of the respective species behave similarly. The reason for such a conspicuous difference has not been elucidated, one possibility may, however, be that mouse cells have less efficient mechanisms for DNA repair than human cells. Conceivably mutations could then accumulate at such a high rate that a malignant transformation would ensue before the cells had reached the end of their finite life span. Certain facts argue against this explanation. 1. Human cells from xeroderma pigmentosum with its deficient DNA repair have not been reported to undergo any spontaneous or UV induced transformation. 2. Human embryonic fibroblasts will be able to undergo perhaps as many as 100 doublings in culture before losing capacity for further cell cycles with creation of an enormous number of cells, but still no malignant transformants. Mouse fibroblasts, on the other hand, only have to undergo as few as a dozen doublings until transformation ensues. It is difficult to see how a quantitative difference in DNA repair would explain such a huge difference in behavior.

The species differences with respect to spontaneous transformation have generally been accepted as important facts. It has, however, not always been appreciated that they also pervade aspects of induced malignant transformation. Many examples may be quoted such as the ease by which sarcomas are caused by foreign bodies implanted in mice, whereas such tumors seem to be absent in the human situation, where of course numerous instances exist of inadvertent exposure to implanted solid matter. The readiness by which mineral oil produces rodent plasmocytomas may be another case in point, as may the papilloma to carcinoma sequence in murine chemical skin carcinogenesis. More recently the same difference has been seen with transfection of oncogenes. Up till now no single oncogene or any combination thereof have been sufficient to accomplish full malignant transformation of human or avian cells, whereas this can be done reproducibly with mouse cells.

Because of the ill understood vagaries of rodent and other unstable species it seems prudent to concentrate a discussion of essential facets of the malignant phenotype to human and other stable species.

In this setting a dividing line can be drawn between benign and malignant tumors, where human pathologists and oncologists have assembled abundant empirical material. In terms of table 1 data may be summarized as follows. Benign tumors only show unrestrained growth transformation - all the other features of the "malignant tetrad" seem to be absent, contrary to the impression sometimes gained from observation of rodent neoplasias. Few experiments have been performed on the transformability of benign neoplastic cells compared to normal ones; there are no positive data to show that the former would be particularly prone to undergo malignant transformation. Again the stable benign behavior of such common human tumors as fibromas, lipomas, papillomas etc. may reflect the inherent stability of our species.

To understand whether any or all of the feature of table 1 would constitute essential differences between normal and malignant tissues, it would be most desirable to have an experimental system based on stable cells, where all steps could be taken under controlled conditions. This is unfortunately not the case yet. In spite of fierce attempts no reproducible system exists for complete malignant transformation of for instance human cells. Deductions about crucial differences between normal and malignant tissues are therefore uncertain.

Over the years a considerable number of human cancers have been studied either as tissue culture lines or in a more limited fashion as serially transplanted tumors. One major bias is that the capacity for different cancers to form lines in vitro varies enormously. Whereas less than one percent of breast cancers become established virtually all Burkitt lymphomas can be serially propagated in vitro. It is thus impossible to exclude that the lines which have been studied represent malignancies with peculiar but undefined properties which would permit establishment in culture. But if this possibility is left aside abundant evidence exists that all human malignancies (and also those from other mammals) share the properties of table 1. Are then all four equally important or is one of them more crucial than the others? Do they have to be coexpressed or are they linked to each other in any other way ? Recent dissection with oncogenes introduced into human or chicken cells (two stable species) begins to give answers to this question.

Human cells infected with Simian Sarcoma Virus (SSV with v-sis) and Feline Sarcoma Virus (FeSV with v-fes) or chicken cells transformed by Rous sarcoma virus (RSV with v-src) have reacted in a principally similar fashion. They have rapidly developed <u>unrestrained growth and irregular migration transformation</u>, which by the use of temperature sensitive mutants (v-src) has been shown to depend on an intact viral oncogene. In spite of prolonged propagation of the respective transformed cells no evidence has been seen of infinite growth or genetic diversity transformation. In fact, transformation has only a small if any effect on the total number of subsequent possible cells doublings. Also cells remain diploid after transformation by the viruses mentioned. This implies that multiple and apparently random integration of provirus is not sufficient to drive cells from stable species to full malignancy. This multiclonal proliferation instead resembles hyperplasia or multiple benign tumors ("fibromatosis"). If on the other hand rodents are used as targets of for instance RSV or SSV true malignant tumors or fully transformed cells in vitro are formed. The activity of v-sis has been particularly illuminating. This gene is known to be practically identical to the cellular gene (c-sis) coding for the B-chains of the potent growth factor PDGF. SSV has apparently acquired its neoplastic potential by adding one PDGF gene copied from a normal fibroblast genome to its own genome. Comparisons have been carried out between human cells exposed to PDGF from the outside or from within by transformation by sis-gene carrying SSV. Essentially no difference was found in the behavior of the transformed cells. The conclusion will therefore be that SSV - in a stable species - owes its entire transforming potential to its capacity to induce constant overproduction of a growth factor but that this does not suffice to generate the entire malignant tetrad. If the interactions between PDGF and its specific cell membrane receptor (the autocrine circle) is blocked by antibody the transformed cell reverts to normal growth behavior.

A search for expression of oncogenes has disclosed that transcripts of PDGF A and/or B chains exist in a large proportion of human malignant tumors, where gliomas have been particularly well studied. One salient finding has been that the expression of sis and presence of PDGF receptor show clonal variation with all possible combination of presence and absence of receptor/growth factor. The almost inevitable conclusion has been that although expression of this gene may give some growth advantage it cannot be sufficient for the malignant phenotype. This idea is further supported by the inability of PDGF antibody to inhibit growth or influence malignant cells in any other fashion. All other data on oncogene expression in human malignancies seem compatible with this idea, because in no instance have attempts to interrupt such putative autocrine circles led to normalization of cell growth control.

Infinite growth transformation has been difficult to study because it can only be indirectly assessed by the absence of irreversible reproductive sterility upon prolonged serial cultivation. Two facts argue against a primary role. One is the effect of mononucleosis virus infection (EBV) on human B-lymphocytes. Most adults carry EBV in a proportion of their B-lymphocytes. These cells can be shown to be immortal by explantation and serial cultivation in vitro. In spite of this, virtually all malignant lymphomas except Burkitt's are EBV negative. This suggests that the generality of malignant lymphomas even in individuals with immortal B-lymphocytes develop from other cells which were not immortalized prior to the transformation process. The second argument derives from observations of established rodent cell lines such as 3T3 where one can select against unrestrained growth and irregular migration transformation with perpetuation of immortality. Such populations have a strongly reduced tumorigenicity, again suggesting that the immortalization may not be the primary component of the malignant tetrad.

Genetic damage of any kind is not sufficient to cause malignancy. The peculiarity with malignant cells seems to be their genomic instability with creation of new genotypes apparently not only by the acquisition of new point mutations but by minor or major rearrangements within and between chromosomes. Attempts to induce complete transformation of human cells by chemical carcinogens or irradiation have not been encouraging. Altered growth behavior with decreased dependence on serum and/or capacity for anchorage independent growth has been reported, but it has not been convincingly shown that this corresponds to complete transformation as manifested in explanted bona fide human cancers. The only possible experimental mechanisms by which progressive persisting genetic damage can be induced seems to be via infection by SV40. This DNA virus may immortalize human fibroblasts and epidermal cells. Such lines have profound progressive chromosome rearrangements and display unrestrained growth transformation. They resemble explanted human malignant tumor lines in all respects listed in table 1 and may therefore be the only experimental counterpart of spontaneous malignant human neoplasias. We do not know if other genes than early transforming SV40 genes are important for creation of the fully transformed phenotype. The tumorigenicity of SV40 transformed cells seems to be low, it is not known if this depends on their strong antigenicity or other factors.

EVOLUTION OF MALIGNANT TUMOURS

Any theory of carcinogenesis will have to explain the apparent multi-hit nature of human cancers and a long latency time between first exposure to a carcinogen and manifest neoplasia. The task is further complicated by the fact that cancers seem to originate from one single transformed cell. The process is probably very complicated, but a model which would fit current experimental data could be one where genetic damage would be the primary and most essential event. The damage would be such that it would permit cell division and emergence of "new" genotypes.

Preservation of the somatic genotype in spite of mutations, presence of physiologic mechanisms for gene rearrangement i.e. lymphocyte differentiation and the possibly strong tendency for cellular DNA to replicate autonomously ("selfish DNA") must be efficient to prevent accumulation of too many erroneously functioning cells. The most important but entirely non-specific mechanism by which this is accomplished is probably through terminal differentiation. Large numbers of somatic cells are eliminated during the life-span of any animal. This "waste" will in all likelihood contain many severely mutated cells; some of which may be "premalignant".

It is often stated that the probability of any given cell to become malignantly transformed is exceedingly low. Such estimates are based on the assumption that virtually all somatic cells persist long enough to be at risk. I find it more logical also to calculate with the fact that a cell has to persist for many decades after its first insult in a human being to have a chance to develop into a cancer cell. Such long lived "stem-like" cells may in fact be rare and malignant transformation therefore not as uncommon on a per cell at risk basis as conventionally thought.

Little is known about mechanisms for DNA rearrangements. Theoretically, there need not be any requirement for cells to enter the s-phases of the cell cycle. Much speculation has centered around the importance of "transposable elements" from findings in bacteria, yeast, maize and Drosophila. The signals which govern the transpositions of these mobile genes are not well elucidated, an interesting fact about them is, however, that they frequently produce deletions of adjacent stretches of nucleotides and therefore cause the arrangement of the DNA sequences in chromosomes to be unstable. Dramatic DNA changes of probable evolutionary significance have been observed in certain plants, which may have been caused by transposable elements. These profound and fleeting genomic have centered around the role of endogenous retroviral DNA coding for reverse transcriptase. Via RNA transcripts genes may be copied and reinserted in foreign places. From observations of proto-oncogenes and their corresponding viral oncogenes it is well known that cellular genes, at least if they become involved in the replication of RNA viruses, may change structurally and functionally. Cycles of removal and reinsertion of such altering genes could conceivably manifest themselves as "genetic instability". The stability of the somatic genome in normal cells, early and late cancers should hopefully be possible to analyse with the aid of rapidly evolving molecular techniques.

Any cell where altered genotypes are constantly created would run considerable risk of losing important proliferation and differentiation controls. Once unrestrained growth supervenes the stage is set for replication of the altered genotype. Conceivably all links of the complicated chain which checks cell proliferation would be susceptible to an alteration which leads to permanent escape from growth control. Current data suggest that this often involves any of the proto-oncogenes. The pure deletions which seems to characterize certain heritable cancers such as retinoblastoma indicate that not only activation of preexisting genes but also loss of genes may cause unrestrained cell proliferation. From the common coexistence of unrestrained growth and irregular migration transformation it seems likely that both have to be disabled in malignant cells and that there may be common pathways. This latter possibility is supported by the fact such growth factors as PDGF and EGF not only affect proliferation but always also migration.

The maximal size which a malignant neoplasm may reach in the absence of infinite growth transformation is probably determined by the growth potential of the "founding" normal cells. RSV transformed chicken and bovine fibroblasts reach total population sizes which correlate with the corresponding maximal size of the respective normal cells.

Malignant neoplasms which have not been immortalized, should become stationary once a certain size has been reached. Such a phenomenon would explain one of the paradoxes of human pathology - the discrepancy between number of microscopic and clinically manifest cancers in such organs as prostate, thyroid and breast. Maybe those small carcinomas, which have all microscopic hallmarks of malignant tumors (altered amount of DNA, pleomorphism, invasive growth) only lack the capacity for infinite growth - a feature which would be morphologically undetectable.

The final essential component of malignancy would then be infinite growth - a property which human in contrast to many other species have great difficulty to acquire.

THE GLIOMA EXAMPLE

To give a concrete example of a plausible chain of events, the following outline is given of how a human glioblastoma multiforme may have arisen. The model is speculative. Other chains may occur in other malignancies, but at least part of the suggested series of steps should be possible to check experimentally.

1. Genetic (or epigenetic) alterations will occur in an astrocyte potentially capable of entering the cell cycle and provided with receptors for PDGF (imperfectly differentiated remnant from an embryonic cell lineage?). These may be caused by chemicals or be 'spontaneous'.

2. At some stage any of the two genes for the A- or B-chain of PDGF are (by chance?) permanently activated creating an autonomous autocrine loop in the 'founder' cell.

3. Normal multiplication inhibition is partially lifted

("unrestrained growth transformation") and the affected clone transformation will therefore grow as a benign circumscribed astrocytoma grade 1-2. Particulary in children its growth potential will be limited with spontaneous regression as a result (benign cerebellar astrocytoma is the typical example). At this stage the tumor is cytogenetically diploid.

4. The multiplying clone runs an increased risk of acquiring 'genetic instability transformation'. Once this has occurred Darwinian evolution takes place with emergence and disappearance of new clones. One of those will undergo "infinite growth transformation". Because of the unstable genotype aneuploid pleomorphic cells characteristic of glioblastoma multiforme are created.

5. In this process other more efficient mechanisms for unrestrained growth than the original autocrine loop may take over. Synthesis of PDGF will then be a biochemical atavism which now lacks an essential function for the tumor cells themselves but may still be responsible for the excessive endothelial and fibroblast stroma proliferation which is characteristic for this type of malignancy.

The tumor is now fully malignant, but careful search may reveal traces of its benign astrocytoma forerunner as has often been noted by neuropathologists.

CONCLUSION

The essential malignant features can be sorted into four categories:

Unrestrained growth, irregular migration, capacity for indefinite multiplication and presence of unstable evolving genotypes. Only if all four are present will malignancy exist. Benign tumors are principally different in their lack of irregular migration, infinite growth and genetic instability. The four components of the malignant tetrad have been partially dissected with the aid of transfection by oncogenes or infection by oncogenic viruses. All four are essential and cooperate to produce the full malignant phenotype. The order by which they occur may be different from case to case. This speculative review with its emphasis of human neoplasia suggests two principal avenues towards malignancy a) the common direct route and b) the unusual route via benign precursors. In the second case creation of autocrine loops with induction of unrestrained growth is suggested as the primary step which will then produce benign overgrowth. Subsequently genetic instability, irregular migration and infinite growth may be added thus creating a clone with its characteristic malignant tetrad.

TABLE 1
FOUR TYPES OF OPERATIONNALLY DISTINGUISHABLE NEOPLASTIC TRAITS

Type of transformation	defining feature	clinical consequences
unrestrained growth	continued net increase of cell number; "plus growth"	increase in tumor volume
irregular migration	abnormal migration; capacity to settle and grow at abnormal locations	invasion, metastasis
infinite growth	indefinite expansion of net cell number	progressive increase of tumor burden until patient dies
genetic diversity	creation of new abnormal genotypes	tumor progression, development of drug resistance?

HEREDITARY FACTORS
AND CARCINOGENESIS AGENTS

© 1987 Elsevier Science Publishers B.V. (Biomedical Division)
Concepts and theories in carcinogenesis. A.P. Maskens et al. eds.

GENETICS AND CANCER - MECHANISMS OF SUSCEPTIBILITY

D.G. HARNDEN

Paterson Laboratories, Christie Hospital & Holt Radium Institute, Manchester M20 9BX, U.K.

THE CONCEPT OF AN INHERITED COMPONENT IN CANCER

In the study of any biological parameter it is axiomatic that there will be an interaction between genetic and environmental factors. The phenotype is the resultant of this interaction, and for normal characteristics of plants and animals this is accepted without question. The borderline between normal and abnormal is however ill defined. Variation is tolerated as normal within certain limits but if these limits are exceeded variation becomes abnormality. Dietary deficiency may result in an individual failing to reach the stature for which a potential exists by virtue of the genes that are inherited. That is normal. But if the deficiency is such that, say, bone development is specifically affected and rickets develop, that is abnormal. The way in which environmental effects are manifest will, of course, differ with the nature of the stimulus and the particular genetic system involved. In some cases, as with these examples just quoted, the environmental influence is preventing the expression of normal gene function. There are more dramatic examples of such an interaction; for example the effect of thalidomide exposure at specific times during morphogenesis on normal limb development. Note that here timing is critical as well as the nature of the stimulus and the nature of the at-risk tissues. An entirely separate type of interaction arises from the exposure of genetically variant individuals to an external stimulus. In the case of glucose-6-phosphate dehydrogenase deficiency the individual carrying the mutant gene is frequently apparently normal and may remain so throughout life. If, however, one of a number of specific environmental stimuli is encountered, in this case, some infections, certain drugs, or the toxin from the broad bean (_Vicia fava_), a severe haemolytic anaemia may develop. There are many well documented examples of such interactions in the causation of a variety of diseases.

We should accept, therefore, a priori, that genetic factors are likely to be important in carcinogenesis and moreover that what we need to consider is an interaction between environmental stimuli and variation in the population a large part of which is likely to be genetically determined. Such ideas are well accepted in other fields e.g. drug metabolism and pharmacokinetics (28).

GENETIC ENVIRONMENTAL INTERACTION

Somehow the concept of genetic susceptibility to cancer has met with considerable resistance. This is due, in large measure, to the clear evidence of a major contribution to the causation of cancer by environmental factors. It is quite mistaken, however, to think of genetic and environmental causes as being mutually exclusive. It does not make sense to talk of 80% (or any other percentage) of cancers being due to "the environment". This means that 20% of cancers are not due to the environment and would they, therefore, be wholly genetic in origin? It is much more satisfactory to consider that, in all cancers, both genetic and environmental influences will play some part. What we have to determine is the nature of the interaction. It is clear that in many cases the environmental component will be the more important influence but only in a very small proportion will it be so overwhelming that genetic factors play little or no part. Equally there are a few cases where the genetic element alone is so strong that environmental factors can confidently be said to contribute little, but a lesser but nevertheless important genetic influence is likely in the vast majority of cancers.

EVOLUTIONARY CONSIDERATIONS

Another argument that is often used is that, since cancers are by and large diseases of older people there can be little genetic element in cancer. In evolutionary terms a disease which has its major impact in the post-reproductive years is unlikely to be a major selective force in Darwinian evolution. However, the pattern of cancer incidence with age that we now see is the resultant of evolution and not the starting point. It can be argued that the present age distribution of cancer is precisely the result that one would expect if genetic factors predisposing to cancer had had a major impact on the evolution of the human population. Any mutant gene which conferred susceptibility to cancer occurring during the years of active reproduction and child rearing would have a severe selective disadvantage. This would be true of dominant genes but equally true of recessive cancer susceptibility genes unless they also confer some unrecognised heterozygote advantage (as in G6PD deficiency and sickle cell anaemia). Thus only those susceptibility genes which exert their influence in later life would be tolerated in the population. It can be further argued that in a society where food and perhaps shelter were in short supply, as with early man, it would have proved helpful for the survival of the community if a disease removed the older individuals shortly after their offspring had established themselves. Burnet (5) has argued that cellular instability is preprogrammed in the genome and that cancer is an expected consequence which is biologically useful. This is an interesting idea but one can broaden this concept and accept that this may be only one of a variety of mechanisms by which variation in the population leads to a high proportion developing cancer in the post reproductive years.

DOMINANCE VERSUS RECESSIVITY

One corollary of this argument is that any gene which prevents the expression of a cancer susceptibility gene is likely to be a powerful positive selective force during the reproductive years. One would therefore expect virtually all cancer susceptibility genes to be recessive. In other words, what is normally inherited is cancer resistance. Resistance is therefore likely to be dominant over susceptibility and there are a number of lines of evidence which now strongly support this idea (see below). It is important in passing to note that the concepts of dominance and recessivity are purely relative. In a series of alleles a particular allele may be dominant to one member of the series but recessive to another. This is particularly well documented for the mouse. In man we usually are comparing a mutant gene to the "wild type" i.e. what we consider to be normal. Furthermore, the decision on whether a condition or disease is thought to be dominant may depend entirely on our ability to observe what is normal. Without the help of typing sera the blood groups and histocompatibility antigens cannot be observed and could be said "not to exist". Correlations of disease with blood groups or HLA type would then not be detectable. If we do not know what to look for, we will not be able to see it. This may be true for many situations where genetic susceptibility to cancer may exist. The interaction of a genetic factor with an environmental agent may be hard to recognise simply because we do not yet know what to look for. Some specific examples are given below but I attribute the following cryptic anecdote to my former colleague, Professor J.H. Edwards of Oxford. He once assured me that the current state of cancer genetics is well illustrated in the study of skin cancer in cows in Australia by a blind man. When I expressed bewilderment, his explanation was that without sight the blind man could only decide by touch which cows were affected and he would determine only that some cows had cancer and some did not and that the occurrence of skin cancer did not correlate with any parameter he could measure. His sighted colleague, however, could tell at a glance that only white cows had skin cancer and the possibility of an interaction between exposure to UV light and the genes determining coat pigmentation was immediately apparent. The moral is that one may only be able to recognise a genetic element when equipped with the appropriate means of detection. Absence of the means of detection does not mean that the genetic effect does not exist.

PENETRANCE

It is undoubtedly true that syndromes, diseases or traits which follow a clear cut Mendelian pattern of inheritance account for a very low proportion of the total number of cases of cancer and this is another reason why it is often thought that genetic factors are of little importance. However, if one bears in mind the need for an interaction with environmental factors, the small number of clearly Mendelian diseases conferring susceptibility to cancer may not be surprising. Cancer per se cannot be inherited. If an inherited mutant gene caused a cell to become malignant whenever that gene was expressed, all cells with that genotype would, at a specific point in morphogenesis, or when called upon to function in post natal life, change into cancer cells which would be incompatible with either morphogenesis or normal function.

One must suppose, therefore, that subsequent events are required for the latent susceptibility to be expressed. Only if the probability of such an event approaches 100% will it be possible to recognise a Mendelian trait for cancer susceptibility. The probability of such secondary events occurring will be controlled both by other genes (the genetic background) and interaction with other environmental stimuli. This is really another way of saying that Mendelian traits are easily recognised if "penetrance" is high but if "penetrance" is low or very low it may not be possible to recognise the genetic nature of the disease susceptibility.

THE FOCAL NATURE OF THE DISEASE

Often with inherited disease the pathological state is expressed by all the cells required during morphogenesis or during post natal life to carry out a specific function. Thus, in achondroplasia specific cells required for the production of normal cartilage growth plates all malfunction to give a generalised bone dysplasia. Similarly in phenylketonuria, the enzyme defect affects all cells leading to the widespread manifestations of the disease. But in cancer because of the nature of the disease the abnormality which leads on to cancer need only be expressed in one or a small number of cells. This focal nature of the disease helps considerably to define the nature of the abnormal event. As we have seen above expression of an inherited cancer gene in a normal or developing tissue would be incompatible with normal function. It must be supposed, therefore, that the secondary event that occurs only in one or a small number of cells is likely to be mutational in nature. We are therefore considering genes which increase the probability of a mutational event occurring or else the probability of such an event progressing to give a fully developed malignancy. The cellular phenotype which gives rise to this increased probability may or may not be recognisable at the cellular level. Even if recognisable, it may not be immediately apparent that the phenotype is associated with an increased malignant potential.

THE NATURE OF INHERITED SUSCEPTIBILITY

It is possible to envisage several different mechanisms by which a genetic susceptibility might be manifest.

1. The inherited abnormal gene may itself be part of the necessary changes which occur within the cellular genome during the process of carcinogenesis. It is now widely accepted that genomic changes, almost certainly in several steps, are an integral part of the development of neoplasia. If an inherited mutant gene provided one of these steps and the probability of the other steps remains the same then the likelihood of a cancer developing will be enhanced.

2. The inherited gene may not itself be part of the neoplastic process but its function may be such that it makes one or more of the necessary steps more likely to occur in a proportion of the cells affected and expressing the gene.

3. It is also possible that a susceptibility gene does not alter by any means the probability of an abnormal cell arising. It may act by increasing the probability with which that abnormal cell may progress to give a clinically recognisable cancer. For example hormonal influences, immune response and possibly intercellular interactions as yet undefined will all influence the way in which a potentially malignant cell will behave and hence the probability of progression.

SPECIFIC MODELS OF INHERITED SUSCEPTIBILITY

1. The two mutation model of Knudson. Knudson (18) noted that the age incidence curves of familial childhood cancers, especially retinoblastoma, differed from those of the non-familial forms of the same cancers. Essentially the inherited cancers fitted a "one-hit" curve while the non-inherited ones fitted a "two hit" curve. On this basis he proposed that cancers require two mutational events in the genome for cancer to occur. He proposed that, in the non-familial cases, two sequential somatic mutations would be required (and the event would therefore be improbable) while in familial cases one of the mutational events was inherited and the other acquired by somatic mutation. The event would therefore be highly probable because of the known frequency of

"spontaneous" mutational events in mammalian cells and the number of cells at risk. This would fit with the "direct pathway" type of susceptibility described above. If one also takes into consideration the requirement that these events will only be of neoplastic significance if occurring in a defined population of retinoblasts, this type of hypothesis fits well with observed facts about age of occurrence, number of tumours and bilaterally.

Recently this hypothesis has received strong experimental support from the observation that in retinoblastoma tumours the region around chromosome 13q14 is frequently and unexpectedly hemizygous or apparently homozygous for gene markers, esterase D or polymorphic DNA probes (6,7).

This would be compatible with the idea that one gene is or becomes abnormal but that it is not expressed in the presence of a normal allele (i.e. is a cellular recessive) but that if the normal allele is mutated or else removed by deletion, translocation or chromosome loss the abnormal gene can then express its abnormal function or the gene product will be totally absent.

Familial retinoblastoma, which is clearly inherited in a Mendelian dominant fashion would, therefore, be revealed as a recessive disease which expresses in only a tiny minority of cells because of the loss of the normal allele; the probability of the loss is so high that expression of the gene is almost inevitable and the inheritance pattern appears to be dominant.

There has been a lot of speculation about the nature of the retinoblastoma gene. Knudson, for example, has suggested that it may be a gene which plays a vital role in the morphogenesis of the eye and which has for one of its normal functions the regulation of the expression of one of the onc genes concerned with cellular proliferation. He has coined the term "anti-oncogene" (19). While this is an interesting idea, it still lacks experimental confirmation.

2. Delayed Mutation. There are some features of retinoblastoma which are hard to fit to the two-mutation hypothesis. For example, in bilateral (i.e. familial cases) the cancer appears in both eyes at approximately the same age. As Matsuanga (25) has pointed out, it is difficult to envisage randomly occurring mutations always

giving rise to simultaneous tumours when the age span of the disease is 0-10 years. Furthermore some families exist where the gene appears to be expressed only in the third or subsequent generations (4). These observations are consistent with the idea that a "premutational" event arises in the germ line of an individual but that expression of that gene requires a further change to convert it into a full mutation. Furthermore, differences in expression could be due to gonadal mosaicism for conversion to the active state in different family members. A similar, but conceptually quite different idea is that expression of a "premutation" may depend upon its transfer to a different genetic environment. This latter idea is very comparable to the case of the spotted dorsal gene in platyfish where repeated backcross to a swordtail parent permits the gene to express not as a distinctive colour marker but as a gross hyperpigmentation over large areas of the body, including areas of melanoma (1).

One should not, however, think of such concepts as being incompatible with the two mutation hypothesis. It would be quite consistent for the two mutation model to be essentially correct but subject to modification or refinement as a consequence of other considerations such as genetic environment.

3. <u>Chromosomal Hypotheses</u>. It has been known since the turn of the century (2) that chromosomal changes were present in cancer cells. There has been argument, until recently, as to whether those changes were causal, secondary but important, or unimportant consequences of neoplastic change. While this is not the place to consider in detail the nature of genomic changes in cancer, it has now become clear that chromosome abnormalities in cancer and leukaemia cells are of two types (i) random changes which appear to be a consequence of loss of stability of the genome and (ii) highly specific rearrangements which are associated with a particular subgroup of a cancer or leukaemia (13). The best known example of the latter is still the Philadelphia (Ph1) chromosome in chronic myeloid leukaemia. In other instances, the specificity is not always obvious if all cases of a particular disease are all grouped together and it may only emerge when cases are grouped by specific pathology, cell surface markers or are in some other way sub-typed.

Such specific chromosome changes in the genome of somatic cells may of course occur in individuals who do not have any recognised proneness to cancer but as we learn more about the possible mechanisms by which these chromosomal rearrangements may exert their effect in transforming cells into cancer cells it is becoming apparent that (a) chromosome loss, deletion or translocation may reveal cancer susceptibility genes and (b) that any individual in whom, for any reason, chromosomal rearrangement is more probable may be more likely to develop a neoplasm.

(a) <u>Chromosome deletion and other gene changes.</u> The observation that chromosome deletion in tumour cells may play a part in revealing cancer susceptibiblity genes on the homologous chromosome was first made, as already mentioned, in the case of retinoblastoma. Subsequently there have been a number of reports of hemizygozity or apparent homozygozity in a number of different types of cancer. Some have been in situations where a genetic susceptibility was already known or suspected.

Possibly the best example is the group of cancers known to be associated with the Weideman-Beckwith syndrome of hemihypertrophy and macroglossia, where there is an unusual susceptibility not only to Wilms' tumour but also to rhabdomyosarcoma and hepatocellular carcinoma. Koufos et al.(22,23) have demonstrated that there is unexpected homozygozity for genes on chromosomes 11 (11p13) in all three types of tumours. Deletions at this location are well recognised as a constitutional abnormality in patients with Wilms' tumour and the aniridia, genitourinary, retardation (AGR) syndrome, and have been found in the tumour cells of spontaneous Wilms' tumours. It thus appears that in these cases, the acquired somatic deletion reveals on the chromosomally normal homologue a gene which when hemizygous, can give rise to a variety of different types of neoplasm presumably depending on the tissue in which the deletion takes place. It is also implicit in this observation that the gene or genes on the normal homologue are cancer susceptibility genes which did not express in the majority of the cells. In some cases the mutant gene will be acquired in somatic cells but in others it will be inherited. Similar deletions, recognized by loss of polymorphic restriction fragments have been found in malignant melanoma (9).

So far attempts to link these deletion sites with known oncogenes have not been successful and in the best documented case it is clear that c-Ha-ras 1 gene is outside the deletion on chromosome 11 associated with aniridia - Wilms' tumour (8). Nevertheless, it does now look highly probable that one mechanism of carcinogenesis or at least one part of that mechanism will be the unmasking of recessive cancer susceptibility genes by loss of the dominant homologue in the progenitor tumour cell. The normal allele, therefore, could be considered a dominant cancer resistance gene.

Such concepts are consistent with experimental work which shows that the characteristic of cellular "immortality" is recessive in the fusion of an "immortal line" with a normal human fibroblast which gives rise to a hybrid cell which has a limited life span (26) and older work on the suppression of tumorigenicity in hybrid cells formed by the fusion of tumorigenic cell lines with normal cells (17).

Thus, any individual carrying such a recessive gene could be unusually liable to develop cancer. If the number of cells at risk is large the probability of an "unmasking" deletion will be so high that a clear Mendelian pattern will be evident. However if the number of cells at risk is low or the probability of meeting a significant environmental influence is low it may not be easy to recognize the genetic component.

Mechanisms of loss of the normal allele other than deletion are of course possible. Cavanee et al. (6) demonstrate somatic cell crossing-over and chromosome loss. Mutation and gene conversion are other possibilities but are hard to demonstrate in individual cases.

(b) Proneness to chromosome rearrangement. Good evidence has accumulated over the past ten years or so that, in some individuals at least, increased chromosome instability is associated with an increased susceptibility to cancer. In particular spontaneous chromosome instability has been observed in Bloom's syndrome, Fanconi's anaemia and ataxia-telangiectasia (A-T) (27). Each syndrome has its own characteristic pattern of chromosome abnormality and moreover in each instance cells from patients with these diseases are unusually sensitive to exposure to specific environmental agents. Taking A-T as an example (3), it is clear that patients with this recessively inherited disease show (i) chromosome instability characterised by specific clonal rearrangements, (ii) unusual sensitivity to the lethal and clastogenic effects of ionising irradiation and radiomimetic chemicals (iii) a predisposition to cancer, particularly lymphoid leukaemia and lymphoma. How these features, attributable to a single gene, are related to each other is not clear but recent evidence (21) shows that the most specific of the the breakpoints (14q12) in the chromosome rearrangements in A-T patients is at the locus of the alpha chain of the T cell receptor using in situ molecular hybridisation techniques. This could suggest that the specific rearrangements seen in the clonal proliferations which occur in A-T are similar to those which occur in true neoplasms and which have been shown to be instrumental in relocating significant genes in new sites which influence the expression of the gene product or the nature of that product. Again the best example is the rearrangement of the c-abl gene which occurs during translocation from chromosome 9 to chromosome 22 (Ph1) in CML and which results in the expression of a modified c-abl product which has a newly acquired tyrosine kinase activity (20,29). If this link between the chromosomal instability in A-T and the specific rearrangements seen in tumours is valid it could suggest that genetic variation in response to environmental agents could be important in generating the specific genetic rearrangements which are important in establishing clones of unlimited growth potential and eventually neoplasia.

SUSCEPTIBILITY TO ENVIRONMENTAL AGENTS

In addition to these rather clear cut examples of environmental interactions with genetic constitution there are other examples of a response to environmental stimuli which are not easily explained on the basis of increased chromosomal instability. For example in basal cell naevus syndrome (BCNS or Gorlin's syndrome) the evidence for radiation induction of basal cell carcinomas is good (30), but there is little evidence for either chromosomal sensitivity or unusual sensitivity to cell killing following exposure to ionizing radiation (10). None of the studies carried out so far, however, exclude a tissue dependent sensitivity. Likewise in retinoblastoma patients there is clear clinical evidence of radiation induction of osteosarcoma (11), but the evidence for an unusual radiosensitivity in cells from retinoblastoma patients is conflicting and on the whole not convincing. On the other hand there is evidence for the deletion of sequences in the 13q14 region in osteosarcoma (12) which could suggest that similar mechanisms are operating in osteosarcoma as in retinoblastoma. This is strengthened by the finding that similar deletions do not occur in other embryonal tumours or sarcomas.

We must nevertheless leave open, at present, the possibility that totally different mechanisms of susceptibility to environmental agents remain to be discovered.

CANCER, DEVELOPMENT AND DIFFERENTIATION

The processes of development and differentiation are under genetic control and some cancers are associated with errors of these processes. Some genetic defects which confer cancer susceptibility may do so as part of a wide spectrum of effects the most obvious of which are developmental abnormalities. The association of Wilms' tumour in some patients with aniridia, abnormalities of the genitourinary tract and mental retardation is such an example. It is known that, in the development of the mouse, some genes which function for very short periods during embryogenesis may also be expressed in specific tumours - e.g. the int-1 and int-2 genes which are intimately associated with the development of mammary carcinoma in mice and which are expressed in mammary tumours, are also expressed transiently but each at a different stage during embryogenesis (15). Any failure of such a finely-tuned development mechanism could be very important in the genesis of neoplasia. In man, Beckwith's syndrome, already mentioned, is an example of the association of specific developmental abnormalities with a range of different neoplasms - Wilms' tumour, hepatoblastoma and rhabdomyosarcoma. Basal cell naevus syndrome again combines multiple congenital malformations with a proneness to a specific cancer.

On the other hand some of the inherited cancer susceptibilities do not appear to be associated with any developmental abnormality. Rather they are associated with focal dysplasias which could suggest local failure of the normal control of differentiation. In neurofibromatosis, polyposis coli and dysplastic naevus syndrome, the cancers arise out of a pre-existing, widespread but focal, abnormal pattern of development. It seems very probable that errors or blocks in differentiation are critical in the development of some cancers. While we do not know the precise mechanisms it does appear that in some individuals genetic control over these processes is less stringent than in others leading to a cancer proneness.

VARIABLE DNA

There is growing evidence that certain DNA variations occur for which the population are highly polymorphic. Jeffreys and his colleagues have shown that certain of these highly variable DNA's may be used to identify a single individual from a "DNA fingerprint" (16). Attempts are currently being made to determine whether or not such variation can be used to identify cancer susceptible individuals in the population. Other DNA sequences do not show this hyper-variability but do show polymorphism in the population. Krontiris et al. (24) have shown a highly polymorphic region located a short distance "downstream" from the oncogene c-Ha-ras 1. There are four common alleles and a large number of rare ones. Krontiris and his colleagues have suggested that these rare alleles are common in patients with certain neoplasms. However, Thein et al. (31) find no excess of the rare alleles in patients with myelodysplasia. A rather different finding by Heighway et al. (14) is that one of the common alleles (A4) shows a markedly different distribution in patients with small cell carcinoma of the lung as compared to non-small cell carcinoma of the lung. This difference is highly significant in statistical terms but its significance in biological terms is not known. This observation does however raise the possibility that the human population is polymorphic for DNA sequences which are in some way associated with the development of neoplasia. Even though there is at present no indication of possible mechanisms this does raise the possibility of screening populations using DNA polymorphisms to locate sub-groups susceptible to specific neoplasms.

CONCLUSIONS

1. Genetic factors may be important in a wide variety of neoplasms.

2. In effectively all cases cancer will arise from interaction between genetic and environmental factors.

3. Evolutionary processes may have resulted in strong selection in favour of genes which, when acting normally, suppress the expression of genes which confer cancer susceptibility.

4. "Dominant" cancer genes may in some cases at least be recessive at the cellular level and depend for expression on secondary events which are almost inevitable.

5. There are at least three main mechanisms of cancer susceptibility (a) direct inheritance of part of the cellular lesion (b) increase in probability of mutational events occurring (c) increase in probability of progression to cancer.

6. Some specific mechanisms have been recognised at the cellular level, e.g. deletion and chromosomal translocations, but other mechanisms which are suggested by the association of cancer with abnormalities of differentiation and development are yet to be elucidated.

7. It is possible that genetic techniques may be used to recognise high risk groups.

REFERENCES

1. Anders F (1967) Experientia 23: 1-10

2. Bovery T (1914) Zur Frage der Enstehung maligner Tumoren. Gustav Fisher, Jena

3. Bridges BA, Harnden DG (1982) Ataxia Telangiectasia: a Cellular and Molecular Link between Cancer, Neuropathology and Immune Deficiency. John Wiley, Chichester

4. Bundey S, Morten JFN (1981) Human Genetics 59: 434-436

5. Burnet M (1974) In: Intrinsic Mutagenesis: A genetic approach to ageing. MTP Co. Ltd. Lancaster

6. Cavanee WK, Dryja TP, Philips RA et al. (1983) Nature 305: 779-784

7. Cavanee WK, Hansen MF, Nordenskjold M, Kock E, Maumenee I, Squire JA, Philips RA, Gallie BL (1985) Science 228: 501-503

8. de Martinville B, Francke U (1983) Nature 305: 641-643

9. Dracopoli NC, Houghton AN, Old LJ. (1985) PNAS 82: 1470-1474

10. Featherstone T, Taylor AMR, Harnden DH (1983) Am J Hum Genet 35: 58-66

11. Francois J (1977) Ophtalmologica 175: 185-191

12. Hansen MF, Koufos A, Gallie BL, Philips RA, Fodstad Ø, Brøgger A, Gedde-Dahl T, Cavanee WK (1985) PNAS 82: 6216-6220

13. Harnden DG (1986) In: Genetic rearrangements in leukaemia and lymphoma (ed. J.M. Goldman and D.G. Harnden) Churchill Livingstone, Edinburgh. pp. 1-26

14. Heighway J, Thatcher N, Cerney T, Hasleton PS (1986). Br J Cancer 53: 453-457

15. Jakobivits A, Shackleford GM, Varmus HE, Martin CR (1986) Cell (in press)

16. Jeffreys AJ, Brookfield JFY, Semeonoff R (1955) Nature 317: 818-819

17. Klinger HP (1982) Cytogenet Cell Genet 32: 68-84

18. Knudson AG (1971) Proc Natl Acad Sci USA 68: 820-823

19. Knudson AG (1985) Cancer Res 45: 1437-1443

20. Konopka JB, Watanabe SM, Singer JW, Collins SJ (1985) PNAS 82: 1810-1814

21. Kennaugh AA, Butterworth S, Hollis R, Baer R, Rabbits TH, Taylor AMR (1986) Human Genetics , in press

22. Koufos A, Hansen MF, Lampkin BC, Workman ML, Copeland NG, Jenkins NA, Cavanee WK (1984) Nature 309: 330-334

23. Koufos A, Hansen MF, Copeland NG, Jenkins NA, Lampkin BC, Cavenee WK (1985) Nature 316: 330-334

24. Krontiris TA, Di Martino WA, Colb M, Parkinson DR (1985) Nature 313: 369-374

25. Matsunga F (1979) J Nat Cancer Inst 63: 933-939

26. Pereira-Smith OM, Smith JR (1983) Science 221: 964-966

27. Ray JH, German J (1981) In: The chromosome changes in Bloom's syndrome ataxia-telangiectasia and Fanconi's anaemia. Raven Press Books Ltd., New York, pp 351-378

28. Rowlands M, Sheiner LB, Steimer JL (1984) (eds). Variability in drug therapy, description, estimation and control

29. Shtivelman F, Lifshitz B, Gale RP, Canaani E (1985) Nature 315: 550-554

30. Strong LC (1977) Cancer 40: 1861-1866

31. Thein SL, Oscier DG, Flint J, Wainscoat JS (1986) Nature 321: 84-85

© 1987 Elsevier Science Publishers B.V. (Biomedical Division)
Concepts and theories in carcinogenesis. A.P. Maskens et al. eds.

RADIATION CARCINOGENESIS

G.E. ADAMS

Medical Research Council Radiobiology Unit, Chilton, Didcot, Oxfordshire, England.

INTRODUCTION

Although mankind has always been exposed to low levels of natural radiation, there is considerable doubt whether this has had much role to play in the aetiology of human cancer. Radiation carcinogenesis is a problem of the twentieth century as is the case with some other environmental hazards to which the public may become exposed. Cancers induced by radiation are generally indistinguishable from those occurring naturally or arising from other causes. Their occurrence can only be inferred from a statistically-significant excess over the natural incidence. Almost all direct evidence of human radiation carcinogenesis has been obtained therefore from epidemiological sources. Much indirect evidence has been accumulated from experimental animal studies but often, results are confounded by problems such as species differences, the complex dose-response relationships which are often observed and the numerous assumptions that must be made in extrapolating from laboratory results to human cancer.

Until recently, it was assumed that epidemiological sources of information on radiation carcinogenesis will soon disappear and that improvements in risk assessment would eventually have to rely on laboratory studies including those employing the new techniques of cell and molecular biology. Regrettably however, the recent events at Chernobyl are likely to provide material for epidemiological studies well into the twenty first century.

As in other fields of carcinogenesis, knowledge of events at the cellular and molecular level is essential to an understanding of radiation carcinogenesis. The many separate but inter-related effects of radiation cover a vast time scale ranging from the very early physical and chemical events to some late sequelae (including cancer induction) that may only appear many years later.

The energies of photon or particulate radiation that emanate from radionuclides, X-ray sets, particles accelerators etc., are vastly in excess of those of the chemical bonds in biological molecules. Ionization i.e. electron ejection from the atoms with which the radiation interacts, is the major primary event. This occurs in times of the order of 10^{-17} seconds. The subsequent train of events involving other physical and radiation chemical phenomena are too complex to be reviewed in a short review paper. They are however reasonably understood in terms of their time scales and inter-relationships. It is well known for example that the immediate chemical consequences of the initial physical processes of ionization and excitation involves breakage of chemical bonds i.e. the formation of _free radicals_. Above all other modes of cancer induction therefore, there can be little doubt that the initiating events in radiation carcinogenesis involve the participation of free radicals. Nevertheless the precise identification of such processes and the understanding of the subsequent chain of events that lead to cancer induction many years later, is a complex undertaking.

RADIATION DOSE AND RADIATION RISK

Estimates of the risk of cancer from radiation can be made in various ways. _Additive_ risk is the increased incidence of a particular cancer expressed per unit absorbed radiation dose for a given population size. The _multiplicative_ or _relative_ risk model expresses the ratio of the risk in an irradiated population to that in a matched control population. The former model is the approach favoured by UNSCEAR (United Nations Scientific Committee on the Effects of Atomic Radiation) and has the advantage of specifying the absolute number of individuals involved. For example, a risk of 10^{-4} implies 10 excess cancers in a population of 100.000 individuals each of whom has received an average dose of 1 Gray.

Radiation is unique in comparison to other carcinogenic agents in that the dose to tissue - even to microscopic regions of tissue - can often be expressed precisely. (Remarkably, the dose received by many individuals who suffered the effects of the atomic weapons released over Japan in World War II is now known to a fair degree of precision). Carcinogenic potential depends upon absorbed radiation dose and is substantially greater for densely ionizing radiations such as neutrons and alpha-particles than it is for sparsely ionizing radiations i.e. X and gamma rays. The availability of precise methods for measuring absorbed radiation dose has contributed greatly to both the understanding of mechanisms of radiation carcinogenesis and the interpretation of dose-response relationships.

Epidemiological studies on populations exposed to radiation through occupational practices have provided useful information. These include miners of uranium ore and other metal-containing ores, radiation diagnosticians and painters of luminous watch dials. Risk estimates are complicated by the long latency period of induction of excess cancers, often over twenty years, and the difficulties of assessing the dose received over the usually protracted period of exposure.

Exposure to radiation emanating from natural sources is very low although there are some concerns about possible risks arising from exposure to radon gas slowly emanating from building materials. In earlier times, radon levels were small due to normal ventilation: more recently however improvements in insulation methods in modern dwellings has led to an increase in indoor radon levels.

Substantial exposure to select groups of individuals has occurred from man-made sources of radiation. One example is the detection of excess thyroid cancer in a small group of Marshall Islanders exposed to fall out from atmospheric weapons testing in the fifties. The Chernobyl disaster is another. By far the main source of data in exposure to man-made environmental radiation has come from the Life-Span Study of the survivors of the atomic bombs dropped on Hiroshima and Nagasaki. This study (1) has followed about 80.000 exposed individuals and cancer incidence is compared with that in an age-matched control population of about 26.000 individuals. About 180 excess cancers occurred over the period up to 1974. This figure is misleading however since the large majority of the population received low doses of radiation relative to that received by the remainder. Excess cancer has occurred mainly in the group who received a whole-body dose of 1 ray or greater.

An analysis in 1974 found that leukaemia showed the greatest excess incidence although excess was found for a variety of other cancers. Results from an additional four-year follow-up showed that the excess incidence of leukaemia was no longer significant. Remarkably however there was evidence of increased incidence of other cancers including for the first time colonic and stomach cancer. These data illustrate the extraordinarily long induction periods in some types of radiation-induced cancers.

Valuable information has been obtained from groups of individuals who received radiation during medical treatment. This is too substantial to review here but a few general points can be made. In earlier years fairly high doses of radiation were given to patients suffering from various non-malignant conditions. These included enlarged tonsils in children and young adults, patients with ring-worm of the scalp and some naso-pharyngeal disorders. Other studies have involved patients given the alpha-emitting radionuclide radium-224 (2,3) and a large group treated with X-rays to ameliorate the painful symptoms of ankylosing spondylitis (4). In particular, the latter has shown an excess incidence of leukaemia as well as some other tumours. The average, but non-uniform dose to the bone marrow was 3.4 Gray, a substantial amount of radiation. Similarly excess leukaemia incidence has been observed in women treated with radiation to the pelvic region for non-malignant gynaecological conditions. Studies such as this have indicated a surprising phenomenon. While radiation is hardly ever used for treatment of non-malignant conditions, higher doses are routinely given in the treatment of primary cancer by radiotherapy. There are no clear indications of excess leukaemia occurring in patients successfully treated by radiotherapy for carcinoma of the uterine cervix. This suggests that in some circumstances, carcinogenic risk may be less at higher doses than it is at lower but still substantial doses. This can be clearly demonstrated in the laboratory by the so-called "bell-shaped" dose-response curves.

DOSE - RESPONSE RELATIONSHIPS

Radiation dose-response relationships can be complex particularly at the high dose level. The epidemiological data on human radiation leukaemogenesis, the relatively short latency period compared to that for other cancers and the substantial data from experimental studies combine to make leukaemia a suitable model for studying dose-response studies. Some data on the induction of leukaemia in experimental mice are shown in figure 1.

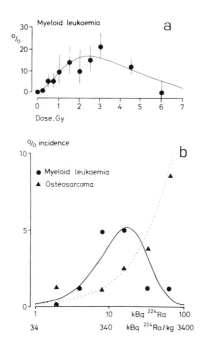

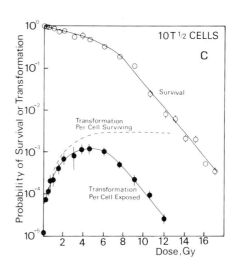

Fig. 1. Some dose-response relationships. a) Induction of myeloid leukaemia in male CBA/H mice after brief exposure to 250 kVp X-rays (from ref. 5). b) The relationship between percentage incidence of myeloid leukaemia and osteosarcoma and amount of ^{224}Ra injected. Combined single and multiple injection experiments (from ref. 7). c) Radiation survival and transformation data for C3H 10T1/2 cells exposed to ^{60}Co gamma-rays (data from ref. 16)

The data reproduced in figure 1a shows the dose-response curve for the induction by X-rays of acute myeloid leukaemia (AML) in Harwell CBA mice (5). This model has some advantage in that firstly, the disease in the mouse resembles human AML in several respects. Secondly, the natural spontaneous incidence of the disease in this strain of mouse is very low. This means that realistic estimates of leukaemogenic risk can be obtained for a fairly low radiation dose provided sufficient numbers of mice are used in the experiment. The incidence curve rises from zero to a peak value and falls thereafter. The overall response is influenced by two factors. Firstly, it would be reasonable to suppose that the probability of malignant transformation at the <u>cellular</u> level rises with increasing dose. However as the dose increases into the range where cell-killing occurs, the number of surviving cells that are still capable of transformation begins to fall. The counter-balancing of these two effects results in the overall response curve for cancer induction. This model first proposed by L.H. Gray (6) would explain for example, the lack of excess leukaemias following high-dose radiotherapy to the pelvic region for treatment of Ca cervix referred to earlier. For the experimental data of Mole (5) (figure 1a) the curve fits reasonably well, the expression $P = \alpha D^2 e^{-\lambda D}$ where P is the probability of leukaemia induction, D is the radiation dose and α and λ are constants.

Figure 1b shows some data on the induction of AML by alpha-particles emanating from plutonium administered to CBA/H mice (7). This isotope is retained in growing bone and is capable therefore of heavily irradiating regions of bone marrow. The data although still rather sparse, indicate a response curve qualitatively similar to that found for the low LET X-rays (Linear Energy Transfer, LET, is the rate at which energy is imparted to the absorbing medium per unit distance of track length). Induction of AML may be significant at doses below those required for the induction of osteosarcoma (dotted line in figure 1b). The significance of high LET radiation is discussed later in relation to mechanisms as is the relevance to radiation carcinogenesis of cellular transformation studies.

CELLULAR AND SUB-CELLULAR PROCESSES

Radiation is a "weak carcinogen" in that the dose range for which substantial carcinogenic risks exists, overlaps the dose range where cell-kill occurs. This, and the precision of dosimetric procedures, provide unique opportunities for investigating any quantitative inter-relationships between the lethal and sub-lethal effects of radiation action at the cellular level.

A radiation dose of about one ray produces some 2×10^5 ionizations within the mammalian cell. Of these, about 1% occur in the genomic material which in turn lead to about 1000 strand breaks. Almost all disappear within a few hours either by spontaneous rejoining or by enzyme-mediated repair. Some breaks remain however as "aligned" or double-strand breaks and these are undoubtedly the critical lesions that are responsible for loss of cell viability - cell death. Nevertheless, a dose of about 1 ray leaves about 40% of the irradiated cells still capable of cell division indicating that much of the initial chemical damage is of little consequence to the fate of the cell - at least as far as lethality is concerned.

a) <u>Cell Inactivation</u>:

Figure 2 shows survival data for Chinese hamster V79 cells irradiated with low LET X-rays and/or high LET alpha-particles (8). Clearly the latter type of radiation is much more cytotoxic, an effect generally observed throughout experimental radiobiology. Further high LET dose-response relationships are usually exponential (linear on the semi-log plot in figure 2) whereas the low LET

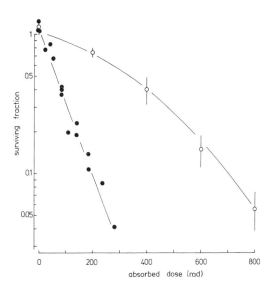

Fig.2 Survival curves for Chinese hamster V79 cells irradiated with low LET gamma-rays (o) and high LET alpha-particles (●) (from ref.8)

response plot often shows curvature on such a plot. This phenomenon has been associated with the cell's capacity to "repair" some of the damage imparted by the radiation and is commonly invoked to explain some dose-rate effects. The efficiency of radiation-induced cell-kill and indeed effects such as chromosomal changes and mutation usually falls if the radiation is delivered at a low dose-rate or in multiple fractions separated by intervals of several hours or longer. The implications of this in radiological protection are commented on later.

The greater effectiveness of high LET radiation for inducing cell-killing relative to that for low LET radiation, is understandable in terms of the properties of the radiation tracks (shown schematically in figure 3a). Typical radiation tracks from high LET alpha-particles and low LET X-rays are shown traversing a segment of the DNA helix. Some typical alpha-particles deposit energy at rates of the order of 100 kilo-electron volts per micron of track length which implies that many ionizations will occur as each particle passes through the DNA. Conversely, for X-rays, the energy deposition rate is very much less. There is therefore, a greater probability of double strand break formation from a single alpha-particle track than there is from either a single X-ray track or from chance alignment of two single strand breaks arising from 2 X-ray tracks. Many physical models have been invoked to account for

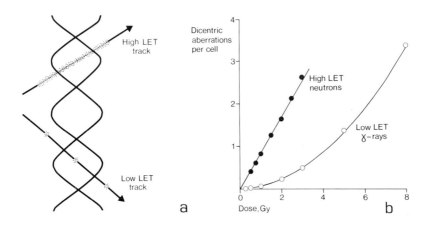

Fig. 3 a) Schematic illustration of different patterns of energy deposition from low and high LET radiation tracks traversing a section of the DNA helix. b) The different efficiences of high LET fission neutrons and low LET gamma-rays in causing dicentric chromosome aberrations in human lymphocytes (data from refs. 9, 10)

the shapes of the cell survival curves based on for example, accumulation of damage or "interaction" of sub-lesions. There are however, alternative explanations.

b) Chromosomal Changes

Radiation produces a variety of aberrations in the mammalian chromosome not all of which are necessarily lethal. Most aberrations appear to arise from interactions between two or more lesions and involve various types of exchange as well as breaks and discontinuities. At metaphase, chromosome-type exchanges including both sister chromatid are observed as well as chromatid-type exchanges involving only one chromatid. This is an important difference between radiation and chemical agents that cause chromosomal damage where, as a general rule, only chromatid type damage is observed. Since cell sterilization and chromosomal damage both involve primary damage at the DNA level, one might expect some degree of commonality between the respective dose-response relationships. This is indeed the case. Figure 3b illustrates the effect of radiation quality on the induction of dicentric chromosome aberrations in human lymphocytes (9,10). As is the case for radiation lethality, there is a substantial effect of radiation quality on the efficiency of dicentric formation. The high LET fission neutrons are substantially more effective than low LET gamma-rays particularly in the low dose region.

c) Single-gene Mutation

Inter-relationships between different types of radiation effects are even more clearly illustrated by the data of Thacker, Goodhead, Stretch, Cox and others reproduced in figure 4. Radiation can induce cellular resistance to the toxic effects of thioguanine. This is due to reduction in activity of the enzyme hypoxanthine guanine phosphoribosyl transferase HGPRT which permits cells to incorporate purines from the growth medium. The coding gene is located on the X-chromosome and therefore alteration of a single gene will reveal the mutant behaviour. This allows the mutation to be studied at reasonably low radiation doses.

Figure 4a (from Thacker (11)) plots the mutation frequency as

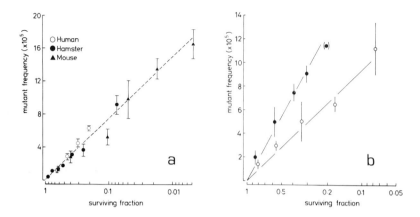

Fig. 4 a) Relationship between mutation and survival for X-ray induction of thioguanine resistance in cells from different mammalian species (from ref. 11). b) Comparison of induction of thioguanine resistance for X-rays and plutonium alpha-particles for different surviving fractions (from ref. 8).

a function of the fraction of cells that survive the <u>same</u> dose of radiation. The slopes are linear, extrapolate through the origin and somewhat surprisingly, are similar for three different cell types. It is difficult to reconcile these data in terms of <u>independent</u> lesions leading to cell death and repair. Thacker (11) has proposed that endogenous repair mechanisms utilised by the cell to deal with some of the initial radiation lesions are not entirely free of error. If the probability of the repair system for changing the genetic material (mutation) to that for elimination of the defect to give normal survivors is fixed, this would explain the relationship shown in figure 4a. Figure 4b compares this inter-relationship with that found in experiments using high LET alpha-particle radiation (8). Again, the mutation frequency at the HGPRT locus is proportional to the cell-killing efficiency of the radiation. However, the slope of the linear plot is greater than that found for low LET X or gamma radiation. This might suggest on the basis of the error-prone hypothesis, that whatever repair processes take place following high LET irradiation, they occur with less <u>fidelity</u> compared with damage induced by low LET-irradiation.

ONCOGENIC TRANSFORMATION

a. In vitro models

Some in vitro models are now available for investigating mechanisms of radiation carcinogenesis (12,13). Apparent neoplastic transformation can be induced in some cell lines by a variety of agents including radiation. Such transformed cells can induce tumours when implanted into appropriate animal hosts and also often display other characteristics such as loss of anchorage dependence, loss of contact inhibition and changes at the DNA level. All such systems have limitations but some allow a direct quantitative examination of radiation dose-response relationships. Radiation-induced transformation was first observed in 1966 by Borek and Sachs using short-term cultures of Syrian hamster embryo cells (14). Transformation is readily detected by appearance of "piled-up" colonies on the culture plates. The C3H mouse 10T1/2 established cell line (15) is also frequently used for radiation studies (papers in ref. 12). These fibroblast-like cells exhibit normal contact inhibition when a monolayer reaches confluence. When irradiated however, some cells give rise to colonies which overgrow the confluent layer. These cells can induce tumours after innoculation into an appropriate animal host.

An example of a dose-response curve for radiation-induced transformation of the 10T1/2 cell line is shown in figure 1 (data from Elkind and co-workers (16)). The bottom curve which expresses transformation frequency per exposed cell shows the familiar "bell shape" discussed earlier for carcinogenesis in vivo. However, correction of this curve to take account of cell-loss by radiation induced inactivation gives the transformation curve for the fraction of cells at risk. Unexpectedly, the curve reaches a plateau value where higher doses show no increase in transformation efficiency. The precise reasons for this are nor yet clear.

b. The reversed dose-rate effect

Studies with the 10T1/2 system and other cell lines show the expected increase in transformation efficiency with increasing values of LET in line with the trends for cell lethality mutagenicity etc. Further, for low LET, X or gamma radiation, transforming efficiency <u>decreases</u> with decreasing radiation dose-rate (17). This would also be expected on the basis of dose-rate effects observed for the cell-killing and mutagenic effects previously observed in numerous cell lines. Such effects are reasonably interpreted in terms of the increased effectiveness of repair process which can be fully expressed when the radiation is given low dose-rates or in multiple fractions separated by appropriate time intervals. The protection effects of at low dose-rate are usually observed for cell killing and mutagenesis for high LET also but <u>not</u> for transformation of 10T1/2 cells by fission neutrons (18). Particularly at low doses, the transformation efficiency of fission neutrons significantly <u>increases</u> on reduction of the dose-rate. It has been proposed (18) that this is due to a mis-repair, or "error-prone" repair phenomenon.

Interestingly an apparent reverse dose-rate effect has been observed <u>in vivo</u> in regard to the induction of osteosarcoma in NMRI mice (19). The bone-seeking isotope radium-224 which emits alpha-particles, induces more tumours when the isotope is administered in multiple injections over a protracted period than it does when the same total amount of isotope is administered in a single injection. Calculation of carcinogenic risk from low doses of radiation accumulated over a protracted period is a major problem in the field of radiological protection. Investigation of the reverse dose-rate effect and analysis of its relevance to human carcinogenesis is an important research priority.

c. <u>Molecular aspects of radiation carcinogenesis</u>

Radiation deposits energy randomly throughout the genomic material although much of the chemical damage that results is of little consequence to the fate of the cell. This complicates the problem of identifying the initial lesion or lesions that <u>are</u> important in initiating the chemical and biological processes that lead to transformation.

Mutagenic processes caused by some agents e.g. ethyl methanesulphonate, involve, in some instances, point mutations. Here, changes in a single base, or a small number of bases, are sufficient to cause the change in cellular character. In contrast, evidence is accumulating that <u>radiation</u> mutagenesis involves deletions of large segments of genetic material. Thacker (20) has analysed by hybridization techniques, the DNA from 58 independent HPRT-deficient mutants from V79 hamster cells induced by gamma-radiation. Almost half of the mutants showed loss of all functional hprt gene sequences hybridizing to the cDNA probe. Others showed partial loss. Molecular genetic analysis of some radiation-induced mutants in mice has also indicated the presence of gross deletions (21).

<u>Oncogene amplification</u>: Probes for investigating amplification of proto-oncogenes in tumours are becoming increasingly available.

Thymic lymphomas are produced in some strains of mice by X-irradiation. While such tumours are not really appropriate models for human radiation carcinogenesis, molecular studies are producing useful information. Radiation leukaemia virus (Rad LV) is a class of viruses first isolated as a "leukaemogenic activity" in cell-free extracts from these thymic lymphomas. The tumours express the virus in both the primary tumour and in serial transplants in syngeneic mice.

Oncogene activation has been observed in these radiation-induced thymic tumours. DNA extracts from the tumour cells when transfected into NIH 3T3 cells, transform the cells and cause amplification of one of the ras oncogenes (22). Similar oncogene studies with other radiation-induced experimental tumours are in progress in several laboratories including the MRC Radiobiology Unit. These include investigations in the acute myeloid leukaemia model using CBA/H mice described above (Cox, Breckon and Silver - work in progress). Radiation induces various cytogenetic changes in these mice and notwithstanding the karyotypic instabililty, some of the changes tend to predominate in both primary and transplanted myeloid tumours. In particular gross translocations from chromosome 2 are often observed in addition to trisomies at chromosome 15. Currently the DNA from these, and other cytogenetic changes are under direct investigation using a battery of oncogene probes.

Applications of such methods in other radiation-induced tumours are obviously a high priority and already underway in several laboratories. Other priorities include investigation of any promotional activity of radiation (most studies in the past have concentrated on radiation as an initiator), the interaction of radiation with other types of carcinogenic agents and basic studies on the involvement of free radical processes in the overall mechanism of cancer induction by radiation.

REFERENCES

1. Kato H, Schull WJ (1982) Radiation Res 90: 395-432

2. Mays CW, Spiess H (1984) In: Radiation Carcinogenesis. Epidemiology and Biological Significance, Boice JD, Freumeni JF (eds), Raven Press, New York.

3. Gössner W, Gerber GB, Hagen U, et al (eds) (1985) The Radiobiology of Radium and Thorotrast, Urban and Schwarzenberg

4. Smith PG, Doll R (1982) Brit Med J 284: 449-460

5. Mole RH, Papworth DG, Corp MJ (1983) Brit J Cancer 47: 285-291

6. Gray LH (1965) In: Proceed. of the XVIII Ann Symp on Fundamental Cancer Res Williams and Wilkins, Baltimore, pp 7-25

7. Humphreys ER, Loutit JF, Major IR et al (1985) Int J Rad Biol 47: 239-247

8. Thacker J, Stretch A, Goodhead DT (1982) Radiation Res 92: 343-352

9. Lloyd DC, Purrott RJ, Dolphin GW, et al (1975) Int J Rad Biol 28: 75-90

10. Lloyd DJ, Purrott RJ, Dolphin FW, et al (1976) Int J Radiat Biol 29: 169-182

11. Thacker J (1979) In: Radiation Res: Proc 6th Int Congress Rad Res, Tokyo 1979, Japanese Association for radiation Research, pp 612-620

12. Nygaard OF and Simic MG (eds) (1983) Radioprotectors and Anticarcinogens, Academic Press, New York - collected papers

13. Cox R, Adams GE (1986) Int J Rad Biol 49: 501-547

14. Borek G, Sachs L (1966) Nature 210: 276-278

15. Reznikoff CA, Brankon DW, Heidelberger C (1973) Cancer Res 33: 3231-3238

16. Elkind MM, Han A, Hill CK, et al (1983) In: Proc 7th Int Cong Rad Res, Broerse JJ, Barendsen GW, Kal HB et al (eds), Martinus Nijhoff, Amsterdam, pp 33-42

17. Han A, Hill CK, Elkind MM (1984) Br J Cancer 49, Suppl. VI: 91-96

18. Hill CK, Buonaguro FM, Myers CP, et al (1982) Nature 298: 67-69

19. Muller WA, Gössner W, Hug O, et al (1978) Health Physics 35: 33-55

20. Thacker J (1986) Mutation Res 160: 267-275

21. Rinchik EM, Russell LB, Copeland NG, et al (1986) Genetics 112: 321-342

22. Guerrero I, Calzada P, Mayer A, et al (1984) Proc Nat Acad Sci USA 81: 202-205

MECHANISMS IN CHEMICAL CARCINOGENESIS: ENZYMATIC CONTROL OF REACTIVE
METABOLITES

F. OESCH

Institute of Toxicology, University of Mainz, Obere Zahlbacher
Strasse 67 D-6500 Mainz

Since most of the chemical carcinogens _per se_ are chemically
relatively unreactive, the first step in chemical carcinogenesis is
usually the metabolic activation of such a precursor compound
("pre-carcinogen") into an electrophilically reactive metabolite
("ultimate carcinogen") which on the grounds of this property can
react with nucleophilic moieties in DNA and can thereby alter the
genetic information. If DNA replication is faster than the repair of
such a lesion or if the chemical or topographical properties of the
damage are such that it will neither enzymically nor spontaneously
be repaired, the lesion becomes persistent. Quite obviously,
depending on where in the genome damage takes place, the normal
control of cell proliferation may be disturbed.

One of the most frequently occurring structural element in
environmental xenobiotics as well as in clinically used drugs is the
aromatic moiety. Compounds possessing this structural element as
well as olefinic compounds can be transformed to epoxides by
microsomal monooxygenases. By virtue of their electrophilic
reactivity such epoxides may spontaneously react with nucleophilic
centres in DNA, RNA and protein. Such alterations of critical
cellular macromolecules may lead to cytotoxic, allergenic, mutagenic
and/or carcinogenic effects. Whether such effects will be manifested
depends on the chemical reactivity as well as other properties such
as geometry and lipophilicity of the epoxide in question on the one
hand, and on enzymes controlling the concentration of such epoxides
on the other (31). Several microsomal monooxygenases exist which
differ in activity and substrate specificity. With respect to large
substrates, some monooxygenases preferentially attack at one
specific site different from that attacked by others. Some of these
pathways lead to reactive products; others are detoxification
pathways (42). Moreover, enzymes metabolizing such epoxides

represent a further important factor (13,17,23,28). Finally, enzymes which sequester precursors of complex epoxides play an important role (9) which is often not taken into account. In the following the role of these groups of enzymes will be discussed. At the same time they may serve as prototypes for further analogous enzymes which are important in the control of reactive metabolites derived from other structural elements.

EPOXIDE GENERATING ENZYMES

Epoxides are metabolically formed from aromatic and olefinic precursor compounds by the action of microsomal monooxygenases (24,31,32). Enzymes which are responsible for the further metabolism of epoxides can play dual roles (3) in the control of metabolically-formed epoxides dependent on the pattern of microsomal monooxygenases present in the situation under consideration. This is caused by the fact that several of the individual monooxygenases differ substantially from each other by their preferential site of oxidative attack in substrate molecules. This leads to various sets of reactive metabolites, some of which may be detoxified by second-step enzymes whilst others are converted to even more reactive secondary or tertiary metabolites by the same second or third-step enzyme(s). Benzo(a)pyrene is metabolized by monooxygenases to the reactive 7,8-oxide and this reactive compound is inactivated by microsomal epoxide hydrolase to the corresponding 7,8-dihydrodiol. This is, however, the precursor molecule for a second monooxygenation step, which reintroduces an epoxide moiety leading to a dihydrodiol bay-region epoxide. According to chemical quantum calculation by Lehr and Jerina (23), this is especially chemically reactive and has been proven to be an ultimate carcinogen (21,22,24,35,36). Thus, a single enzyme can play a multiple role in inactivating some metabolites but producing precursors for other reactive species. To generate information for risk estimation, we therefore need not only information on the relative efficiencies of these enzyme activities but also on the precise role which they play in the situation under consideration. To study this question we have used in vitro systems which are capable of monitoring quantitatively a corresponding genotoxic effect, e.g. bacterial mutagenicity (32).

The role of enzymes with a characteristic co-factor can be studied by either removal or addition of that co-factor. Enzymes which share their co-factor whith others can only be monitored for their relative importance by isolating them to apparent homogeneity. This applies also to enzymes which do not have a characteristic co-factor, such as epoxides hydrolyses, which merely adds the elements of water (28,31). A further factor which frequently is not taken into account is that several reactive metabolites are frequently involved in a given toxic response. They can be toxicologically fundamentally different from one another and since they are reactive and short-lived it is in many cases difficult or impossible to quantify or characterize them chemically. Therefore, we monitored with various strains of bacteria the potency of certain synthetically prepared reactive metabolites to cause mutations. When the K-region epoxide, benzo(a)pyrene 4,5-oxide, was monitored with TA 98 and TA 1537, the strain 98 was somewhat more efficiently mutated, by a factor of 1.6. After in situ bioactivation of the chemical synthesized 7, 8-dihydrodiol to the corresponding very short-lived dihydrodiol bay-region epoxide, the strain TA 98 was much more efficiently reverted than TA 1537, by a factor of 15. This ratio was again different from that observed after in situ bioactivation of the 9, 10-dihydrodiol. So there are ratios of how various strains of bacteria are reverted which are characteristic for the individual reactive metabolites derived from the same parent compound.

The importance of these considerations becomes clear from the fact that the effect of microsomal epoxide hydrolase was essentially opposite depending on the kind of cytochrome P-450 predominantly present. This was investigated by adding this enzyme which had been purified to apparent homogeneity (1) to benzo(a)pyrene activated by liver microsomes. When these microsomes were from untreated mice the mutagenicity was decreased to 1-2% of the original rate by the addition of purified microsomal epoxide hydrolase. This small remaining mutagenicity could not be further reduced by adding more enzyme being due to the epoxide hydrolase-resistant portion of reactive metabolites. It was shown by means of the ratios of the mutagenic potency towards various detector strains (see above) that the K-region 4,5-oxide was predominantly responsible for the major (i.e. epoxide hydrolase-sensitive) portion of the mutagenic effect under these conditions. The situation was fundamentally different when liver microsomes from mice pretreated with 3-methylcholanthrene were used, producing a different pattern of monooxygenase isoenzymes. These create a different pattern of primary reactive metabolites and in this situation epoxide hydrolase has first a weak but activating effect (3). This is because now dihydrodiol epoxides are predominantly responsible for the mutagenic effect. The microsomes used for creating the metabolites do themselves possess epoxide hydrolase and can generate dihydrodiol epoxides, but addition of more epoxide hydrolase leads to a (small but significant) increase of the mutagenicity, since more of these dihydrodiol epoxides are produced. If the amount of epoxide hydrolase is further increased a small decrease and then a small increase of the mutagenicity is observed (3). The effect is multiphasic since several metabolites are contributing to the mutagenicity. This situation - induction by 3-methylcholanthrene - is especially important, because benzo(a)pyrene as well as other carcinogenic polycyclic aromatic hydrocarbons show their carcinogenic effects at doses which produce 3-methylcholanthrene-type induction of monooxygenase isoenzymes. Thus not only the quantity but even more the quality of the cytochrome P-450 present represent a fundamental factor in the control of reactive metabolites and the biological effects produced by them.

ENZYMES WHICH CONTROL EPOXIDES BY INACTIVATION OR PRECURSOR SEQUESTRATION

Many of the inactivating enzymes are much less efficient for epoxides which carry hydroxyl groups close to the epoxide rings, whilst a hydrophobic center near the oxiran ring is generally favorable (12,28,29,42). Therefore vicinal dihydrodiol epoxides are in the majority of cases investigated to-date the metabolites of polycyclic hydrocarbons that are responsible for most of the carcinogenic and mutagenic effects induced by these compounds (16, 18,24,25,27,33,34,38,41). Mutagenicity and DNA-binding experiments

with benzo(a)pyrene-7,8-dihydrodiol 9,10-epoxide indicate that some
inactivation is caused by the presence of glutathione (8,10,14) but
not by microsomal epoxide hydrolase (3, 7,10,42). These negative
findings may result from the short half life of the diol epoxide in
an aqueous environment, although this may not necessarily be the
same in a biological membrane. Not all vicinal diol epoxides are of
low stability. The non-bay-region vicinal dihydrodiol epoxide,
benz(a)anthracene 8,9-dihydrodiol 10,11-epoxide (BA-8,9-diol
10,11-oxide), has a half life of many hours and is therefore useful
for metabolic studies. It is mutagenic (26,43) and is often the
major DNA-binding species formed from benz(a)anthracene in vivo and
in vitro (4,25,38) and it serves as a model for less stable diol
epoxides. The results reported below show that a diol epoxide can be
metabolically inactivated by dihydrodiol dehydrogenase but not by
microsomal or cytosolic epoxide hydrolase. If one assumes that the
activities of the investigated enzymes in vivo are comparable to
those that are present in our experiments in vitro, inactivation of
the diol epoxide by dihydrodiol dehydrogenase would be slower than
the rate of inactivation of the K-region oxide by microsomal epoxide
hydrolase, but still sufficiently rapid to substantially affect diol
epoxide concentrations in mammalian systems. To study their role in
metabolic inactivation, the three enzymes, microsomal and cytosolic
epoxide hydrolase and cytosolic dihydrodiol dehydrogenase , were
purified and bacterial mutagenicity was used as an indication of
their effects on the mutagenicity of BA-8,9-diol 10,11-oxide and
benz(a)anthracene 5,6-oxide (BA 5,6-oxide), the K-region epoxide. As
expected from its substrate specificity (2,20), microsomal epoxide
hydrolase readily inactivated BA 5,6-oxide. No significant effect on
the mutagenicity of BA-8,9-diol 10,11-oxide was obtained even with a
100-fold excess over that required for complete inactivation of the
K-region oxide. Relatively large amounts of cytosolic epoxide
hydrolase were required to inactivate BA 5,6-oxide. BA-8,9-diol
10,11-oxide was not inactivated by cytosolic epoxide hydrolase.

Dihydrodiol dehydrogenase, on the other hand, inactivated this
diol epoxide. Relatively high amounts of dihydrodiol dehydrogenase
were needed for this inactivation, whereas a low amount of
microsomal epoxide hydrolase was sufficient for the inactivation of

BA 5,6-oxide. A 50 % inactivation of 1 microgram of BA 5, 6-oxide was achieved with either 0.4 units of purified rat microsomal epoxide hydrolase, equivalent to 1.3 milligram of liver, or with 7 units of purified rabbit cytosolic epoxide hydrolase, equivalent to 28 milligrams of liver. These are relatively small quantities of enzymes. Microsomal epoxide hydrolase equivalent to 330 milligrams of rat liver and cytosolic epoxide hydrolase equivalent to 200 milligrams of rabbit liver did not inactivate this mutagen, whereas with dihydrodiol dehydrogenase an amount equivalent to 200 milligrams of liver was required to obtain a 50 % inactivation. The effective, but moderate rate of inactivation of vicinal diol epoxide suggests that differences in susceptibility are - at least in substantial part - caused by differences in dihydrodiol dehydrogenase activity between species, organs, and physiological states.

At least 7 glutathione transferases exist in the rat liver cytosolic fraction. They were named AA, A, B, C, D, and E in the reverse order of their elution from a carboxymethylcellulose column (15). A seventh form has been named glutathione transferase M because of its ability to react with menaphthylsulfate (6). We have recently discovered and purified an additional enzyme with distinct properties, that we have termed glutathione transferase X (5). This form and the glutathione transferases A, B, and C, which are the most abundant forms present in rat liver in terms of amounts of protein (19), have been purified to apparent homogeneity and investigated for their abilities to inactivate the two prototype epoxides discussed above, BA 5,6-oxide and BA-8,9-diol 10,11-oxide. Mutagenicity and DNA-binding experiments that have been carried out using trans-7,8-dihydro-7,8-dihydroxy-benzo(a)pyrene and an activating system have shown that in the presence of glutathione some inactivation takes place (8,10,17). Both prototype epoxides, the K-region epoxide and the diol-epoxide were inactivated by glutathione transferases A, B, C and X. About 1000-fold higher concentrations of glutathione transferase were required for inactivation of the diol-epoxide than for inactivation of the K-region epoxide. This was independent of the enzyme form used. These similarities in the ratio of inactivation of the two epoxides by the three enzymes were remarkable because the enzymes differed substantially from each other in efficiency with which they inactivated the epoxes. Interestingly, the newly discovered form X was much more efficient than form C, which in turn was clearly more active than form A and this latter form clearly more active than form B.

EFFECT OF THE DICUSSED ENZYMES FOR TWO PROTOTYPE EPOXIDES

In order to gain a perspective from the results discussed above, the amounts of the various purified enzymes which are required for a 50 % inactivation of the mutagenicity of the two prototype epoxides BA 5,6-oxide (a K-region epoxide) and BA-8,9-diol 10, 11-oxide (a vicinal dihydrodiol non bay region epoxide) are presented in Table 1. When intrinsic enzyme activities and the relative amounts of enzymes present in the liver are considered and subcellular compartmentalization is disregarded, the glutathione transferases can play a more important role in the inactivation of both prototype epoxides, BA 5,6-oxide and BA-8,9-diol 10,11-oxide than dihydrodiol dehydrogenase or the epoxide hydrolases, although the latter are specific enzymes for the hydrolysis of epoxides. Amongst the glutathione transferases, large differences in efficiency of detoxification occur and this even holds true for the immunologically closely related forms A, C and X (5,19), which differ in efficiency by more than an order of magnitude. With regard to the enzymes present in rat liver the forms C and X appear to be able to contribute most to the inactivation of the two epoxides examined here; form C because of its quantitative abundance in rat liver, and form X because of its high efficiency in inactivating these epoxides. Such an estimate is rather crude, when different types of enzymes are compared, because of differences in cofactor concentration, in pH optima and in other environmental factors which may lead to substantial differences between enzyme activity _in vivo_ and under our experimental conditions. Microsomal epoxide hydrolase was tested in the mutagenicity experiments as the free purified enzyme, whereas _in vivo_ it is situated in the endoplasmic reticulum and in other membranes (37). This may be of great advantage in comparison with cytosolic enzymes, since it increases the

Table 1. Relative importance of various purified enzymes for the inactivation of two prototype epoxides[a]

Enzyme	Enzyme concentration in liver[b] (µg/mg tissue)	Amounts of enzyme required for a 50 % reduction in mutagenicity			
		BA 5,6-oxide[c]		BA-8,9-diol 10,11-oxide[d]	
		µg/incubation	mg liver equivalents	µg/incubation	mg liver equivalents
Microsomal epoxide hydrolase	.5	.7	1.3	inactive (>> 170)	>> 300[e]
Cytosolic epoxide hydrolase	.16	4	30	inactive (>> 30)	>> 200[e]
Glutathione transferase A	.5	.11	.2	110	200
Glutathione transferase B	2.2	.5	.2	130	60
Glutathione transferase C	1.1	.02	.017	30	20
Glutathione transferase X	.25	.003	.011	6	20
Dihydrodiol dehydrogenase	.45	inactive (>> 3)	>> 1000[e]	70	170

a   Data taken from (11,12).
b   Values refer to untreated, adult males of the species from which the enzyme was purified.
c   BA 5,6-oxide: benzo(a)anthracene 5,6-oxide
d   BA-8,9-diol 10,11-oxide: benzo(a)anthracene-8,9-dihydrodiol 10,11-epoxide
e   Only determinable as an upper limit from the experiment.

opportunities for reaction with epoxides, which are generated in these membranes and tend to stay there because of their relative lipophilicity (8). Dihydrodiol dehydrogenase may not only inactivate diol epoxides, but may also sequester precursor dihydrodiols, an effect that has not been taken into account in the experimental model used. In spite of these limitations, the data presented here on the more efficient _in vitro_ inactivation of epoxides by glutathione transferases than by the other enzymes indicate that it is quite likely that glutathione transferases also play an important role in the _in vivo_ inactivation of epoxides and that glutathione transferase X is especially important. Such basic information is of crucial importance for the extrapolation of experimental findings to man and thus for the distinction between overwhelming and negligeable cancer risks which is the most important prerequisite for any effective primary cancer prevention by a rational exposure limitation.

ACKNOWLEDGMENTS

This work was supported by the Bundesministerium fur Forschung und Technologie.

REFERENCES

1. Bentley P, Oesch F (1975) FEBS Letters 59: 291-295

2. Bentley P, Schmassmann HU, Sims P, et al (1976) Europ J Biochem 69: 97-103

3. Bentley P, Oesch F, Glatt HR (1977) Arch Toxicol 39: 65-75

4. Cooper CS, MacNicoll AD, Ribeiro O et al (1980) Cancer Lett 9: 53-59

5. Friedberg T, Milbert U, Bentley P et al (1983) Biochem J 215: 617-625

6. Gilham B (1971) Biochem J 121: 667-672

7. Glatt HR (1976) Die Bedeutung verschiedener aktivierender und inaktievierender Stoffwechselschritte fur die Mutagenitat des Karzinogens Benzo(a)pyren. Thesis of University of Basel

8. Glatt HR, Oesch F (1977) Arch Toxicol 39: 87-96

9. Glatt HR, Vogel K, Bentley P et al (1979) Nature 277: 319-320

10. Glatt HR, Billings R, Platt KL et al (1981) Cancer Res 41: 270-277

11. Glatt HR, Cooper CS, Grover PL et al (1982) Science 215: 1507-1509

12. Glatt HR, Friedberg T, Grover PL et al (1983) Cancer Res 43: 5713-5717

13. Guenthner TM, Oesch F (1981) In: Polycyclic Hydrocarbons and Cancer. Gelboin H and P.O.P. Ts'o (eds), Vol. 3, Academic Press, New York, pp 183-212

14. Guenthner TM, Jernstrom B, Orrenius S (1980) Carcinogenesis 1: 407-418

15. Habig WH, Pabst MJ, Jakoby WB (1974) J Biol Chem 249: 7130-7139

16. Hecht SS, LaVoie E, Mazzorese R et al. (1978) Cancer Res 38: 2191-2198

17. Hesse S, Jernstrom B, Martinez M et al. (1980) Biochem Biophys Res Commun 94: 612-617

18. Huberman E, Sachs L, Yang SK et al. (1976) Proc Acad Sci USA 73: 607-611

19. Jakoby WB, Ketley JN Habig WH (1976) In: Glutathione: Metabolism and Function. Arias I & Jakoby WB (eds), Raven Press, Vol. 6, New York, pp 213-223

20. Jerina DM, Dansette PM, Lu AYH et al (1977) Mol Pharmacol 13: 342-351

21. Kapitulnik J, Wislocki PG, Levin W et al (1978) Cancer Res 38: 354-358

22. Kapitulnik J, Wislocki PG, Levin W et al (1978) cancer Res 38: 2661-2665

23. Lehr RE, Jerina DM (1977) Arch Toxicol 39: 1-6

24. Levin W, Wood AW, Wislocki PG et al (1978) In: Polycyclic Hydrocarbons and Cancer. Gelboin & Ts'o (eds), Vol. 1, Academic Press, New York, p 189

25. MacNicoll AD, Cooper CS, Ribeiro O et al (1981) Cancer Lett 11: 243-249

26. Malaveille C, Kuroki T, Sims P et al (1977) Mutat Res 44: 313-326

27. Newbold RF, Brookes P (1976) Nature 261: 52-54

28. Oesch F (1973) Xenobiotica 3: 305-340

29. Oesch F (1974) Biochem J 139: 77-88

30. Oesch F (1976) J Biol Chem 251: 79-87

31. Oesch F (1979) Arch Toxicol Suppl 2: 215-227

32. Oesch F and Glatt HR (1976) In: Tests in Chemical Carcinogenesis, Montesano R, Bartsch H, Tomatis L (eds), IARC Scientific publications Nx 12, Lyon, pp. 255-274.

33. Sims P, Grover PL, Swaisland A et al (1974) Nature 25: 226-228.

34. Slaga TJ, Viaje A, Berry DL et al (1976) Cancer Lett. 2: 115-122.

35. Slaga TJ, Viaje A, Bracken WM (1977) Cancer Lett. 3: 23-30.

36. Slaga TJ, Bracken WJ, Gleason G et al. (1979) Cancer Res. 39: 67-71

37. Stasiecki P, Oesch F, Bruder G et al (1980) Europ J Cell Biol

21: 79-92.

38. Vigny P, Kindts M, Duquesne M et al (1980) Carcinogenesis 1: 33-41.

39. Vogel K, Bentley P, Platt KL et al. (1980) J Biol Chem 255: 9621-9625.

40. Walker CH, Bentley P, Oesch F (1978) Biochem Biophys Acta 539: 427-434.

41. Wislocki PG, Wood AW, Chang RL et al (1976) Biochem Biophys Res Commun 68: 1006-1012.

42. Wood AW, Levin SW, LU AYH et al (1976) J Biol Chem 251: 4882-4890.

43. Wood AW, Chang RL, Levin W et al (1977) Proc Nat Acad Sci USA 74: 2746-2750.

DNA VIRUSES AND HUMAN CANCER

L. GISSMAN

Deutsches Krebsforschungszentrum, Institut für Virusforschung,
Im Neuenheimer Feld 280, 6900 Heidelberg, Fed. Rep. Germ.

DNA tumor viruses are able to transform cells in vitro, to induce tumors in experimental animals and are natural causes of certain animal cancers. Therefore, it appears justified to assume that they may play a role in the etiology of human cancer as well.

Five individual families of DNA tumor viruses have been identified so far, i.e. the Polyomaviruses, Adenoviruses, Papillomaviruses, Herpesviruses and Hepadnaviruses. Although members of the first two families, e.g. Simian Virus 40 (SV40), or Adeno type 2 are tumorigenic only in their non-natural hosts a substantial part of our present knowledge about transforming genes has been

TABLE 1

VIRUS	VIRUS FAMILY	NATURAL HOST	TUMORS IN
SV 40	Polyoma	African green monkey	Rodents
Adeno 5	Adeno	Man	Rodents
Cottontail rabbit papillomavirus	Papilloma	Cottontail rabbit	Natural host
Marek's disease virus	Herpes	Chicken	Natural host
Woodchuck hepatitis	Hepadna	Woodchuck	Natural host

accumulated by studying these viruses. In contrast, animal viruses of the Papilloma-, Herpes- and Hepadna-family can (experimentally as well as under natural conditions) induce tumors in their natural hosts (see Table 1). There are members of these virus families, too, which are associated with particular types of human cancer and are very likely causatively involved in the development of these tumors:
- Epstein Barr Virus and Burkitt's lymphoma as well as Nasopharyngeal carcinoma

- Hepatitis B Virus and hepatocellular carcinoma
- Papillomaviruses and genital cancer, particularly squamous cell carcinoma of the uterine cervix.

In the following the evidence for such a link will be summarized and possible mechanisms for transformation be discussed.

I. CHARACTERISTICS AND EPIDEMIOLOGY OF THE DISEASE
Burkitt's lymphoma (BL)

BL was initially described as a tumor occurring at a high frequence in children in Central Africa. Characteristically it originates near the jaw and metastasizes to the kidney, liver and lymphoid tissue of the gut. BL cells are characterized by specific reciprocal translocations involving the long arm of chromosome 8 in all cases. It represents a poorly differentiated malignant lymphoma consisting of a clonal proliferation of immunoglobulin producing B-lymphocytes. While it is one of the most frequent cancers in African children (5-15/100.000/year), it represents only 3% of childhood cancers outside Africa (0.2-0.5/100.000/year). In Africa, there is a strong geographical correlation between the incidence of BL and the occurrence of malaria.

Nasopharyngeal carcinoma (NPC)

It originates from nasopharyngeal epithelium and is usually anaplastic or poorly differentiated growing aggressively and metastasizing to regional lymph nodes. NPC occurs worldwide with an annual frequency of 1 per 100.000 except in southern provinces of China and in Chinese people in South East Asia where up to 30 cases/100.000/year are diagnosed.

Primary hepatocellular carcinoma (HCC)

The incidence of HCC varies tremendously with geography: Whereas in industrialized countries approximately one case/100.000/year is recorded it is the most frequent cancer in many areas of South East Asia and Africa with an annual death rate of 100 per 100.000. It has been estimated that worldwide liver cancer may be the cause of half a million deaths per year.

Cervical cancer

Cancer of the uterine cervix usually originates at the squamous-columnar junction and is in the majority of the cases of the squamous cell type. In developing countries the annual incidence rate can be more than 10 fold higher (100-200/100.000) than in Europe and the U.S. Even within the same country there are remarkable differences within the population: personal hygiene as well as sexual habits strongly influence the frequency of cervical carcinoma; already in the last century it had been suggested that a venereally transmitted infectious agent may be involved in the development of this tumor. Interestingly there is a good correlation between the incidence of cervical and penile cancer in individual countries, although in all geographic areas the absolute rate of penile carcinomas is 10-20 fold less compared to the incidence of cervical carcinomas.

II. ASSOCIATION BETWEEN VIRUS AND TUMOR
Epstein Barr Virus (EBV)

Epstein Barr Virus is a member of the Herpes Virus family and is widespread in nature: the vast majority of adults have been in contact with this virus as monitored by the presence of persisting antibodies against structural proteins. Usually the infection is silent but is accompanied in a small proportion of cases with the clinical symptoms of infectious mononucleosis, a limited proliferation of B-lymphocytes followed by a strong reaction of T-cells. The virus is then persisting life-long in one in 10^5 to 10^7 B-cells as calculated from the frequency at which permanently growing B-lymphoblastoid cell lines can be established from EBV positive healthy individuals.

Burkitt's Lymphoma

EBV DNA as well as a particular viral protein(s) (EBNA) are detected in the nuclei of 96% of the tumor biopsies and in tumor cell lines obtained from high-incidence areas. However, in the remaining 4% and in approximately 80% of tumors occurring in low-incidence areas the malignant cells are devoid of viral markers. It is interesting to note that the incidence of EBV-negative BL in Africa is almost identical to the overall rate of BL in low-incidence countries, i.e. 0.2. to 0.5/100.000/year. Thus the high frequency of BL in Africa is only due to the EBV positive cases. Interestingly, the specific chromosomal translocations seen in BL cells are independent of the presence of EBV. BL patients have elevated antibodies to early and late viral proteins.

Naropharyngeal carcinoma

EBV DNA and the nuclear antigen are present in all undifferentiated carcinomas analyzed so far. As shown by in situ hybridization the viral DNA persists in the epithelial tumor cells and is absent in the infiltrating lymphocytes. As in BL, the viral genome is present in multiple copies as circular closed episomal DNA. Beside the presence of elevated levels of antiviral IgG antibodies in the sera of NPC patients also IgA antibodies against viral proteins are measurable. Since the latter occur already before the clinical manifestation of the disease serological tests can be used for early tumor diagnosis.

Hepatocellular carcinoma

Epidemiological studies most strongly suggest that Hepatitis B virus (HBV) is causatively related to HCC. Worldwide there is a good correlation between the prevalence of chronic carriers of HBV surface antigen (HBsAg) and the incidence of HCC. In a prospective study performed in Taiwan it was shown that the relative risk of HBsAg carriers to develop HCC was 217 compared with non-carriers. Furthermore, 40% of deaths among the carriers were because of HCC which was the reason for less than 1% of deaths in the control population. There is not a simple correlation between HCC and Hepatitis B Virus infection and the high tumor incidence is related to the HBsAg chronic carrier state since among the non-carriers 90% had antibodies against HBV proteins (HBsAg and HBcAg).

In tumor biopsies as well as in cell lines established from HCC varying copy numbers of the viral DNA can be detected in an integrated form. There are usually no virus replication measurable in the tumor cells.

Cervical carcinoma

The association between virus infection and tumor growth has been shown by the presence and expression of Human Papillomavirus (HPV) DNA in tumor biopsies, in precancerous lesions as well as in cell lines derived from cervical cancers (e.g. HeLa). In fact using molecularly cloned viral DNA as probe for hybridization more than 90% of cervical carcinomas harbor HPV DNA. Amongst them HPV types 16 and 18 make up approximately 60% and 20%, respectively. Other types like HPV (10,11,31,35) as well as additional not yet clearly identified virus types individually constitute only a few percent of the HPV positive tumor biopsies although some of them are found in a very high proportion of benign genital warts. So far, only HPV 16 or HPV 18 have been found in tumor cell lines. The viral DNA molecules can be present as single or as multiple copies and are usually integrated into the human genome. In a similar frequency as the cervical cancer biopsies, penile or vulval carcinomas also contain either HPV16 or HPV18 DNA. In case of other squamous cell carcinomas the association with human papillomaviruses is less well established but there is some support that HPV may also be involved in cancer of the lung, the oesophagus or the larynx.

Because of the lack of an in vitro system for virus replication and because of the heterogeneity of human papilloma viruses up to now it has been impossible to establish serological tests to screen for HPV antibodies in the population. It is a very recent development that fusion proteins between prokaryotic peptides and viral proteins are becoming available.

III. POSSIBLE MECHANISMS OF CARCINOGENESIS
Burkitt's lymphoma

As mentioned above the common feature of BL cells (with or without the presence of EBV) is the specific translocation of the long arm of chromosome 8 at position q24 where the c-myc oncogene has been mapped. Since it has been shown in different systems that c-myc is involved in malignant transformation if it is aberrantly expressed through the cell cycle, it is tempting to speculate that the removal of c-myc from its natural environment by translocation may lead to a dysregulation of the c-myc expression. It has been suggested that malaria infection which is holoendemic in the high incidence areas of BL leads to an expansion of the B-cell population which shows a high frequency of recombinational events necessary for immunoglobulin rearrangement. Interestingly, in all cases of BL beside c-myc either the human immunoglobulin heavy chain gene (chromosome 14) or one of the light chain genes (chromosome 2 or 22, respectively) are involved in the rearrangement. How does EBV participate in this process? It has been suggested recently by Lenoir and Bornkamm that EBV has to interact with c-myc in order to induce the fully transformed phenotype as it has been shown by in vitro experiments that c-myc needs the cooperation of other oncogenes (e.g. c-ras) for malignant transformation of a cell. The activation of a second oncogene should be required in the case of EBV-negative BL.

Nasopharyngeal carcinoma

Almost nothing is known about possible mechanisms of carcinogenesis in case of NPC. As mentioned before, EBV markers are present in all biopsies of poorly differentiated NPC. Unlike in BL none of the known cellular oncogenes have been found to be modified in this tumor. However, because of the particular geographical accumulation (see above) one has to anticipate that additional factors are participating here as well. In fact it has been suggested that there is a correlation between certain HLA haplotypes and an increased development of NPC among Chinese. Additionally, a variety of environmental exposures like certain herbs as used in traditional Chinese medicine, smoke and ingestion of cured fish are implicated as risk factors. It is interesting to note that some of these substances have been shown to possess tumor-promoting activity.

Hepatocellular carcinoma

There is no conserved HBV sequence seen in individual HCC biopsies arguing against the presence of an HBV specific tumor gene which is required for transformation. It is in line with this assumption that transformation experiments with HBV have so far been unsuccesful. Moreover, integration of HBV DNA in HCC cells can occur at different sites of the host genome which excludes the activation of a particular cellular oncogene by promotor-insertion.

As suggested by Tiollais et al., HBV may act by inducing liver necrosis and regeneration. Integration of the viral DNA resulting in a cell which no longer expresses viral antigens and thus escapes the immune system would be a prerequisite that this cell becomes a target for further events in carcinogenesis.

Cervical carcinoma

As in HCC there is no specific site in the human genome for

integration of human papillomavirus type 16 or 18 DNA. However, unlike in Hepatitis B virus, in all tumor biopsies and cell lines analyzed so far integration of the circular DNA occurs in the 3' half of the early region leaving the E6, E7 and E1 open reading frames intact. As became apparent mainly by the analysis of cervical carcinoma cell lines these putative exons are transcribed into mRNAs which very likely are also translated into protein. One of these exons (E6) of the bovine papillomavirus (BPV) type 1 has been shown to be sufficient for transformation of a mouse cell line of epitheloid origin (C127).

Although the mechanism of transformation is of course completely unknown one can speculate that the activity of particular viral genes is required for initiation and/or maintainance of the transformed state of the cell. Integration of the viral DNA may not only guarantee the permanent transmission to the daughter cells but at the same time prevent a down-regulation of the "transforming gene(s)" by other viral functions: actually by integration the 3'part of the early region (open reading frames E2-E5) as well as the late genes are separated from the single viral promotor region which in the replicative cycle of the virus forms the common 5'part of all mRNA transcribed from the circular viral genome.

What could be the events leading to integration? It is clear from epidemiological studies that other factors have to be active in the carcinogenesis of cervical cancer, e.g. smoking has been shown to represent a strong risk factor for tumor development. Since the compounds of the cigarette smoke can be identified in the vaginal fluid of smoking women one can assume that such substances are of actual importance. As known from many experimental systems carcinogens are inducing DNA repair and recombinational events.

IV. STRATEGIES FOR INTERVENTION

As discussed in the preceding chapters DNA tumor viruses cannot be considered as single cause for human malignancies but only as risk factors acting in concert with other events in the multistep process of carcinogenesis. Nevertheless the involvement of an infectious agent offers the possibility to interfere (by vaccination) with one step of this process thus preventing the final product or at least limiting the frequency of its appearance.

Restraining of the virus infection is not only of great importance in public health if the primary disease itself represents a serious problem (like in the case of Hepatitis B) but can also be taken as formal proof for an etiological role of this virus in tumor-formation if the incidence of this particular type of cancer gradually decreases within a vaccinated population. It is possible that a DNA tumor virus is still carcinogenic even if its ability to replicate has been abolished. Therefore the development of subunit vaccines is of great importance.

Hepatitis B virus

In case of HBV sera from chronic carriers of the surface antigen (HBs) which are free of infectious virus are used as source for vaccine preparation. Immunization with HBs antigen proved to protect against the infection with the complete virus as shown by a decrease of the hepatitis B incidence in a vaccinated high risk population. This vaccine is now used in a first trial in order to reduce the number of HCC cases in Central Africa. Recombinant HBs antigen produced in yeast has also become available but its usefulness has still to be shown.

Epstein Barr Virus

A large glycoprotein (gp340) of the envelope of Epstein Barr Virus seems to elicit neutralizing antibodies against the whole virus in infected people. Since it is very difficult to purify the gp340 free of infectious virus production of this antigen by recombinant DNA technology seems to be the method of choice to provide a vaccine to be used in the high incidence areas of BL and NPC.

Human Papilloma Virus

As pointed out above there is no serological test available to screen for the presence of antibodies against HPV proteins. Therefore so far nothing is known which viral antigen can be used for immunization. It is questionable, however, whether the infection with an epitheliotropic virus like HPV without intimate contact with the immmune system can be prevented by humoral antibodies against the viral capsid. On the other hand, the increased incidence of cervical carcinomas as well as of their precursor lesions in immunosuppressed women clearly indicate that the immune system participates in the control of tumor growth. Thus it is tempting to speculate that non-structural HPV proteins expressed in the plasma membrane of a malignant or premalignant cell could be the target of a cell-mediated immune response. Individual viral proteins which became available by recombinant DNA technology now offer the possibility to tackle this question.

ACKNOWLEDGEMENT

I am grateful to Drs Harald Zur Hausen and Michael Pawlita for helpful suggestions.

REFERENCES (Only review articles are quoted here)

1. Klein G and Klein E (1985) Nature 315: 190-195

2. Lenoir G and Bornkamm GW (1986) In: Advances in Viral Oncology, Vol. 7. Klein G (ed) Raven Press, New York, in press

3. Miller G (1985) In: Virology. Fields BN (ed), Raven Press, New York, pp 563-589

4. Tiollais P, Pourcel C and Dejean A (1986) Nature 317: 489-495

5. Zur Hausen H (1986) In: Leukemia and Lymphoma Research, Vol. 3. Goldman JM and Epstein MA (eds) Churchill Linvingston, Edinburgh, in press

FROM ONCOGENES TO CANCER CELL

© 1987 Elsevier Science Publishers B.V. (Biomedical Division)
Concepts and theories in carcinogenesis. A.P. Maskens et al. eds.

LEUKEMOGENESIS BY TRANSACTIVATING RETROVIRUSES: BOVINE LEUKEMIA VIRUS AS A MODEL SYSTEM

A. BURNY (1),(2), Y. CLEUTER (2), C. DANDOY (1), R. KETTMANN (1),(2), M. MAMMERICKX (1),(3), G. MARBAIX (2), D. PORTETELLE (1),(2), A. VAN DEN BROEKE (2), L. WILLEMS (1),(2)

(1) Faculty of Agronomy, 5800 Gembloux, Belgium

(2) Department of Molecular Biology, University of Brussels, rue des Chevaux 67, Rhode-St-Genèse, Belgium

(3) National Institute for Veterinary Research, Groeselenberg 99, 1180 Brussels, Belgium

SUMMARY

Bovine leukemia virus (BLV) is the etiological agent of a chronic lymphatic leukemia in cows, sheep and goats. Human T lymphotropic virus type I (HTLV-I) induces a T cell leukemia and its type II counterpart has been found in dermatopathic lymphadenopathy, hairy cell leukemia and prolymphocytic leukemia cases. Moreover, HTLV-I and II are apparently involved in neurological diseases of the degenerative type.

BLV, HTLV-I and HTLV-II share many genomic and structural characteristics. Their most striking feature is the existence of an X region located between the env gene and the long terminal repeat (LTR) sequence. The X region encompasses several genes, among which tat (for transactivator of transcription) is now identified. The tat product probably plays a role in the induction process of the tumor phase. BLV system is an adequate model for studies of cell-virus interplay leading to transformation.

The most frequent malignant tumor of the bovine species is a chronic lymphatic leukemia, also called bovine malignant lymphoma or lymphosarcoma (1). Field observations and experimental transmission experiments have established the infectious character of the disease. The agent was identified as a retrovirus, exogenous to the bovine species. Until the discovery of HTLV-I and HTLV-II in 1980 and 1982 (2,3), BLV seemed to be a curiosity often referred to as a non-typical type-C virus. BLV, HTLV-I and HTLV-II have very similar genomic and structural features. They obviously derive from a common ancestor (4-6). More recently, primate viruses closely related to HTLV-I were identified (7-10). The proviral DNA of these viruses contains the long terminal repeats (LTRs), the gag (for group specific antigen), pol (for polymerase and endonuclease) and env (for envelope) sequences, charasteristic of all retroviruses. Moreover, a region called X by Seiki et al. (11) is located between env and the 3'LTR in HTLV-I. A similar X region is present in HTLV-II and BLV genomes. The longest open reading frame identified in X codes for a protein (tat) that trans-activates the viral LTR. In the presence of tat, transcription of viral genes is greatly enhanced. It is believed that tat plays a major role in tumor induction by HTLV-I, II, or BLV. Tat-1 (tat gene of HTLV-I) codes for a 42kD protein; tat-2 (tat gene of HTLV-II) encodes a 37 kD protein product whilst the BLV equivalent is a 34 kD protein.

HTLV-III/LAV-1 (or HIV) (12,13), the protopype virus inducing the immune deficiency syndrome (AIDS) and the more recently discovered HTLV-IV (20) and LAV-2 (21) are morphologically and structurally related to lentiviruses (14-16). Again, a simian counterpart has been discovered (17-19). It is apparently more closely related to HTLV-IV/LAV-II than to HTLV-III/LAV-I observations (S. Wain-Hobson, personal communication) indeed indicate that LAV-2 is quite remote from LAV-1. It is also of significant interest to note that STLV-III does not exert pathogenic effects in its host, the African Green Monkey and that HTLV-IV seems to be a weak pathogen for man (20).

The HTLV-I/II/BLV and HTLV-III(LAV-I)/HTLV-IV(LAV-II)/STLV-III virus groups share the striking peculiarity to code for transactivating proteins (4,5,22-32) acting upon either transcription (HTLV-I/II/BLV) (group I viruses) or at a post transcriptional step (HTLV-III(LAV-I)/HTLV-IV(LAV-2)/STLV-III/Visna) (group II viruses). It follows that the transactivating proteins from the group I viruses are found in the nucleus where they interact with the viral LTR and perhaps regulatory sequences of normal genes. The transactivating proteins from group II viruses seem to mostly act at a post-transcriptional level (33) perhaps believed that the modes of action of HTLV-I and II is very similar and comparable to BLV. The AIDS-related viruses (group II here above) induce increased frequencies of some neoplasms such as Kaposi sarcomas. Their mode of action is however very indirect and barely understood at this writing.

Infection by BLV occurs by close contact between the infected donor and the non-infected recipient. Cases of natural infection by BLV are known in domestic cattle, sheep, capybara and water buffalo (1,34). Experimentally, infection can be transmitted to goats (35), pigs (36), rabbits (D. Portetelle, C. Altaner, personal communication), rhesus monkeys (37) and chimpanzees (1). Body secretions and blood are the vehicles of infection and it is overwhelmingly evident that transfer of infected cells is the major route of propagation of BLV. In numerous cases, transmission is iatrogenic being linked to husbandry and veterinary practices (stables too densely populated, repeated use of contaminated syringes and needles,...). In warm climates, it is possible (but not demonstrated experimentally) that transmission can occur through bites of hematophageous insects especially when the donor is an animal in persistent lymphocytosis. In the latter case, successful transmission of BLV is achieved with as little as 0,1 μl of blood (Mammerickx et al., in press).

ASYMPTOMATIC INFECTION

The only characteristics of these animals is the presence of antibody to BLV proteins. Anti-envelope gp51 antibodies appear first closely followed by the anti p24 response. In general anti BLV antibody titer rises with time, reaching very high values (up to 10^6) at the animal's death. BLV persists in B cells (1, Djilali et al., in press) and perhaps in other tissues. In the former targets, BLV is maintained latent due to the presence in the plasma of a repressor protein, distinct from the immunoglobulin family (38,39). The interplay between BLV repression and BLV transactivation is an intriguing facet of BLV latency that deserves in depth investigations. The majority of BLV-infected animals remain in good health conditions with no significant adverse effect on production traits. In some herds, especially where animals are kept up to an advanced age, tumor cases appear. The potential role of the genetic make-up of the animal in onset of the tumor is presently unresolved.

BLV INFECTION AND PERSISTENT LYMPHOCYTOSIS (PL)

Development of persistent lymphocytosis is under the control of very poorly defined parameters, among which genetic traits are probably important. In this condition (PL) the total number of circulating lymphocytes increases spectacularly and the proportion of B cells becomes highly dominant (40-80%) in strong contrast to the low B/T ratio (1/4) prevailing in the normal individual (1, Fossum et al., in preparation). Furthermore, the number of blastoid B lymphocytes is increased up to 30 fold in the blood from BLV-infected animals (Fossum et al., in preparation). In general, PL is rather stable and may last for years. It does not seem, however, to be a necessary step towards development of the tumor. The tumor stage can break out without any obvious change in the number of circulating lymphocytes. Among PL lymphocytes, about 30% carry the BLV provirus; the remaining 70% are reactive cells (the majority of the B-type) with no trace of BLV information. As mentioned above, repression of BLV expression depends upon the presence of a non-immunoglobulin protein present in the blood plasma. Short term culture of BLV provirus-carrier lymphocytes in the absence of the repressor or transfer of such lymphocytes to a naive recipient results in the lifting of repression and induction of virus expression. Allogenic lymphocytes will produce virus in the contaminated host until they will be rejected by the immune system.

BLV INFECTION AND THE TUMOR PHASE

A fraction only (0,1 to 10%) of infected recipients will develop the tumor phase during the normal lifespan of a domestic animal. The major properties of tumor cells are as follows:

(1) All tumors contain at least a fragment of the provirus. This suggests that some viral functions are strictly required for initiation of the neoplastic process.

(2) Tumors are made of an homogeneous population of cells harbouring up to four copies of the provirus. Tumors are monoclonal

This suggests that some viral functions are strictly required for initiation of the neoplastic process.

(2) Tumors are made of an homogeneous population of cells harbouring up to four copies of the provirus. Tumors are monoclonal with respect to the integration site of the provirus (40). Integration sites, however, are not conserved from one animal to the other.

(3) Whether unique or multiple, proviral copies are complete or deleted. All deleted copies examined have shown preservation of the tat region, stressing again its probable essential role in the tumoral process.

(4) BLV information is totally or almost completely silent, even in tumor cells grown in vitro (41). The 6 cell lines that we developed so far have not been cloned however. Therefore we cannot decide whether the slight BLV expression is due to some contaminating non-transformed cells or to leakage of the leukemic block in some transformed cells leading to cell differentiation and virus expression.

(5) The apparent lack of expression of viral functions suggests that virus expression is necessary to initiate the neoplastic process. Once a stage of no return has been reached, the virus can be switched off.

(6) As the virus replicates in B cells, it is customary to consider that tumor cells are of the B lineage. None of our 6 cell lines, however, expresses immunoglobulins neither in the culture medium, nor at the cell surface nor in the cytoplasm. Two bovine tumor cell lines show very high expression at the cell surface of class II molecules of the major histocompatibility complex. Obviously availibity and use of very specific reagents is mandatory in order to unravel the identity of the tumor cell.

The mode of cell transformation by BLV, HTLV-I and HTLV-II remains conjectural. Beyond any doubt, the viral tat gene plays a key role within a given cellular background. The virus-cell interplay leads the cell to a given stage where it can stay for ever being blocked in its differenciation pathway. For certain the virus is necessary but by no means sufficient. Given sets of circumstances rarely encountered or rare secondary events must contribute to push the cell across barriers beyond which an irreversible state towards full malignancy has been achieved. We know nothing about the nature and number of circumstances and events involved to lead a cell to transformation.

Considering that the virus is mandatory in the initial steps of the process and apparently dispensable later on, we hypothesize that the transient expression of viral functions can lead to permanent expression of critical cellular genes. We foresee two possible explanations:

(1) Expression of the viral tat protein induces with very low frequency (development of the tumor being a very rare event) expression of a cell protein that positively modulates its own production and represses production of the tat protein. In the absence of tat, all viral functions are suppressed. The cell protein stimulates its own production in an autocatalytic way. Similar situations (positive regulatory loops) have been demonstrated in the bacteriophage lambda system, for example.

(2) Expression of the viral tat protein induces chromosomal abnormalities, that definitely stabilize the transformed stage. Examples of chromosomal rearrangements in neoplasia are numerous , such as the translocation of the Philadelphia chromosome in CML (42), the various translocations affecting the myc oncogene in Burkitt lymphoma (43) and the chromosome breaks bcl1 and bcl2 in B cell lymphomas (44,45). Taking as an example a situation recently described in yeast (46), we could imagine that tat expression leads with low frequency to an imbalance of histone class proteins which in turn induces chromosomal abnormalities.

Evidently, many biochemical pathways could be susceptible to deregulation by the tat protein of HTLV-I/II/BLV. The initial event of transformation by these viruses is uncovered; the road to better understanding of cell transformation is wide open.

ACKNOWLEDGEMENTS

The work performed in the authors' laboratory was helped financially by the "Fonds Cancérologique de la Caisse Générale d'Epargne et de Retraite" and by the Ministry of Agriculture. R.

Kettmann and G. Marbaix are "Maitre de Recherche" and L. Willems is "Aspirant" of the "Fonds National de la Recherche Scientifique", A. Van Den Broeke is a Fellow of the Lady Tata Memorial Trust.

REFERENCES

1. Burny A, Bruck C, Chantrenne H, Cleuter Y, Dekegel D, Ghysdael J, Kettmann R, Leclercq M, Leunen J, Mammerickx M, Portetelle D (1980) In: Viral Oncology. G. Klein, ed., Raven Press, New York, pp 231-289

2. Poiesz BJ, Ruscetti FW, Gazdar AF, Bunn PA, Minna JD, Gallo RC (1980) Proc Natl Acad Sci USA 77:7415-7419

3. Kalyanaraman VS, Sarngadharan MG, Robert-Guroff M, Miyoshi I, Blayney D, Golde D, Gallo RC (1982) Science 218:571-573

4. Rice NR, Stephens RM, Couez D, Deschamps J, Kettmann R, Burny A, Gilden RV (1984) Virology 138:82-93

5. Sagata N, Yasunaga T, Ohishi K, Tsuzuku-Kawamura J, Onuma M, Ikawa Y (1984) EMBO J1 3:3231-3237

6. Rice NR, Stephens RM, Burny A, Gilden RV (1985) Virology 142:357-377

7. Miyoshi I, Yoshimoto S, Fujishita M, Taguchi H, Kubonishi 1, Niiya K, Minezawa M (1982) Lancet 1982-II:658

8. Yamamoto N, Hinuma Y, zur Hausen H, Schneider J, Hunsmann G (1983) Lancet I:240-241

9. Homma T, Kanki PJ, King NM, Hunt RDJr, O'Connell MJ, Letvin NL, Daniel MD, Desrosiers RC, Yang CS, Essex M (1984) Science 225:716-718

10. Seiki M, Watanabe T, Komuro A, Miyoshi I, Hayami M, Yoshida M (1985) In: Retroviruses in human lymphoma/leukemia. Miwa M, Sugano H, Sugimura T, Weiss RA, eds. Japan Sci Soc Press, Tokyo/VNU Science Press, Utrecht, pp 241-249

11. Seiki M, Hattori S, Hirayama Y, Yoshida M (1983) Proc Natl Acad Sci USA 80:3618-3622

12. Barre-Sinoussi F, Chermann JC, Rey F, Nugeyre MT, Chamaret S, Gruest J, Dauguet C, Axler-Blin C, Vezinet-Brun F, Rouzioux C, Rozenbaum W, Montagnier L (1983) Science 220:868-870

13. Popovic M, Sarngadharan MG, Read E, Gallo RC (1984) Science 224:497-500

14. Gonda M, Wong-Staal F, Gallo RC, Clements JE, Narayan O, Gilden RV (1985) Science 227:173-175

15. Sonigo D, Alizon M, Staskus K, Klatzmann D, Cole S, Danos O, Retzel E, Tiollais P, Haase A, Wain-Hobson S (1985) Cell 42:369-382

16. Shaw GM, Harper ME, Hahn BH, Epstein LG, Gajduzek DC, Price RN, Navia BA, Petito CK, O'Hara CJ, Groopman JE, Cho ES, Oleske JM, Wong-Staal F, Gallo RC (1985) Science 227:177-182

17. Kanki PJ, Kurth R, Becker W, Dreesman G, McLane MF, Essex M (1985) Lancet I:1330-1332

18. Kanki PJ, McLane MF, King NW, Letvin NL, Hunt RD, Sehgal P, Daniel MD, Desrosiers RC, Essex M (1985) Science 228:1199-1201

19. Letvin NL, Daniel MD, Sehgal PK, Desrosiers RC, Hunt RD, Waldron

LM, McKey JJ, Schmidt DK, Chalifoux LV, King NW (1985) Science 230:71-73

20. Kanki PJ, Barin F, M'Boup S, Allan JS, Romet-Lemonne JL, Marlink R, McLane MF, Lee TH, Arbeille B, Denis F, Essex M (1986) Science 232:238-240

21. Clavel F, Guetard D, Brun-Vezinet F, Chamaret S, Rey M-A, Santos-Ferreira MO, Laurent AG, Dauguet C, Katlama C, Rouzioux C, Klatzmann D, Champalimaud JL, Montagnier L (1986) Science 233:343-346

22. Lee TH, Coligan JE, Sodroski JG, Haseltine WA, Salahuddin JZ, Wong-Staal F, Gallo RC, Essex M (1984) Science 226:57-61

23. Slamon DJ, Shimotohno K, Cline MJ, Golde DW, Chen ISY (1984) Science 226:61-65

24. Derse D, Caradonna SJ, Casey JW Science 227:317-320

25. Rosen CA, Sodroski JG, Kettmann R, Burny A, Haseltine WA (1985) Science 227:320-322

26. Felber B, Paskalis H, Kleinman-Ening C, Wong-Staal F, Pavlakis GN (1985) Science 229:675-677

27. Sodroski J, Rosen C, Wong-Staal F, Salahuddin SZ, Popovic M, Arya S, Gallo RC, Haseltine WA (1985) Science 227:171-173

28. Hess JL, Clements JE, Narayan O (1985) Science 299:482-485

29. Goh WC, Sodroski J, Rosen C, Essex M, Haseltine WA (1985) Science 227:1227-1228

30. Sagata N, Tsuzuku-Kawamura J, Nagaioshi-Aida M, Shimizu F, Imagawa KI, Ikawa Y (1985) Proc Natl Acad Sci USA 82:7879-7882

31. Sodroski J, Rosen C, Goh WC, Haseltine WA (1985) Science 228:1430-1432

32. Sodroski JG, Rosen CA, Haseltine WA (1984) Science 225:381-385

33. Sodroski J, Goh WC, Rosen C, Dayton A, Terwilliger E, Haseltine WA (1986) Nature 321:412-417

34. Marin C, de Lopez N, de Alvarez L, Castanos H, Espana W, Leon A, Bello A (1982) Current Topics in Veterinary Medicine and Animal Science 15:310-320

35. Olson C, Kettmann R, Burny A, Kaja R (1981) J Natl Cancer Inst 67:671-675

36. Mammerickx M, Portetelle D, Burny A (1981) Zentralbl Veterina ermed B 28:69-81

37. Schodel F, Hahn B, Hu¨bner R, Hochstein-Mintzel V (1986) Microbiologica 9:163-172

38. Gupta P, Ferrer JF (1982) Science 215:405-407

39. Gupta P, Kashmiri SVS, Ferrer JF (1984) J Virol 50:267-270

40. Kettmann R, Cleuter Y, Mammerickx M, Meunier-Rotival M, Bernardi G, Burny A, Chantrenne H (1980) Proc Natl Acad Sci USA 77:2577-2581

41. Kettmann R, Cleuter Y, Grégoire D, Burny A (1985) J Virol 54:899-901

42. Heisterkamp N, Stephenson JR, Groffen J, Hansen PF, de Klein A, Bartram CR, Grosveld G (1983) Nature 306:239-242

43. Taub R, Kirsch I, Morton C, Lenoir G, Swan D, Tronick S,

Aaronson S, Leder P (1982) Proc Natl Acad Sci USA 79:7837-7841

44. Tsujimoto Y, Yunis J, Onorato-Showe L, Erikson J, Nowell PC, Croce C (1984) Science 224:1403-1406

45. Tsujimoto Y, Finger LR, Yunis J, Nowell PC, Croce C (1984) Science 226:1097-1099

46. Meeks-Wagner D, Hartwell LH (1986) Cell 44:43-52

© 1987 Elsevier Science Publishers B.V. (Biomedical Division)
Concepts and theories in carcinogenesis. A.P. Maskens et al. eds.

ONCOGENES

A. HALL

Institute of Cancer Research: Royal Cancer Hospital, Chester Beatty Laboratories, Fulham Road, SW3 6JB, London (United Kingdom)

VIRAL ONCOGENES

The study of avian and mammalian RNA tumour viruses has led to a great deal of information on the types of genes involved in carcinogenesis. The first well characterized tumour virus, Rous Sarcoma Virus, can produce sarcomas in infected chickens within 2 to 4 weeks. A large body of genetic and biochemical evidence has shown that a single gene, the viral oncogene v-src, is responsible for the tumorigenic properties of this virus. Around twenty different viral oncogenes have been characterized on a wide variety of RNA tumour viruses (1). The protein products of these oncogenes fall into six broad classes:

1. <u>Tyrosine Kinases</u>: Typified by the v-src product pp60^{src}, these proteins are located at the inner surface of the cytoplasmic membrane and will phosphorylate tyrosine residues of protein substrates.

2. <u>Serine/Threonine Kinases</u>: Two cytoplasmic protein kinases, the products of the v-mos and v-raf oncogenes, have been identified.

3. <u>Nuclear proteins</u>: The proteins encoded by v-myc, v-myb, v-fos, and v-ski are located in the nucleus. No function has yet been assigned to them.

4. <u>Growth factor receptor-like</u>: v-erbB and v-fms have been shown by sequencing to be closely related to epidermal growth factor receptor and macrophage colony stimulating factor-1 receptor respectively.

5. <u>Growth factor-like</u>: By sequence analysis v-sis has been shown to code for a protein very similar to platelet-derived growth factor (PDGF).

6. <u>GTP/GDP binding</u>: Viral Harvey <u>ras</u> (v-Ha-<u>ras</u>) and viral Kirsten <u>ras</u> (v-Ki-<u>ras</u>) are two distinct but closely related oncogenes which encode 21,000 dalton proteins (p21s) that bind GTP and GDP. These will be discussed in more detail later.

It appears then that a wide range of biochemical activities can be associated with the products of viral oncogenes. However, they all seem to be involved in growth control mechanisms and it can be imagined that they are likely to disturb in some way the normal mitogenic responses of cells.

PROTO-ONCOGENES

In 1976, Stehelin and Bishop used nucleic acid probes specific for the v-src oncogene and found related sequences in the genome of normal chicken cells (2). These sequences represented the first identification of a proto-oncogene, in this case cellular src or c-src. Since then proto-oncogenes, corresponding to each of the twenty viral oncogenes have been found and in all vertebrate species so far looked at. It should be clear then that normal human cells contain around twenty genes each of which is closely related to a viral oncogene! The identification of these genes led to much speculation that they might be the sites of action for chemical carcinogens; perhaps an accumulation of lesions in a group of cellular proto-oncogenes could eventually lead to malignancy. A great deal of effort has gone into examining this possibility.

PROTO-ONCOGENES AND HUMAN CANCER

The role of RNA tumor viruses in the etiology of human cancer is thought to be very small. One virus, human T-cell lymphotrophic virus (HTLV-1), does cause a rare form of T-cell leukemia in adults and will transform normal T lymphocytes in culture (3). This virus does not contain a viral oncogene, nor does it affect a cellular gene by cis-insertional activation. It is believed that the integrated provirus produces a protein which can act in trans to activate some, as yet unknown, cellular gene products (4).

In the absence of viruses, three general mechanisms can be envisaged that would lead to activation of cellular proto-oncogenes.

1) Gene Amplification: Double minute chromosomes and homogeneous staining regions have long been associated with human tumors. These are thought to be sites of gene amplification and it is possible these could be proto-oncogenes.

2) Gene Rearrangement: Translocations and deletions have also

been well characterized cytologically in human tumours, specific translocations being especially easy to detect in leukemias. The breakpoints could affect the expression or control of cellular proto-oncogenes.

3) Point Mutations: Changes in single amino acids of proteins can drastically alter their function.

Examples of known genes affected by these three general mechanisms are known.

Amplification of a new gene, N-myc, so called because it is related to c-myc, has been found in a large percentage of late stage neuroblastomas (5). More recently, L-myc (another c-myc related gene), N-myc and c-myc have been found amplified in small-cell lung carcinomas (6) and in one report 21/31 cases have either amplified c-myc (9 cases), N-myc (7 cases) or L-myc (5 cases). Others have reported that the EGF receptor is over-expressed in a large number of squamous cell carcinomas and, in some cases at least, this is known to be due to gene amplification. Examples of other proto-oncogenes amplified in a handful of tumours are known but whith the exceptions just mentioned, there is so far no consistent widespread pattern of amplification.

Dramatic results have been obtained with the characterization of translocation breakpoints; in particular the 8;14 translocation associated with Burkitt's lymphoma. It has been shown that the c-myc gene which is normally located at the tip of chromosome 8 is translocated to a locus that is normally highly expressed in B-cells, namely the immunoglobulin heavy chain genes on chromosome 14 (7). The biological consequences ot this translocation are not totally understood. In most cases the result is over-expression of the myc protein but changes in the regulation of transcription and translation also play a part.

A second striking example is chronic myeloid leukemias with associated 9;22 Philadelphia chromosome. In this case the c-abl gene, normally on 9, is translocated to a previously unknown locus, bcr on chromosome 22 (8). The result is the production of a fusion protein; the amino terminus being derived from the bcr gene and the rest of the molecule from c-abl.

DNA TRANSFECTION ASSAY

In 1980, two groups led by Weinberg and by Cooper reported a biological assay capable of detecting oncogenes in human tumour DNA (9, 10). They were able to introduce DNA, isolated from the human bladder carcinoma cell line, EJ, into a non-transformed mouse fibroblast cell line, NIH/3T3, and transform the cells. When the experiment was repeated with normal DNA no effect was observed. Since then many groups, including ourselves, have used this assay and it appears that overall around 20% of human tumour DNAs can be analysed in this way. The oncogenes responsible for this transformation have in most cases been identified as one of the three members of the ras gene family. A few other oncogenes have been detected but none is nearly so widespread as is ras.

There are three known functional members of the human ras gene family, c-Harvey-ras1, c-Kirsten-ras2, and N-ras (11, 12). The protein products of these genes, p21^{ras}, are expressed in most normal cells, though at low levels. Clearly there must have been some activation event occurring in the tumours. Cloning and sequencing of ras genes from human tumours revealed that the mechanism of activation was a single point mutation. This resulted in a single amino acid change either at position 12 or 61 in the protein (13, 14). Since then oligonucleotides have been used to probe ras genes in tumour DNA and changes at a further position, amino acid 13, have been shown to activate the gene (15). In a handful of examples a normal ras gene appears to have been amplified and we and others have shown that over-expression of the normal product can lead to transformation (16).

THE ROLE OF p21^{ras}

The reason why point mutations at these positions are sufficient to convert a normal proto-oncogene into an oncogene is not known. In fact we know very little about the function of this protein in cells though it is clear it must have a very important part to play in the control of normal cellular growth. The three ras proteins are each capable of binding GTP or GDP (17) and they have an associated GTPase activity (18). Their biochemical properties and some sequence homology to other known GTP-binding proteins has led to the hypothesis that they act like regulatory G-proteins (19).

CONCLUSIONS

New mutations are being found in _ras_ genes using oligonucleotide probes and this obviates the need for the biological assay. We should soon have a more clear and statistically accurate picture of the extent of _ras_ gene involvement in human cancer. However, it is unlikely to account for much more than 20% of tumours and clearly other genes must be involved. In addition, even in tumours containing an activated _ras_ gene other additional genes are almost certainly involved and new assays to identify these will be of the utmost importance.

However altered _ras_ genes have been detected in many human cancers and the activation event is likely to have been an important one in the development of these tumors. It is, therefore, essential to achieve an understanding of the biochemistry of the _ras_ protein and why it is such a crucial protein for normal cell behaviour. When we understand this we might be able to think of ways of interfering with the process of transformation in these cells.

REFERENCES

1. Bishop JM (1983) Ann Rev Biochem 52: 301-354

2. Stehelin D, Varmus HE, Bishop JM, Vogt PK (1976) Nature 260: 170-173

3. Popovic M, Sarin PS, Robert-Guroff M, Kalyanaraman VS, Mann D, Minowada J, Gallo RC (1983) Science 219: 856-859

4. Sodroski JG, Rosen CA, Heseltine WA (1984) Science 225: 381-385

5. Schwab M, Alitalo K, Klempnauer KH, Varmus HE, Bishop JM, Gilbert F, Brodeur G, Goldstein M, Trent J (1983) Nature 305: 245-247

6. Nau MM, Brooks BJ, Carney DN, Gazdar AF, Battey JF, Sansville EA, Minna JD (1986) Proc Natl Acad Sci USA 83: 1092-1096

7. Klein G (1983) Cell 32: 311-315.

8. Heisterkamp N, Stam K, Groffen J, Klein A, Grosveld G (1985) Nature 315: 758-761

9. Shih C, Padhy LC, Murray M, Weinberg RA (1981) Nature 290: 261-264

10. Krontiris TG, Cooper GM (1981) Proc Natl Acad Sci USA 78: 1181-1184

11. Chang EH, Gonda MA, Ellis RW, Scolnick EM, Lowy DR (1982) Proc Natl Acad Sci USA 79: 4848-4852

12. Hall A, Marshall CJ, Spurr N, Weiss RAW (1983)   Nature 303: 396-400

13. Tabin CJ, Bradley SM, Bargmann CI, Weinberg RA, Papageorge AG, Scolnick EM, Dhar R, Lowy DR, Chang EH (1982)   Nature 300: 143-149

14. Brown R, Marshall CJ, Pennie SG, Hall A (1984) The EMBO J. 3: 1321-1326

15. Bos JL, Toksoz D, Marshall CJ, Vries MW, Veeneman GM, van der Eb AJ, van Boom JM, Janssen JWG, Steenvoorden ACM (1985) Nature 315: 726-730

16. Chang EH, Froth ME, Scolnick EM, Lowy DR (1982) Nature 297: 479-483

17. Finkel T, Der CJ, Cooper GM (1984) Cell 37: 151-158

18. McGrath JP, Capon DJ, Goeddel DV, Levinson AD (1984) Nature 310: 644-649

19. Hurley JB, Simon MI, Teplow DB, Robishaw JD, Gilman AG (1984) Science 226: 860-862

© 1987 Elsevier Science Publishers B.V. (Biomedical Division)
Concepts and theories in carcinogenesis. A.P. Maskens et al. eds.

THE BIOCHEMISTRY OF TRANSFORMING PROTEINS

JC BELL* and JG FOULKES

*McGill University, Dept. Biochemistry, 3655, Drummond Street, Montreal, Quebec, Canada H36146.

Laboratory of Eukaryotic Molecular Genetics, National Institute for Medical Research, The Ridgeway, London NW7 1AA, England, UK.

INTRODUCTION

Originally defined by analysis of acutely transforming retroviruses, it is now apparent that the genomes of all eukaryotic species contain a set of genes capable of transforming cells to the malignant state. Around 40 transforming genes, termed oncogenes, have been isolated so far and current estimates suggest that as many as 200 may be found to exist (1).

Generation of oncogenes, from their non-transforming homologues, may be brought about in a variety of ways. These include transduction into a viral genome, gene amplification, insertional mutagenesis, point mutations and chromosomal translocations (2).

Regardless of the mechanism of proto-oncogene activation, the most important question for our laboratory is how a single gene, and hence a single protein, can actually transform cells? This clearly necessitates an understanding of the biochemisty of the transforming proteins. A single protein product capable of inducing the multitude of cellular alterations characteristic of the transformed phenotype must be capable of pleiotropic interactions. Although we understand little of the detailed biochemistry of such interactions, it appears that transforming proteins may be divided into at least three functional categories: 1. nuclear proteins ; 2. guanine nucleotide binding proteins; 3. protein kinases and their modulators .

Oncogene products have been the subject of numerous , recent reviews (e.g. 1, 3, 4), and there seems little point in an extensive reiteration of these articles. Instead, we have tried (i) to outline the salient features of each oncogene class; (ii) to review the evidence for proto-oncogenes in differentiation (iii) to suggest ways whereby an understanding of protein phosphorylation might lead to significant advances in cancer chemotherapy.

NUCLEAR TRANSFORMING PROTEINS

The oncogene products of myc, myb, ski and fos are found in the nuclear matrix of the cell. The mechanism whereby these nuclear proteins induce transformation is unknown, although their subcellular localisation suggests that they may act at the level of transcription, DNA synthesis or RNA processing. These proteins have been shown to bind to double stranded DNA in vitro but specific binding sequences have not yet been demonstrated. A number of mitogens, such as the platelet-derived growth factor (PDGF) and the epidermal growth factor (EGF) induce a rapid but transient transcriptional activation of both the fos and myc proto-oncogenes following the addition of these hormones to normal, untransformed cells (5).

GUANINE NUCLEOTIDE BINDING PROTEINS

A second class of oncogenes is the ras gene family which express a 21,000 molecular weight protein, p21ras. The human cellular ras family consists of at least five proto-oncogenes (which includes 2 pseudogenes). Activation of ras oncogenes in human tumors is most commonly due to point mutations at one of several "hot spots" in the ras coding sequence. Activated ras oncogenes have been detected in human tumours as diverse as carcinomas, sarcomas and haematopoietic malignancies (2).

The first biochemical activity described for a p21ras protein was the ability to phosphorylate itself on a threonine residue. This appears to be an intrinsic activity but it is also a dispensible one, as certain actively transforming versions of p21ras lack a threonine residue at the phosphorylation acceptor site. Although many protein kinases are capable of carrying out an autophosphorylation reaction, all attempts using the ras protein to phosphorylate exogenous substrates have ,so far, proved unsuccessful.

A second biochemical activity described for proteins in the ras family is the ability to bind GTP. Mammalian ras gene products are associated with the inner face of the plasma membrane, bind GTP and exhibit a low GTPase activity. On the basis of sequence homology and biochemical properties it has been suggested that ras proteins may be members of the G protein family, which serve to transduce information from cell surface receptors to internal effector molecules in a variety of systems e.g. hormonal regulation of adenylate cyclase or phosphoinositide turnover (6,7). In yeast one role of the ras proteins may be to integrate nutritional information with intracellular cAMP levels although in mammalians systems present evidence suggests that p21 does not interact with adenylate cyclase (8).

The GTPase activity of the oncogenic versions of p21ras is considerably reduced compared to the normal product. As the GTP-G protein complex is the active version of the G protein family, this could imply that the oncogenic version of p21 would transmit a continuous signal rather than a regulated, transient one. Recently, however, several mutants of the ras protein have been isolated which have revealed that the GTPase activity of p21 (at least as determined in vitro) shows a very poor correlation with the ability of this protein to transform cells (9).

PROTEIN-TYROSINE KINASES AND THEIR MODULATORS

The idea that a transforming protein might act via protein phosphorylation was a particularly attractive one as it provided a mechanism whereby a single protein could induce the multitude of altered cell parameters characteristic of the transformed phenotype. Since the discovery of the cAMP-dependent protein kinase in 1968, reversible protein phosphorylation is now established as the major mechanism for the regulation of protein function in eukaryotic cells (10, 4). The first evidence that oncogenes might directly encode protein kinases originated from the work described in Erikson's laboratory, for the transforming protein of the Rous sarcoma virus, pp60^{src} (11). Shortly after this discovery, Munter and Sefton(12) identified tyrosine as the novel phosphate acceptor.

Phosphotyrosine is a rare modification in the normal cell (0.02% of total phosphoamino acids) but it is implicated as having an important role in the regulation of cell growth by a number of recent findings (reviewed in 4). First, one-third of all known oncogenes have now been shown to encode protein-tyrosine kinase activities. Second, the plasma membrane receptors for several growth simulating hormones, namely epidermal growth factor (EGF), platelet-derived growth factor (PDGF), insulin-like growth factor-1, insulin and colony stimulating factor-1 (CSF-1), have been demonstrated to be protein-tyrosine kinases. Third, the oncogene of the Simian sarcoma virus, sis, has been shown to be derived from the cellular gene which encodes PDGF and the oncogene of the avian erythroblastosis virus erb-B has been found to be homologous to the kinase domain of the EGF receptor. Finally, the McDonough feline sarcoma virus oncogene encoded glycoprotein, fms, has recently been shown to be related to the CSF-1 receptor (13). Thus, protein-tyrosine kinases appear to be essential components in the regulation of both normal and abnormal cell growth.

Transformation of cells by tyrosine kinases is most easily visualized as resulting from a constitutive over - expression of the kinase activity. This would increase the degree of phosphorylation of those proteins which are substrates for the related, non-transforming proto-oncogene product. Phosphorylation of a protein can alter its conformation to either activate or inhibit that protein and so lead to a change in some physiological process. There is a good evidence which indicates that at least the initial event in malignant transformation is a dynamic reversible process, dependent on the balance of the kinase-phosphatase activities (14). To date, little is known about phosphotyrosyl-protein phosphatases but there appear to be multiple forms , all of which are distinct from the better characterized phosphoseryl-phosphothreonyl phosphatases (14).

Recently, there has been considerable interest in the idea of anti-oncogenes, whereby transformation would result from the functional loss of a gene product rather than the activation of a gene e.g. in Wilm's tumour and hereditary retinoblastoma. The DNA sequences encoding phosphotyrosyl-protein phosphatases may, therefore, represent a group of genes awaiting identification as anti-oncogenes.

SUBSTRATES OF PROTEIN-TYROSINE KINASES

To understand how protein-tyrosine kinases regulate cell growth necessitates the identification of their substrates. The various approaches have include the use of 1- and 2-dimensional gel electrophoresis to compare phosphoproteins found in normal and transformed or growth factor stimulated cells; the development of both poly- and monoclonal antibodies directed towards phosphotyrosine or an analogue thereof; immunoprecipitation or isolation of specific proteins based on a priori prediction of their involvement and the phosphorylation of candidate substrates in vitro. However, to date, no targets have been firmly established for any protein-tyrosine kinase.

There are several reasons for the slow progress in this area. Foremost is the complexity of the processes under investigation, namely growth control and transformation. The best model for protein phosphorylation as a regulatory mechanism is that of glycogen metabolism. To date, at least 6 protein kinases, 4 protein phosphatases and 4 heat stable regulatory proteins have been isolated by analysis of this system (10). If the cell employs such measures to control glycogen levels, it is daunting to imagine the networks which regulate cell growth. Secondly, phosphotyrosine is a rare modification, accounting for only 0.02 to 2.0 % of the total phosphoamino acids even in cells containing highly active protein-tyrosine kinases. The detection of such minor species is inherently difficult. Thirdly, it is now clear that protein kinases, at least those found in association with retroviral oncogenes, are promiscuous, even in vivo, and phosphorylate proteins which are unrelated to the transformation event. Therefore it is necessary to distinguish between in vivo substrates and physiological targets. Recently we have written an extended review of the published literature in this area as well as defined a set of criteria which must be satisfied before establishing a protein as a physiological target (4). There seems little point in reiterating the analysis which led to this conclusion. Instead, we would like to outline one approach our laboratory has adopted in the search for targets of the protein-tyrosine kinase encoded by the abl oncogene.

REGULATION OF RIBOSOMAL PROTEIN S6 PHOSPHORYLATION ON SERINE BY THE ABL PROTEIN-TYROSINE KINASE

Although all protein-tyrosine kinases appear to be specific for tyrosine residues in vitro, the addition of EGF, PDGF or insulin to responsive cells also results in the increased phosphorylation of certain proteins on serine residues. Similarly, in cells transformed by either the abl or src oncogenes, both of which encode protein-tyrosine kinases, an increase in protein-bound phosphoserine has been observed. Among these phosphoseryl-proteins, ribosomal protein S6 is of particular interest because its phosphorylation is correlated with growth promoting stimuli in a wide variety of systems (15). We decided, therefore, to use the phosphorylation of S6 on serine as a defined biochemical endpoint, and then work backwards to determine how this process is regulated by the abl kinase. As a starting point, it was axiomatic that the abl kinase must either activate an S6 protein-serine kinase and/or inactivate an S6 phosphatase. Previously, we had observed that the tumour promoter, TPA (4-B-phorbol 12-beta-myristate 13-acetate) which is known to directly activate the enzyme protein kinase C and induce S6 phosphorylation, induces phosphorylation of the same five S6 phosphopeptides as found in abl transformed cells (15). We tested a variety of models, therefore, whereby the abl kinase might regulate S6 phosphorylation by activation of protein kinase C.

The most direct mechanism whereby the abl kinase could activate protein kinase C would be the direct phosphorylation of this enzyme on tyrosine, so activating it, which in turn would phosphorylate S6 on serine. However, protein kinase-C isolated from abl transformed cells does not contain phosphotyrosine (16).

In recent years, considerable attention has been focused on the hydrolysis of phosphatidylinositol 4, 5, biphosphate (PIP_2) a reaction which is stimulated by a wide variety of factors, including neurotransmitters and growth hormones (7, 17). Hydrolysis of PIP_2 by phospholipase C generates two potential second messengers, diacylglycerol which activates protein kinase C and inositol triphosphate, which stimulates the release of calcium to activate calmodulin dependent pathways. If the abl kinase activated this pathway this could lead to an increased steady state level of diacylglycerol and to a constitutive activation of protein kinase C. To this end, we next examined PI metabolism in abl transformed cells and observed a constitutive activation of PI turnover in these cells

(16). We are now determining the steady state level of each of the phosphoinositide metabolites in these cells which may indicate which step(s) is activated by the abl kinase. The next step will be to examine the phosphotyrosine content of the enzyme regulating that step. Finally, this work suggests that a valuable approach in studying the mechanism of cell transformation by protein-tyrosine kinases will be to identify the physiological substrates of both protein kinase C and the Ca^2-calmodulin dependent kinases/phosphatases, as these may also represent key targets in the transformation process.

PROTEIN-TYROSINE KINASES AND DIFFERENTIATION

A large proportion of all human tumours occurs in tissues that are involved in constant self-renewal and differentiation (18). Such observations led to the idea that malignancies arise as a result of aberrations in the normal cellular differentiation pathways (e.g. 19). Perhaps proto-oncogene products are components of networks involved in the regulation of normal differentiation with oncogene products exerting their biological effects through disruption of these networks. Two independent but complementary sets of evidence support this hypothesis. First of all, it is becoming evident that some proto-oncogenes are expressed in a developmentally regulated fashion. Secondly, mutated proto-oncogenes can profoundly alter the outcome of normal differentiation programmes.

a) The c-src gene

The c-src protein-tyrosine kinase is detectable in all embryonic tissues. In human embryos it reaches its highest levels in the neural tube, brain and heart (20). Similarly, in rodent embryos the highest levels of c-src kinase have been detected in astrocytes and post-mitotic neurons (21). In early chick embryos and developing cerebellum, c-src is expressed in two distinct phases. The first wave of c-src kinase activity is observed transiently in proliferating neural plate cells and is followed later in differentiation by a constitutively high level of c-src expression in non-dividing neurons (20).

This distinctive pattern of c-src synthesis shows an interesting correlation with the observed effects of v-src on the developing nervous system. Introduction of v-src into neural plate cells results in transformation and a block in their normal differentiation programme (22). On the other hand, RSV infection of PC12, a cell line which appears to represent a latter stage in neuronal development, results in differentiation of the PC12 progenitors into non-proliferative neuronal cells (23). Together, these observations suggest that the c-src gene product may fulfill distinct functions at various stages in development, including the initiation of at least certain differentiation programmes. The v-src gene product has also been demonstrated to interfere with the differentiation of myogenic cells, chondroblasts and melanoblasts (24) suggesting that some v-src (and possibly c-src) specific substrate(s) play an integral role in a regulatory network involved in the differentiation of a wide variety of tissues.

Not only is c-src regulated in terms of its expression during differentiation, but recent work suggests that post-translational modifications of the c-src protein may generate tissue specific forms of the gene product (21).

b) The c-abl gene

The normal c-abl protein-tyrosine kinase transcript, also shows an interesting pattern of expression in both embryonic and adult tissues. RNA blot hybridization demonstrates that c-abl transcripts first become detectable at day 5 of murine embryonic growth, peak at around day 9 and eventually decline to a stable level of expression at day 17 (25). In the adult mouse, c-abl is expressed at the highest levels in haematopoietic tissues and testes (26). The testes show a particularly intriguing form of c-abl expression, where a unique size class of the mRNA has been shown to be expressed only in the haploid cell types of mature testes but not in oocytes or immature testes. In Drosophila, c-abl transcripts show developmental regulation both in quantity of transcript made and in size of c-abl mRNA (27, 28). One mRNA species is synthesized during oogenesis, stored in oocytes and then apparently utilized only during the first few hours of embryogenesis. Other forms of c-abl transcripts are expressed at variable levels in embryos, pupae and adult tissues with highest levels of expression roughly correlating with rapidly proliferating tissues. The developmentally regulated splicing patterns of c-abl mRNA suggest that different forms of the c-abl protein are expressed at discrete stages in differentiation. Indeed, recent cDNA sequence data predicts at least three c-abl proteins which share common C-termini but differ in their amino terminal 20-40 amino acids as a consequence of alternate splicing patterns (29).

In vitro, v-abl can affect a broad range of cells, but relevant to this discussion is the observation that in vivo it generates leukaemias by blocking normal B cell differentiation (30). Furthermore, a mutated form of human c-abl with elevated kinase activity (26) has been implicated in the generation of chronic myelogenous leukaemia suggesting that inappropriate c-abl kinase activity can interfere with normal haematopoietic differentiation.

c) The EGF receptor gene

The receptor for the epidermal growth factor (EGF) also shows developmentally regulated expression. For instance, at day 10 of gestation EGF receptors appear on both embryonic and extra embryonic tissues of the mouse (31,32). The EGF receptors expressed on embryonic cells have a higher affinity for EGF than those found on adult liver. Although EGF is generally associated with induction of cell proliferation, it has been shown to effect both cell growth and differentiation in foetal rabbit lung (33).

The v-erb-B gene of avian erythroblastosis virus (AEV), codes for a polypeptide that is homologous to the EGF receptor and has an intrinsic tyrosine kinase activity (34, 35). The v-erb-B protein contains segments related to the transmembrane and cytoplasmic kinase domains of the EGF receptor, but lacks the regulatory extracellular ligand binding domain. It is possible that the erb-B protein can interact with intracellular growth and differentiation regulatory networks in the absence of ligand through a constitutively active tyrosine kinase. Infection of chicken progenitor cells with AEV result in leukaemogenesis as a consequence of a block in erythroid differentiation (36), suggesting that the normal erb-B homologue (ie EGF receptor) may be involved in the regulation of the differentiation.

d) The c-fms gene

The c-fms gene, the cellular homologue of the McDonough feline

sarcoma virus oncogene (v-fms), is expressed in a tissue specific
fashion being detectable in spleen, liver, brain and bone marrow
(37). Recent evidence shows that c-fms codes for a protein-tyrosine
kinase that is highly homologous, if not identical, to the receptor
for mononuclear growth factor, CSF-1 (13) a factor that promotes
both the proliferation and differentiation of macrophages (38). Thus
c-fms is a clear example of a protein-tyrosine kinase that is
directly linked to a pathway involved in the regulation of
differentiation.

e) Other proto-oncogenes

The c-fos gene is transcribed in a developmentally regulated
fashion in a wide variety of tissues including extraembryonic
membranes, liver and bone marrow derived cells (39). One report
suggests that the expression of the c-fos gene can result in the
differentiation of F9 teratocarcinoma cells (40). Expression of the
c-myc and c-myb genes is reduced following in vitro differentiation
of both HL-60 and F9 cells (41, 42). Constitutive expression of the
myc gene prevents the terminal differentiation of Friend cells (43).
Taken together, these observations suggest that nuclear
proto-oncogene proteins also play important roles in the initiation
of differentiation programmes.

The ras oncogene product induces differentiation of the
phaechromocytoma cell line PC-12 (44, 45) and F9 cells (46).
However, ras appears to have no effect on the stem cell
characteristics of the multipotent embryonal carcinoma cell line P19
(47). It is of interest to note that although expression of the ras
gene in P19 cells does not affect their ability to differentiate,
one cell lineage derived from the differentiation of P19 (ras+)
cells appears to be blocked in its terminal differentiation.

APPROACHES TO CHEMOTHERAPY THROUGH PROTEIN PHOSPHORYLATION

Until recently a major approach adopted by many pharmaceutical
companies in developing chemotherapeutic agents involved screening
compounds empirically. This has been unavoidable given the limited
understanding of the transformation process. With the isolation of
oncogenes, however, this situation has changed dramatically. For the
first time we have a single protein with a defined biochemical

activity capable of transforming cells. It should now be possible to develop specific inhibitors of protein-tyrosine kinases, for example, based on substrate analogs. The major difficulty will be to develop compounds which can distinguish between the mutated oncogenic version of a kinase and its normal cellular homologue. Further developments in this area will also require the identification of those human tumours which involve tyrosine phosphorylation. Although one-third of all known oncogenes encode protein-tyrosine kinases, to date there is very little data implicating these enzymes in human cancer. One notable exception is the abl oncogene which appears to be closely linked with chronic myelogenous leukaemia in humans (26). Our laboratory intends to screen human tumours with an anti-phosphotyrosine antibody to detect those tumours which show an elevated level of phosphotyrosine-containing proteins. Another approach will be to study phosphotyrosyl-protein phosphatases as potential anti-oncogenes. As discussed earlier, at least the initial transformation event by tyrosine-specific protein kinases is a dynamic equilibrium process. We need to purify tyrosine phosphatases and find out how they are regulated. Instead of designing tyrosine kinase inhibitors, one could then think about chemotherapeutic agents based on protein phosphatase activators. Once identified, relevant tyrosine kinase substrates could also become the target of chemotherapeutic drug design. Altough we believe it will be possible to develop specific inhibitors of protein-tyrosine kinases which could be designed to have a minimum of non-specific side effects we can also envisage at least three major potential limitations to their widespread use. Firstly, such drugs might only result in transformed cells adopting a normal phenotype as opposed to destroying the cancer cell. Thus, kinase inhibitors might have to be taken continually allowing the development of drug resistance e.g. via gene amplification. Secondly, cancer has been termed a "disease of the genome" (e.g. 48) due to the marked and continual increase in genetic instability following expression of an oncogene product. Cancer cells are frequently aneuploid, with translocations, point mutations and discrete gene amplifications. Thus, inhibition of the initiating protein-tyrosine activity may have little consequence. At the time the patient presents, multiple oncogenes may have been activated. Their final limitation is a financial one. In the light of the current high cost of drug development, pharmaceutical companies may be reluctant to generate specific inhibitors for the ever growing list of tyrosine kinases (current estimate of at least 20 different oncogene products). However, development of a more generalized tyrosine kinase inhibitor may have some clinical value if used in combination therapy with cytotoxic drugs. For instance, if a mutant tyrosine kinase is impeding stem cell differentiation by inappropriate phosphorylation of some regulatory molecule it may be possible to overcome the block by transient treatment with a broad spectrum tyrosine kinase inhibitor. This could result in a non-dividing terminally differentiated cell population refractory to the active oncogene product.

Given the current cancer mortality figures of 1 in 4 people in the Western world, one must hope that such approaches will prove successful.

John C Bell is a posdoctoral fellow of the National Cancer Institute of Canada. This work is supported by the Medical Research Council, UK.

REFERENCES

1. Bishop M (1985) Cell 42: 23-38

2. Hall A (1986) Chapter "The Oncogenes" of this book

3. Weinberg (1985) Sciences 230: 770-776

4. Foulkes JG Rich-Rosner M (1985) Molec Asp Cell Reg 4: 217-252

5. Greenberg M, Ziff E (1984) Nature 311: 433-438

6. Gilman AG (1984) Cell 36: 577-579

7. Berridge M, Irvine RF (1984) Nature 312: 315-321

8. Beckner SK, Hattori S, Shih TY (1985) Nature 317: 71-72

9. Der CJ, Finkel T, Cooper GM (1986) Cell 44: 167-176

10. Cohen P (1982) Nature 296: 613-619

11. Collett MS, Erikson RL (1978) Proc Natl Acad Sci USA 75:2021-2024

12. Hunter T, Sefton BM (1980) Proc Natl Acad Sci USA 77: 1311-1315

13. Sherr CJ, Rettenmeir CN, Sacca R et al. (1985) Cell 41: 665-676

14. Foulkes JG (1983) Curr Top Micro Immun 107: 163-180

15. Maller JL, Foulkes JG, Erikson E et al. (1985)   Proc Natl Acad Sci USA 82: 272-276

16. Fry MJ, Gebhardt A, Parker PJ et al. (1985) EMBO J 4: 3173-3178

17. Downes P, Michell R (1985) Molec Asp Cell Reg 4: 3-56

18. Buick RN, Pollack MN (1984) Cancer Research 44: 4909-4918

19. Pierce GB, Shikes R, Fink LM (1978) A problem of developmental biology. In: Foundations of Developmental Biology Series. Englewood Cliffs, NJ. Prentice-Hall, Inc

20. Fults DW, Towle AC, Lauder JM et al. (1985)   Mol Cell Biol 5: 27-32

21. Brugge JS, Cotton PC, Queral AE et al. (1985) Nature 316:554-557

22. Keane RW, Lipsich LA, Brugge JS (1984) Dev Biol 103: 38-52

23. Alema S, Casalbore P, Agostini E et al. (1985) Nature 316:557-559

24. Moss PS, Honeycutt N, Pacepon T et al. (1979) Exp Cell Res 123: 95-105

25. Muller R, Slamon DJ, Tremblay JM et al. (1982) Nature 299:640-644

26. Konopka JB, Witte ON (1985) Biochem Biophys Acta 823: 1-90

27. Lev Z, Leibovitz N, Segev O et al. (1984)   Mol Cell Biol 5:982-984

28. Telford J, Burckhard J, Butler B et al. (1985) EMBO J 4:2609-2615

29. Ben-Neriah Y, Bernards A, Paskind M et al. (1986) Cell 44:577-586

33. Rosenburg N, Baltimore D (1980) In: Viral Oncology, KLein G (ed), Raven Press, New York, pp 187-203

31. Adamson ED, Meek J (1984) Dev Biol 103: 62-70

32. Hortsch M, Schlessinger J, Gootivine E et al. (1983) EMBO J 3:1937-1941

33. Pratt RM, Kim CS, Grove RI (1984) Current Topic in Dev Biol 19: 81-102

34. Downward J, Yarden Y, Mayes G et al. (1984) Nature 307: 521-527

35. Kris RM, Lax I, Gullick W et al. (1985) Cell 40: 619-625

36. Beug H, Palmieri S, Freudenstein C et al. (1982) Cell 28:907-919

37. Rettemeir, CW, Roussel MF, Quinn CO et al. (1985) Science 22:320-322

38. Dexter TM, Heyworth C, Whetton AD (1985) Bioassays 2: 154-158

39. Muller R, Muller D, Guilbert L (1984) EMBO J 3: 1887-1890

40. Muller R, Wagner EF (1984) Nature 311: 438-442

41. Mitchell RC, Zokas L, Schreiber RD et al. (1985) Cell 40:209-217

42. Muller R, Curran T, Muller D et al. (1985) Nature 314: 546-548

43. Coppola JA, Cole MD (1986) Nature 320: 760-763

44. Bar-Sagi D, Feramisco JR (1985) Cell 42: 842-848

45. Noda M, Ko M, Ogura A et al. (1985) Nature 318: 73-75

46. Muller R (1986) TIBS 11: 129-132

47. Bell JC, Jardine K, McBurney MW (1986) Mol Cell Biol 6: 617-625

48. Sayer R, Gradi IK, Stephens L et al. (1985) Proc Natl Acad Sci USA 82: 7015-7019

© 1987 Elsevier Science Publishers B.V. (Biomedical Division)
Concepts and theories in carcinogenesis. A.P. Maskens et al. eds.

MOLECULAR MIMICRY BY HYBRIDOMA ANTIBODIES AND ITS APPLICATION IN ANALYSIS OF CELL MEMBRANE MOLECULES

C. DUE and L. OLSSON

Cancer Biology Laboratory, State University Hospital (Rigshospitalet), 9 Blegdamsvej, 2100 Copenhagen, Denmark

INTRODUCTION

The biological functions of most cellular molecules are determined by their 3-dimensional (3-D) folding. Current technologies permit establishment of the 2-dimensional (2-D) sequential construction of nucleotides, proteins, carbohydrates, lipids, and combinations thereof, whereas elucidation of the 3-dimensional folding of the molecules are technically very difficult. DNA and protein biochemistry technologies have become sophisticated and analysis of nucleic acid sequences, amino acid sequences, as well as construction of oligonucleotides and peptides have become routine functions in many laboratories. In contrast, methods for analysis of carbohydrate and lipid structures are considerably less developed, and current methods are exercised by only a limited number of laboratories.

In the last decade the focus in cell biology has turned to the study of those regulatory functions, which are displayed through the action of growth factors, receptors, membrane transporters and cystoskeleton systems. It has become apparent that the involved proteins can be modified by two major biochemical processes, glycosylation and phosphorylation. Glycosylation of proteins modulates their conformation, localization, organization, and turnover, but the details in these mechanisms are virtually unknown (1). The carbohydrates are synthesized as secondary gene products through the action of glycolsyltransferases, in contrast to peptides which are primary gene products. More than 70 different saccharide sequences have been described in complex carbohydrates at the cell surface. They are the result of the combined activity or lack of activity of specific glycosyl transferases, which add single glycosyl residues to carbohydrate chains. The expression of these enzymes varies during development and provides thereby a mechanism for the construction of the characteristic carbohydrate structures that occur in different cells and tissues. It is assumed that a single cell potentially can produce hundreds of different glycosyl transferases.

The fluidity of eukaryotic cell membrane provides the basis for changes in the organization of the different molecules in the membrane (2). It has been suggested that 3-D structures defined by the association of different molecules in the membrane exert biological functions such as ligand receptors (3). This assumption was recently substantiated by the experimental demonstration that insulin receptors may associate with the heavy chain of the major histocompatibility antigens (MHC) class I (4,5). Such molecular associations give rise to 3-D structures that only can be identified in situ or by construction of molecules that in their 3D-folding mimic the structures generated through the association of individual molecules in the membrane.

Methods to generate defined molecules mimicking 3-D structures are therefore highly desirable. Such methods may ideally be used to construct protein molecules with homology to carbohydrate structures, and also identify molecules that associate structurally under specific circumstances. We here describe the application of hybridoma technology to generate anti-idiotype molecules with homology to 3-D structures against which Mabs have been generated. Also, a procedure to identify rare cellular variants releasing specific molecules is described, as this procedure may be useful to identify both appropriate anti-idiotype antibodies, but also for a wide range of other experiments such as transfection of specific genes into eukaryotic cells.

The anti-idiotype approach. Antibodies against idiotypic determinants of antibodies with reactivity to tumor associated antigens (TAA) have recently become very attractive tools for several reasons. It has thus been reported that anti-idiotype antibodies may mimic the natural epitope to the extent that active immunization against the tumor cells can be obtained (6,7). However, the possibility to convert a carbohydrate epitope into a protein structure on an Ig-molecule is another highly attractive aspect that may facilitate a number of investigations. The search for cell membrane components that bind the epitope may thus easily be carried out by a simple analysis for antibody binding. The receptor can be characterized and isolated by the use of anti-idiotypic antibody. It therefore seems that this approach may offer attractive possibilities to study cellular receptors for TAA in those cases , where the specific epitope is confined to a carbohydrate structure as illustrated in a recent study on carbohydrate structures associated with human squamous lung carcinoma (8). The anti-idiotype antibodies may also be used to improve the sensitivity of assays for specific antigens in serum, and polyclonal anti-idiotype antibodies may be useful tools to analyze the possibilities for antibody-mediated arrest of tumor growth by elimination of the specific epitope. Examination of the effect on tumor growth of anti-idiotypic antibody mediated blockage/modulation of the corresponding receptor should also be possible.

Application of anti-idiotype approach to identify receptors for carbohydrate structures. Our general strategy for production of anti-idiotypic (anti-id) and anti-α-idiotypic antibodies against Mabs with specificity for TAA is outlined in Fig. 1 . Balb/c mice were immunized with Mab_1 and Ig-producing hybridomas derived by fusion of spleen cells from the immunized mice with the murine, non-Ig-producer X63-Ag8.653 myeloma line. Hybridoma supernatants with reactivity to the Mab_1 corresponding epitope but not to mouse Ig, were further screened for (i) binding to Fab-fragment of the Mab_1 and (ii) their ability to compete with purified antigen in a radioimmunoassay.

Several hundreds of anti-ids with different epitope specificities are normally generated against the variable region of an Ig molecule, but only a few of those have an internal image with high homology to the original epitope. It is therefore necessary to identify those anti-ids that have an internal image with high homology to the epitope. One aspect is here to show high competition activity between the purified epitope and the anti-id, but such analyses obviously only suggest some structural homology. More convincing is the demonstration that anti-ids may mimic the carbohydrate epitope.

110

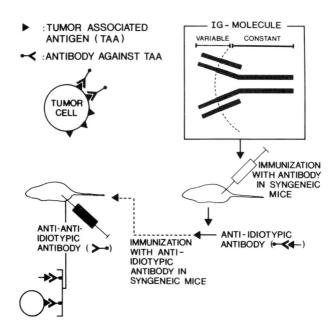

Fig. 1. Strategy for production of Mabs against a Mab (designated Mab$_1$) and analysis of the anti-idiotype Mab for homology to the antigen against which Mab$_1$ is directed. The Mab$_1$ was produced by conventional hybridoma technology. Each mouse received 10 μg Mab$_1$ per subcutaneous injection in Freund's incomplete adjuvant at 10 days interval. After 3 injections, the mice were boosted i.v. with 10 μg Mab$_1$ (contained in 0.1 ml PBS), the spleen removed 4 days later and the splenic cells processed for hybridoma generation (Mabs). The mice were bled at the time of splenectomy, and serum prepared and tested for content of antibodies against Mab$_1$ used for immunization. Polyclonal antibodies against Mab$_1$ were used for immunization. Polyclonal antibodies were prepared from serum of immunized mice. It was found that the immunization with the Mab$_2$ resulted in a polyclonal antibody response against the epitope for Mab$_1$.

Characterization of cellular molecules often includes methods employing specific antibodies. By conversion of carbohydrate structures into proteins, it has become feasible to apply such methods to the characterization of carbohydrate binding molecules (receptors), which largely facilitates the purification and characterization of such receptors.

Other Methods for analysis of ligand receptors. Cellular receptors are a group of glycoproteins with highly specialized functions with molecular weights in the range of 30.000 and 400.000

d. Collectively they are characterized by pronounced selectivity and affinity for their specific ligand and are after interaction with the ligand responsible for initiation of biological activity both in cellular metabolic reactions and eventually in physiological responses observed in the intact organism.

The insulin receptor is a phylogenetically highly conserved molecule which is expressed by almost all eukaryotic cells. It has recently been sequenced and cloned by recombinant DNA-technology. The native cell surface insulin receptor consists of two glycoprotein subunits with molecular weights of about 125.000 dalton (alpha-subunit) and 90.000 dalton (beta-subunit)

The alpha-subunit and the beta-subunit are both derived by proteolytic cleavages from a single polypeptide precursor. The predominant subunit assembly in the native receptor results in a disulphide linked heterotetrameric structure consisting of two alpha- and two beta-subunits. Recently, evidence has accumulated that the insulin receptor is associated with histocompatibility molecules in the surface membrane of cells (4,5,9). A very important advance in receptor biology has derived from the discovery that a number of growth factor receptors are enzymes with phosphokinase activity. This has been shown with receptors of epidermal growth factor (EGF), platelet derived growth factor (PDGF), insulin and insulin like growth factor which all share the same type of kinase activity (tyrosine kinase) as found in several retroviral products. Furthermore, a high degree of homology exists between the EGF receptor and the glycoproteins encoded by the oncogenic avian erythroblastosis virus (10).

Originally, the insulin receptor was defined by physiologic effects in the intact organism or tissue. With the introduction of radiolabeled ligands the definition of receptors, however changed to kinetic characteristics, specificity, saturability, and other phenomena at the cellular level as hexose and aminoacid transport. Thus the ^{125}I-insulin method has given valuable kinetic information of the receptor and has allowed to distinguish between high and low affinity receptors. In the study of diversification of cellular phenotypic characteristics in (malignant) cell population the

112

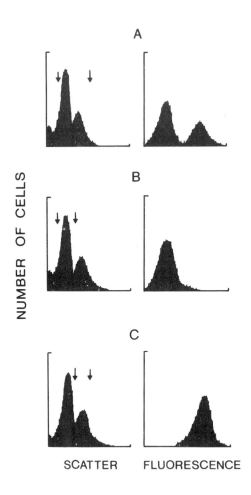

Fig. 2. Fluorescence activated cell sorter analysis of peripheral mononuclear cells stained with fluorescein insulin (0.1 μg/ml) for 90 min at 17°C. The left histograms indicate scatter signals. The right histograms show the fluorescence of cells (log scale) with a scatter signal within the "gates" defined by arrows.
A: Total peripheral mononuclear cells, B: Lymphocytes and C: Monocytes

[125]I-insulin method however cannot evaluate the diversification of insulin receptor expression as the binding of ^{125}I-insulin can only be related to all of the cells tested as a mean receptor expression.

A description of heterogenic phenotypic attributes in otherwise homogeneous cell populations can now be obtained with fluorochrome conjugated specific ligands in connection with fluorescence

activated cell sorter analysis (FACS). Two principal kinds of
ligands are available; (i) Fluorochrome conjugated insulin (11), and
(ii) specific anti-insulin receptor antibodies including,
monoclonal, polyclonal and anti-idiotypic immunoglobulins. The FACS
analysis gives measurements of heterogeneity in receptor expression
at the cellular level and permits identification and isolation of
subsets of cells with differences in receptor expression.

Fig. 2 shows FACS analysis of human peripheral mononuclear
cells incubated with fluorescein insulin. The analysis demonstrates
the well known high expression of insulin receptor in monocytes
compared with lymphocytes.

Immunoblot on viable hybridoma cells. Hybridoma cultures may
lose their Ig-secretion/production, which is often ascribed to loss
of chromosomal fragments or of entire chromosomes. Often, subsets of
cells with intact Ig-production can be identified and expanded by
time-consuming and tedious recloning procedures. In some cases
rescue by recloning may not be feasible. A method to detect (i)
small amounts (e.g. <1%) of Ig-producing cells in an otherwise non
Ig-secreting culture, and (ii) to detect variants secreting Ig of
another subclass than the main culture may be a significant
improvement. It was previously reported that albumin hepatocytes can
be detected by a procedure in which the cells are covered with
teflon and nitrocellulose, whereby the albumin will be released into
the nitrocellulose and thus detectable, whereas the teflon protects
the cells from the toxic effect of the nitrocellulose paper (12). We
adapted this method to hybridoma technology as briefly illustrated
in Fig. 3.

The amount of hybridoma cells seeded per Petri dish may vary
significantly (50×10^4-10^5) according to the purpose of the
experiment. We have hitherto applied the method for 3 purposes:
- detection of a few Ig-secreting variants in an otherwise
  non-Ig-producing culture;
- detection of subvariants that have undergone heavy-chain switch.
  In case of μ-chain secreting hybrids, the nitrocellulose paper is
  blotted with an antibody specific for gamma-chain, and the
  positive clones harvested and expanded. The procedure was recently
  successfully applied to a human IgM-producing hybridoma culture.

114

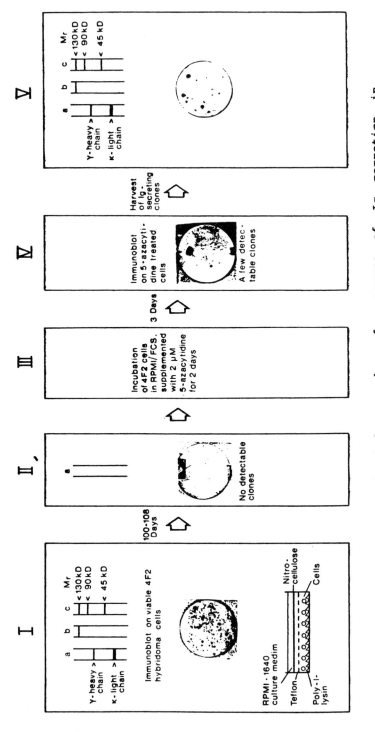

Fig. 3. Experimental procedure for rescue of Ig secretion in hybridoma cultures that for unknown reasons have lost Ig-production. The cells were treated with 5-azaC, seeded into plastic dishes, overlaid with teflon and immunoblotted. Viable hybridoma cells may be harvested after the procedure. For further methodological details, see rf. 12.

Moreover, preliminary experiments aiming to measure the spontaneous frequency of Ig-heavy chain switch ($\mu - \gamma$; $\gamma_1 - \gamma_{2a}$) indicate that these frequencies may be in the range of $10^{-5}-10^{-6}$. Various drugs are now tested for their effects on this frequency; - selection of hybridoma variants with high Ig-secretion.

It is an important feature of the system that relevant hybridoma clones may be harvested viable and therefore expanded in cultures. We consequently consider the system to be a significant adjunct to current hybridoma technology. In addition, it has already been crucial to experimentally demonstrate that the m^5Cyt pattern of Ig related genes affects the expression of such genes in murine and presumably also other eukaryotic cell systems (13). It may also suggest that similar mechanisms are regulating the expression of Ig-genes inserted into prokaryotic genomes by DNA recombinant technology, and that the m^5Cyt pattern should be considered, when eukaryotic vectors are used for expression of cloned Ig molecules.

CONCLUSION

Protein and DNA biochemistry has advanced to the stage, where analysis and construction of such molecules have become laboratory routine. In contrast, carbohydrate and lipid biochemistry technology still seems in its infancy, at least with respect to simplicity and rapidity. It seems therefore advantageous for many purposes, if protein/DNA biochemical procedures can be applied in studies of carbohydrate structures. The generation of antibodies with structural homology to carbohydrate structures may facilitate this approach, and a feasible method is here described. In addition, a procedure to detect rare variants as regard to specific cell membrane features within a cell population is reported, and should facilitate detection of such variants. The techniques may be useful in many areas aiming to dissect biological functions of different cell membrane molecules and structures.

REFERENCES

1. Hakomori S (1985) Cancer Res 45: 2405-2414

2. Cohen RJ and Eisen HN (1977) Cell Immunol 32: 1-9

3. Ohno S (1977) Immunol Rev 33:59-69

4. Simonsen M, Skjodt K, Krone M et al. (1985)   Prog Allergy 36: 151 -176

5. Due C, Simonsen M and Olsson L (1986) Proc Natl Acad Sci USA, in press

6. Nepom GT et al. (1984) Proc Natl Acad Sci USA 81: 2864-2867

7. Lee VK et al. (1985) Proc Natl Acad Sci USA 82: 6286-6290

8. Pettijohn D, Due C, Ronne E et al. (1986) Cancer Res, in press

9. Fehlmann M, Peyron J-F, Samson M et al (1985) Proc Natl Acad Sci USA 82: 8634-8637

10. Downward J, Yarden Y, Mayes E et al. (1984) Nature 307:521-527

11. Due C, Linnet K, Langeland Johansen N and Olsson L (1985) Diabetologia 28: 749-755

12. McCracken AA and Brown JL (1984) Biotechniques 2: 82-87

13. Jones PA (1986) Cancer Res 46: 461-466

© 1987 Elsevier Science Publishers B.V. (Biomedical Division)
Concepts and theories in carcinogenesis. A.P. Maskens et al. eds.

ABERRANT CONTROL OF INTERCELLULAR COMMUNICATION AND CELL DIFFERENTIATION DURING CARCINOGENESIS

H. YAMASAKI

International Agency for Research on Cancer, 150 cours Albert Thomas, 69372 Lyon cedex 08, France

INTRODUCTION

Before a potentially tumorigenic cell meets a carcinogenic stimulus, its proliferation and differentiation and those of its neighbouring cells are under tight control and their functions are well coordinated. In other words, cells in a given tissue form an orderly society, and a cancer cell is a rebel against that society. Therefore, it is important to study how the cellular society is maintained, and how carcinogenic stimuli produce chaos in the society. One of the most important mechanisms by which cellular differentiation and proliferation are controlled is through cell-cell interaction (1). It is reasonable to assume that cellular mechanisms of carcinogenesis involve disturbance of cell-cell interaction.

It is now believed that almost all forms of carcinogenesis involve a multistage process and that each stage can be influenced by a variety of exogenous and endogenous factors (2-4). It is also believed that, during the initiation phase, carcinogens damage DNA, and, during the promotion stage, the initiated cells expand clonally over surrounding normal cells. The activation of certain cellular oncogenes is implicated in the process of carcinogenesis and it is becoming clear that these cellular oncogenes play an important role in the control of cell differentiation and cell proliferation (5,6). Some carcinogenic stimuli, such as chemical carcinogens, have been suggested to activate these cellular oncogenes directly (7). In this article, I will review the available literature that suggests the involvement of aberrant control of cell differentiation and proliferation and of intercellular communication during multistage carcinogenesis, and try to link these events to each stage of carcinogenesis.

118

CELL DIFFERENTIATION AND CARCINOGENESIS

In order for a potential cancer cell to grow into a tumour mass, it must grow more than surrounding normal cells, so that the cancerous cells can expand over the normal tissue. However, it is clear that mere hyperproliferation of cells does not constitute a tumour. For example, psoriasis is a hyperproliferative disease of the skin, but it is not neoplastic because the hyperproliferative cells maintain a programme of epidermal differentiation and such differentiation leads the cells to their death; thus, even if cells proliferate very rapidly, as long as harmony is maintained between cell proliferation and differentiation, a tumor will not occur. In cancer, the harmony breaks down, and there are too many immature proliferating cells. It has been proposed that cancer is a disease in which the programme of differentiation is altered (8). This is schematically presented in Fig. 1.

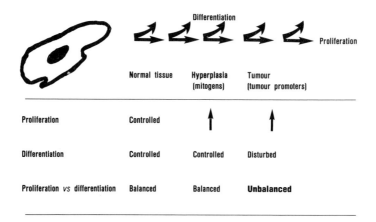

Fig. 1 Schematic view of cancer cells in comparison to normal cells.

Historically, the aberrant differentiation theory of carcinogenesis came from comparative studies of cancer cells and normal cells. Cancer cells usually exhibit more embryonic gene expression than normal cells. However, since tumour cells never produce protein that is completely different from that of normal cell, the essential difference between tumour cells and normal cells is that the former express several genes at the time and place which are not appropriate. In fact, many cancer cells can be induced to differentiate terminally (8,9), strongly suggesting that if a cancer cell is forced to differentiate into the normal pathway of the differentiation programme, the balance of cell proliferation and cell differentiation can be re-established.

Although comparisons of normal and tumor cells provide convincing evidence that transformed cells have an altered programme of cell differentiation, it is difficult to establish whether and when the differentiation programme is altered during carcinogenesis. It is possible that aberrant differentiation is the result rather than the cause of carcinogenesis, reflecting an inherent problem in cancer research. One way of approaching this problem is to study factors that are known to be involved in the causation of cancer, e.g., defined carcinogenic chemicals, viruses or genes that are known to be involved in carcinogenesis, such as oncogenes. Using these tools, it has become clear that the differentiation process is indeed altered during carcinogenesis. Phorbol ester tumour-promoting agents are the tools that have consistently been reported to modulate programmes of cell differentiation in cultured cells as well as in vivo (reviewed in 10). These results are consistent with the idea that aberrant gene expression or an altered differentiation programme play an important role in the tumour promotion process.

The idea that the promotion step is due to aberrant differentiation of initiated cells was extended by Matsunaga (11) to explain the mechanism for the causation of hereditary bilateral retinoblastoma in humans. The initiation step is presumed to be a genetic predisposition, because bilateral retinoblastoma cases usually show autosomal dominant inheritance. His analysis of age-specific incidence data on 244 cases of bilateral retinoblastoma showed a high intraclass correlation of the ages of the patients at the time of diagnosis of the disease in both the right and left eyes. This result argues against the two-mutation theory of the disease proposed by Knudson (12), in which the occurrence of cancers

in both the right and left eyes would not be expected within a short
time interval, since somatic cell mutation is a random and rare
event. Matsunaga suggests that it is more reasonable to assume that
the "expression of the retinoblastoma genes" is largely determined
by host factor common to both eyes. He believes that the promotion
stage in bilateral retinoblastoma constitutes an error in the
process of differentiation. However, his result is also compatible
with the idea that a somatic mutation occurs before the retinoblasts
are separated into two eyes during development.

Another line of evidence suggests that an altered programme of
differentiation may be triggered during the initiation phase. Using
mouse skin epidermal cells, Yuspa's group (13) showed that painting
of mouse skin with chemical carcinogens alters the differentiation
programme of epidermal cells. Usually, when epidermal cells are
cultured, they respond to calcium such that at higher concentrations
they differentiate. When epidermal cells were taken from mouse skin
that had been painted with chemical carcinogens and cultured, they
did not differentiate, even when the concentration of carcinogen was
increased to the dose that usually induces differentiation of normal
epidermal cells (14). Mouse keratinocytes also become resistant to
the differentiation signal of elevated calcium concentration after
they were exposed to carcinogens in vitro (15); and these
calcium-resistant cells were not tumorigenic. These results suggest
that resistance to differentiation signals occurs early in
carcinogenesis, and that an initiating agent may alter the
commitment to cell differentiation.

Changes in the cell differentiation pattern induced as early
events by chemical carcinogens have also been demonstrated in other
systems. Early changes seen during the induction of colon cancer in
mice and rats by chemical carcinogens are alterations of the
proliferation pattern in the colonic mucosa (16). Usually, the outer
layers of epithelial cells do not proliferate in normal colon;
however, after treatment with chemical carcinogens, the outer layers
also proliferate. Familial multipolyposis patients have a genetic
predisposition to intestinal-tract cancer, and examination of non
neoplastic colonic mucosa from these patients indicates that they
have a defect similar to that observed in experimental animals

treated with chemical carcinogens (17). Inhibition of differentiation has also been reported to be the earliest change in chemical induction of rat colon tumours (16).

Recent studies suggest that activation of cellular oncogenes may be responsible for certain cancers (5-7), and it has been proposed that the targets (or substrate) for chemical carcinogens inside cells are particular oncogenes. The normal physiological role of some cellular oncogenes is in the control of cell proliferation and cell differentiation (5,6). Alteration of their normal function by chemical carcinogens may therefore change the differentiation pathway and lead to tumor formation. The clearest example of activation of cellular oncogenes by chemicals was reported by the group of Barbacid, who observed that 100% of mammary tumours induced by a single injection of N-methyl-N-nitrosourea contained activated H-ras oncogene and that the mutation in H-ras occurred at the site in all tumours (7).

Recently, several pedigrees of transgenic mice were produced by introducing recombinant genes into fertilized mouse eggs (18). When new oncogenes are introduced into these transgenic mice, they develop tissue-specific neoplasms. For example, transgenic mice with SV40 T antigen gene always develop tumours of the choroid plexus (19). Mice bearing the myc gene fused to a murine mammary tumour viral promoter always develop mammary tumours after pregnancy (20). When the SV40 T antigen was linked to the regulatory part of a human insulin gene, however, the transgenic mice developed pancreatic-B cell tumours (21). These results suggest that the expression of oncogenes depends on the type of differentiation of the cells. If expression of the inserted oncogene were not regulated by the differentiation state of the cell, the transgenic mice should produce tumours at all sites; furthermore, the oncogenes would have been expressed during development and there would be a high percentage of malformations.

Several strong lines of evidences suggest that the induction of differentiation can suppress malignancy. When highly malignant HeLa cells are fused with normal fibroblasts or keratinocytes, the hybrids are often non tumorigenic in vivo, although they express transformed phenotype in vitro (22). When hybrid cells are induced to differentiate terminally in a host animal into which they are injected, they develop the phenotype of their fibroblast or keratinocyte parent. Toti-potency has been demonstrated during the development of mouse embryonal carcinoma cells injected into mouse blastocysts in several experiments (23), indicating that the experimental restoration of an intact differentiation programme can reverse the malignant phenotype. During liver carcinogenesis, many nodules disappear, and this remodelling of preneoplastic hepatocytes is considered to be the result of re-differentiation of altered cells to mature hepatocytes (24).

GAP-JUNCTIONAL INTERCELLULAR COMMUNICATION

Gap junctions are believed to be the only channels through which molecules can be exchanged between cells (1). Since their discovery, cells have been considered not as individual units but as functionally connected units. Gap-junctional structures can be studied by electron microscopy, and their function can be studied by several methods (1): metabolic cooperation, electric coupling, and dye transfer. Each method has its advantages and disadvantages.

The term "metabolic cooperation" appeared originally in a paper by Shubak-Sharp et al (25), who described a phenomenon whereby variant tissue culture cells, genetically incapable of incorporating a nucleic acid precursor into polynucleotide, could do so when in contact with wild-type cells. Of the methods used to measure intercellular communication, metabolic cooperation methods are probably the most widely used, since the technique involved is relatively simple in comparison with other methods (reviewed in 26). The most common method is measurement of metabolic cooperation between HPRT+ and HPRT- cell combinations. When HPRT+ and HPRT- cells are cocultured in the presence of 6-thioguanine, HPRT cells metabolize 6-thioguanine, and a toxic metabolite, 6-thioguanine monophosphate, is formed and transferred to HPRT- cell via gap junctions. Therefore, not only HPRT+ cells but also HPRT- cells are killed, although the latter cannot metabolize 6-thioguanine and are therefore resistant to it when cultured alone. In an other commonly used assay, one population of cells is labelled with a radioactive nucleoside, for example, ³H-uridine, and cocultured with nonlabelled cells; transfer of radioactive metabolite is determined by grain counting on radioautographed cell layers. Since both of these assays require coculture of two populations of cells, their obvious disadvantage is that they do not allow measurement of intercellular communication capacity in one population of cells. The dye transfer method described below resolves this problem.

In the dye-transfer method, tracer dyes is microinjected into cells and their spread is monitored. The tracer molecules used must not diffuse through the membranes so that one can be sure that their spread into neighbouring cells occurs only through gap junctions. Several suitable molecules have been used: Lucifer Yellow CH is employed widely: others include coloured dyes, radioactively-labelled molecules, heavy metals and enzymes (1). Another method of studying gap-junctional intercellular communication is to measure fluorescence without microinjection technique - for instance, that of fluorescein esters. These esters enter cells readily and are then hydrolysed to free their fluorescein moiety, which is polar and is lost from cells only slowly (27). The microinjection technique has one great advantage, that the tracer dyes can be injected into any type of cells - fibroblasts, epithelial cells, normal cells or transformed cells. In our laboratory, we use this microinjection technique routinely to study the possible involvement of gap-junctional communication in tumour promotion.

The two methods described above can be used to measure only the transfer of molecules (1). If one wants to prove that there is no communication, it is not enough to show that there is no movement of molecules through gap junctions: ion transfer must also be studied. Electrophysiological methods are required for this purpose (1). Proof that there is no ion transfer is good evidence that there is no communication. It is evident that the latter method is relatively sophisticated and is not easy to set up in laboratories.

INHIBITION OF GAP-JUNCTIONAL COMMUNICATION BY TUMOUR PROMOTING AGENTS.

Phorbol ester tumour-promoting agents have been shown repeatedly to inhibit gap-junctional communication of various types of cells in culture, using all three of the methods described above (28-32). To my knowledge, this is the first class of compounds that has been shown repeatedly and reproducibly specifically to inhibit gap junctional communication. Decreased numbers of gap junctions have also been found in cells treated in culture with 12-O-tetradecanoylphorbol 13-acetate (TPA) and in TPA-treated mouse skin by electron microscopy and biochemical methods (33-35).

Inhibition of intercellular communication by TPA was originally shown independently by Trosko's group (29) and by Murray's group (28), using metabolic cooperation between cultured cells. Inhibition of metabolic cooperation by TPA has been confirmed repeatedly by many research groups (36-38). In order to show that the transfer not only of molecules but also of ions is inhibited by tumour-promoting agents, we used the electrophysiological method and have shown successfully that electrical coupling between cultured human amniotic epithelial cells is inhibited by a low concentration of TPA (30). Our results indicate that TPA inhibits not only the initial coupling but also the establishment of intercellular communication between cells.

Since measurement by electrical coupling is laborious, we turned to microinjection of dye and its transfer to surrounding cells, which makes it possible to study the mechanistic aspects of phorbol ester-mediated inhibition of intercellular communication: we have also shown that intercellular communication is inhibited by phorbol ester tumour promoting agents (32). We found a good correlation between the ability of various derivatives of phorbol esters to inhibit dye transfer and their ability to promote tumours on mouse skin. We have also tested repeatedly anti-tumour-promoting agents, such as retinoic acid, dexamethasone, fluocinolone acetamide and cyclic AMP, and found that they all antagonize the effect of TPA on intercellular communication (39). These results are consistent with the idea that phorbol ester-mediated inhibition of intercellular communication is involved in the mechanism of tumour promotion on mouse skin.

Like many other effects of phorbol esters on cells, inhibition of gap-junctional communication is reversible. The effect of TPA can be reversed even in the presence of cycloheximide and/or actinomycin D (32,40), suggesting that TPA-mediated inhibition of communication may not involve total destruction of gap-junctional structures but only closure, so that molecules cannot pass through, or dispersal of the gap-junctional stuctures into small pieces. When TPA is removed, gap-junctional stuctures may open or reassemble. A model of the open and closed state of gap junction has been proposed (41).

It is now clear that phorbol esters bind to specific cellular receptors. Recent, detailed studies have indicated that this receptor is protein kinase C and that phorbol esters can bind directly to and activate this kinase, taking the role of diacylglycerols. Protein kinase C requires calcium, phospholipid and diacylglycerol for maximum activation (42). Since TPA can replace diacylglycerols and activate this protein kinase C (43), it has been suggested that diacylglycerols are functional analogues of phorbol esters. If this is the case, then diacylglycerols should act like TPA, and, in fact, there have been many reports that diacylglycerol can mimic the effects of TPA. We have also found that diacylglycerol can inhibit intercellular communication between BALB/c 3T3 cells (44). It also inhibited intercellular communication between TPA-sensitive, but not TPA-resistant, Syrian hamster embryo cells (unpublished results).

Although phorbol esters are the clearest examples of tumour promoters that inhibit junctional communication, many other such agents have been reported to inhibit communication (45). In addition, tumour-promoting stimuli, such as partial hepatectomy for rat liver carcinogenesis and skin wounding for mouse skin carcinogenesis, also reduce gap junctional activity (46,47). These findings are summarized in table 1. These results stimulated several investigators to use blockage of intercellular communication as an endpoint in a screening test for tumour-promoting agents (45,48).

ROLE OF BLOCKED INTERCELLULAR COMMUNICATION IN CELL TRANSFORMATION

Several lines of evidence suggest that blocked intercellular communication is involved in clonal expansion of initiated cells, i.e., the process of tumour promotion. For example, when phorbol esters were used as tumour promoting agents in two stage transformation of BALB/c 3T3 cells, there was a good correlation between the extent of inhibition of intercellular communication and

TABLE 1.

INHIBITION OF GAP JUNCTIONAL INTERCELLULAR COMMUNICATION BY TUMOR PROMOTING STIMULI

Methods of junctional communication measurement	Promoting stimulus	Target cells or tissue	Reference
METABOLIC COOPERATION			
HPRT+/HPRT-*	Phorbol esters and many other tumor promoting agents	Chinese hamster V79 Human fibroblasts Rat hepatocytes/rat liver epithelial cells	29 61 62
³H-uridine metabolites transfer	Phorbol esters	Mouse epidermal cell line /Swiss 3T3 cells	28
ASS-/ASL- **	Phorbol ester, DDT	Human fibroblasts	63
ELECTRICAL COUPLING	Phorbol esters	Human amniotic membrane epithelial cells	30
		BALB/c 3T3 cells	64
DYE TRANSFER Microinjection	Phorbol esters and some other tumour promoting agents	Human colon epithelial Mouse epidermal cell line BALB/c 3T3 cells Chinese hamster V79	31 65 32 66
	Partial hepatectomy	Rat liver	47
Photobleaching	TPA and dieldrin	Human teratocarcinoma cells	67
GAP JUNCTION STRUCTURE ANALYSIS Electron microscope	Phorbol ester	Chinese hamster V79	33
	Phorbol esters	Mouse skin in vivo	35
	Skin wouding	Urodele skin	46
	Phenobarbital or DDT administration	Rat liver in vivo	68
Gel electrophoresis analysis	Phorbol esters	Chinese Hamster V79	34
Analysis with gap junction antibody	Partial hepatectomy	Rat liver in vivo	69

* HPRT, hypoxantine guanine phosphoriribosyltransferase
** ASS-, argininosuccinate synthetase-deficient; ASL-, argininosuccinate lyase-deficient

enhancement of cell transformation (49). However, in another two-stage transformation system, C3H 10T1/2 cells, no such correlation was found (50).

Rivedal et al (51) have studied the effect of TPA on intercellular communication and enhancement of transformation in Syrian hamster embryo cells. TPA inhibited communication only in a cell line in which it enhanced cell transformation, and had no effect in a TPA-resistant line, suggesting that there is a good correlation between inhibition of communication and enhancement of cell transformation. However, it should be emphasized that this transformation system uses colony formation as its endpoint, whereas the BALB/c 3T3 and C3H 10T1/2 systems are focus assays. In the Syrian hamster embryo cell system, TPA induces morphological transformation of colonies within a day, whereas four to five weeks are required for the other two systems, which use focus formation. Therefore, it is likely that TPA enhances the process of cell transformation in BALB/c 3T3 and C3H 10T1/2 cells, whereas it enhances expression of morphological transformation in Syrian hamster embryo cells. Nonetheless, these results suggest that block of junctionnal communication may be involved both in the process and expression of cell transformation.

Use of BALB/c 3T3 cell variants provided another line of evidence for the involvement of blocked intercellular communication in cell transformation. When variants that are sensitive (clone A31-1-13) were compared to those that are resistant (clone A31-1-8) to induction of cell transformation by ultraviolet radiation or chemical carcinogens, no difference was seen in their ability to metabolize carcinogens, to bind these metabolites to DNA, to repair DNA damage or in their susceptibility to induction of mutation (52,53). However, there was a drastic difference in their intercellular communication capacity: although their communication capacity was similar at the growing phase, transformation-sensitive (A31-1-13) but not resistant (A31-1-8) cells lost this capacity at confluency (54). We interprete these results to indicate that transformation-sensitive cells have an intrinsic ability to express a TPA-like effect (block of the communication) at confluence, leading to enhanced transformation in this cell line.

INTERCELLULAR COMMUNICATION AMONG AND BETWEEN TRANSFORMED AND NONTRANSFORMED CELLS

In the past, much attention was paid to studying and comparing the communication capacity of transformed or tumorigenic cells with that of their normal counterparts (1,55). Although several reports suggest that transformed and tumorigenic cells have a lower communication capacity than non transformed and non tumorigenic cells, this observation does not apply in all cases (1, 55). Previous studies were carried out under the hypothesis that since transformed cells lose their growth control and growth control is mediated _via_ junctional communication, transformed cells should have a lower communication capacity (1).

I should like to propose another hypothesis, that transformed cells have reduced growth control because they are not controlled by surrounding normal cells. Under this hypothesis, communication among transformed cells is not a major problem; the most important determinant is that transformed cells cannot communicate with surrounding normal cells. If they did, the normal cells could transfer growth control signals to the transformed cells and cause them to lose their phenotypes.

In vitro cell transformation focus assay systems, such as the BALB/c 3T3 cell system, provide an ideal tool for testing this hypothesis, since transformed cells can be produced _in situ_ over a non transformed cell layer. Communication among and between transformed and non transformed cells in this system can be studied easily. Using this system we found that transformed and nontransformed cells can communicate among themselves but that there is no communication between the two cell types (56). This selective communication can be induced in cells transformed by chemical carcinogens, ultraviolet radiation or oncogenes (56,57 and unpublished results).

Although we must expand our observation to other systems, especially _in vivo_ and to epithelial cells, these results support our working hypothesis that the selective intercellular communication capacity of transformed cells is important to the maintenance of transformed phenotypes. This hypothesis is shown schematically in Figure 2.

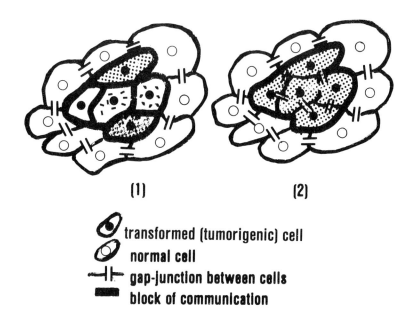

transformed (tumorigenic) cell
normal cell
gap-junction between cells
block of communication

Fig. 2 Selective intercellular communication and maintenance of transformed phenotypes - schematic view. Scheme (1) shows a tumor in which individual cells cannot intercommunicate and thus cannot communicate with the surrounding normal cells. In scheme (2), the cells in the tumor intercommunicate among themselves but not with surrounding cells. In neither case is there communication between the tumour and the surrounding normal cells.

CELL-CELL INTERACTION AND GENE EXPRESSION

In the process of tumor promotion, there is a selective clonal expansion of initiated cells but not of surrounding normal cells. How is this achieved? I have explained that a selective block of communication between initiated and normal cells is one way of isolating initiated cells from normal cells. However, if they are isolated in this way but the genetic information in the initiated and in the normal cells is the same, both would expand clonally and we would see no clonal expansion to a tumor. Since this is not the case, it is reasonable to assume that initiated cells contain different genetic information from that of normal surrounding cells; it is also reasonable to assume that this genetic difference occurs when the cell meets the initiating agent and that isolation of initiated cells from the surrounding normal cells is the way in which expression of the altered genetic information takes place. Here, I should like to give several examples in which we can see that cell-to-cell interaction can modulate gene expression.

During embryogenesis, of course, cell-to-cell interaction is a very important determinant in the process of organogenesis. For example, a recent paper demonstrates that antibodies against gap-junctional proteins can disturb early development of the amphibian embryo (58). Although these results suggest the direct involvement of gap-junctional communication during embryogenesis, the antibody is quite bulky, and antibody treatment of cells may result in their physical dissociation.

When cells are dispersed for monolayer culture, many types lose their differentiating characteristics, whereas after culture in organotypic culture they maintain their characteristics. For example, cartilage cells quickly lose their capacity for making their specific products when dispersed but regain them when they are packed together again (59); however, when the cells are dispersed for more than ten days, they fail to restore their function even after reassociation.

In a more recent study, it was shown that, in order to maintain primary hepatocytes in the differentiated state, they must be in contact with certain epithelial cells that derive from the liver (60). Although it is assumed that these epithelial cells come from the biliary canaliculi, this is not certain. With this system, when hepatocytes are removed from rat liver by conventional perfusion and cocultured with epithelial cells, the specific differentiating function of the hepatocytes can be maintained for more than eight weeks, whereas when hepatocytes are cultured without epithelial cells, they lose their function within 48 h. In this coculture system, it is the direct interaction of epithelial cells with hepatocytes that is important. If there is a layer of collagen between epithelial cells and hepatocytes, hepatocyte function cannot be maintained. It is also interesting to note that, if hepatocytes are in contact with epithelial cells at one point, all other hepatocytes distant from the epithelial cells can also maintain their differentiated state. This suggests that direct interaction between epithelial cells and hepatocytes is necessary for transfer of the message to maintain hepatocyte differentiation, and that the message can be transferred to other hepatocytes through homogeneous membrane interaction. In collaboration with Dr Guguen-Guillouzo, we have recently found that there is apparently no gap-junctional communication between epithelial cells and hepatocytes, implying that the message for maintenance of hepatocyte function is passed by cell-to-cell recognition or membrane-to-membrane interaction.

These results also indicate that junctional communication is only one of several mechanisms of cell-cell interaction for controlling gene expression. Thus, it is necessary to study control of cell-cell interaction not only through gap junctions but also through other means.

ACKNOWLEDGEMENT

I thank Ms E. Heseltine for editing the manuscript and Ms C. Fuchez for various secretarial aids.

REFERENCES

1. Loewenstein (1979) Biochim Biophys Acta 560: 1-65

2. Slaga TJ, Sivak A, Boutwell RK (1978) Mechanisms of Tumor Promotion and Cocarcinogenesis. Raven Press, NY.

3. Hecker E, Fusening NE, Kunz W et al (1982) Cocarcinogenesis and Biological Effects of Tumor Promoters, Raven Press, NY.

4. Börzsönyi M, Lapis K, Day NE et al (1984) Models, Mechanisms and Etiology of Tumor Promotion, IARC Scientific Publications 56, IARC, Lyon

5. Bishop JM (1982) Sci Amer, March: 69-78

6. Weinberg RA (1985) Science 230: 770-776

7. Barbacid M (1986) Carcinogenesis, 7: 1037-1042

8. Sachs L (1986) Sci Amer, January: 30-37

9. Marks PA, Rifkind RA (1978) Ann Rev Biochem 47: 419-448

10. Yamasaki H (1984) In: Mechanisms of Tumor Promotion, Vol IV, Tumor Promotion and Carcinogenesis in vitro, Slaga TJ (ed), CRC Press Inc, Boca Raton, Florida, pp 1-26

11. Matsunaga E (1979) J Natl Cancer Inst 63: 933-939

12. Knudson AG Jr (1971) Proc Natl Acad Sci USA 68: 820-823

13. Yuspa SH, Hennings H, Lichti U (1981) J Supramolec Struct Cell Biochem 17: 245-257

14. Kulesz-Martin M, Koehler B, Hennings H et al (1980) Carcinogenesis 1: 995-1006

15. Yuspa SH, Morgan DL (1981) Nature 293: 72-74

16. Deschner EE (1978) Z Krebsforsch 91: 205-216

17. Deschner EE, Lipkin M (1975) Cancer Res 35: 413-418

18. Palmiter RD, Brinster RL (1985) Cell, 41: 343-345

19. Palmiter RD, Chen HI, Messing A et al (1985) Nature 316: 457-460

20. Stewart TA, Pattendale PK, Leder P (1984) Cell 38: 627-637

21. Hanahan D (1985) Nature 315: 115-122

22. Stanbridge EJ, Der CJ, Doersen CJ et al Science 215: 252-259

23. Brinster RL (1974) J Exp Med 140: 1049-1056

24. Tatematsu M, Nagamine Y, Farber E (1983) Cancer Res 43: 5049-5053

25. Shubak-Sharpe H, Burks RR, Pitts JD (1969) J Cell Sci 4: 353-367

26. Hooper ML (1982) Biochim Biophys Acta 651: 85-103

27. Stewart WW (1978) Cell 14: 741-759

28. Murray WA, Fitzgerald JD (1979) Biochem Biophys Res Comm 91: 395-401

29. Yotti LP, Chang CC, Trosko JE (1979) Science 206: 1089-1091

30. Enomoto T, Sasaki Y, Shiba Y et al (1981) Proc Natl Acad Sci USA 78: 5628-5632

31. Friedman EA, Steinberg M (1982) Cancer Res 42: 5096-5105

32. Enomoto T, Martel M, Kanno Y et al (1984) J Cell Physiol 121: 323-333

33. Yancey SB, Edens JE, Trosko JE et al (1982) Exp Cell Res 19: 329-340

34. Finbow ME, Schuttleworth J, Hamilton AE et al (1983) EMBO J 2: 1479-1486

35. Kalimi GH, Sirsat SM (1984) Cancer Lett 22: 343-350

36. Newbold RF, Amos J (1981) Carcinogenesis 2: 243-249

37. Dorman BH, Boreiko CJ (1983) Carcinogenesis 4: 873-877

38. Kinsella AR (1982) Carcinogenesis 3: 499-503

39. Yamasaki H, Enomoto T, Hamel E et al (1984) In: Cellular Interactions by Environmental Tumor Promoters, Fujiki H, Hecker E, Moore RE et al (eds), Japan Sci Soc Press, Tokyo/VNU Sci Press, Utrecht, pp 221-233

40. Yamasaki H, Enomoto T, Martel N et al (1983) Exp Cell Res 146: 297-308

41. Unwin PNT, Zampighi G, (1980) Nature 283: 545-549

42. Nishizuka Y (1984) Nature 306:693-698

43. Sharkey NA, Leack KL, Blumberg PM (1984) Proc Natl Acad Sci USA 81: 607-610

44. Enomoto T, Yamasaki H (1985) Cancer Res 45: 3706-3710

45. Trosko JE, Yotti LP, Warren ST et al (1982) In: Carcinogenesis - A Comprehensive Survey, Vol 7, Hecker E, Fusening NE, Kunz W et al (eds), Raven Press, NY, pp 565-585

46. Loewenstein WR, Penn RD (1967) J Cell Biol 33: 235-242

47. Meyer DJ, Yancey SB, Revel JP (1981) J Cell Biol 91: 505-523

48. Yamasaki H (1984) Food Addit Contam 1: 179-187

49. Enomoto T, Yamasaki H (1985) Cancer Res 45: 2681-2688

50. Dorman BH, Butterworth BE, Boreiko CJ (1983) Carcinogenesis 4: 1109-1115

51. Rivedal E, Sanner T, Enomoto T et al (1985) Carcinogenesis 6: 899-902

52. Kakunaga T, Crow JD (1980) Science 209: 505-507

53. Lo KY, Kakunaga T (1982) Cancer Res 42: 2644-2650

54. Yamasaki H, Enomoto T, Shiba Y et al (1985) Cancer Res 45: 637-641

55. Weinstein RS, Merk FB, Alroy J (1976) Adv Cancer Res 23: 23-89

56. Enomoto T, Yamasaki H (1984) Cancer Res 44: 5200-5203

57. Yamasaki H, Frixen U, Mesnil M et al (1986) Proc Am Assoc Cancer Res 27: 133

58. Warner AE, Guthrie SC, Gilula NB (1984) Nature 311: 127-131

59. Holtzer H, Abbott J, Lash J et al (1960) Proc Natl Acad Sci USA 46: 1533-1542

60. Fraslin JM, Kneip B, Vaulont S et al (1985) EMBO J 4: 2487-2491

61. Mosser DD, Bols NC (1982) Carcinogenesis 3: 1207-1212

62. Willams GM, Telang S, Tong C (1981) Cancer Lett 11: 339-344

63. Davidson JS, Baumgarten I, Harley EH (1985) Cancer Res 45: 515-519

64. Yamasaki H, Enomoto T, Shiba Y et al (1985) Cancer Res 45: 637-641

65. Fitzgerald DJ, Knowles SE, Balland J et al (1983) Cancer Res 43: 3614-3618

66. Zeilmaker MJ, Yamasaki H (1986) Cancer Res, in press

67. Wade MH, Trosko JE, Shindler M (1986) Science 232: 525-528

68. Sugie S, Mori H, Takahashi M (1984) Int Cell Biol, 1984: 316

69. Traub O, Druge PM, Willecke K (1983) Proc Natl Acad Sci USA 80: 755-759

© 1987 Elsevier Science Publishers B.V. (Biomedical Divison)
Concepts and theories in carcinogenesis. A.P. Maskens et al. eds.

GENETIC ALTERATIONS AND GENETIC REGULATIONS IN EMBRYOGENESIS AND ONCOGENESIS

J.J. PICARD

Laboratory of Developmental Genetics, Place Croix du Sud, 5 (Bte 3), 1348 Louvain-la-Neuve, Belgium.

It is presently broadly accepted that embryogenesis proceeds by a coordinated regulation of genetic expression without irreversible alterations of the genetic material. On the other hand, it is commonly assumed that a genetic alteration is always at the origin of the oncogenic transformation. The present review will discuss some of the basic evidence for these two generalizations. In addition, the last part of the review will analyze the significance of the expression of embryonic genes in malignant cells. Genetic alterations are defined as any change in the primary sequence of DNA, including chromosomal aberrations, translocations, amplifications, deletions, base substitutions and chemical modifications of bases such as methylations. Genetic regulation is defined as all epigenetic processes leading to a modification of the genetic expression without genetic alteration.

EMBRYOGENESIS IS THE RESULT OF COORDINATED REGULATION OF GENETIC EXPRESSION AND NOT THE RESULT OF COORDINATED GENETIC ALTERATION.

A considerable amount of evidence has accumulated indicating that the differential synthesis of mRNAs and proteins in adult cell types is due to the regulation of the genetic expression and not to the specific alteration of the genome. This evidence strongly suggests that embryogenesis results from identical or similar coordinated mechanisms which control a precise sequence of spatial and temporal changes of gene expression. Direct demonstration that embryogenesis is not controlled by gene alterations has been much more difficult to obtain. Two main evidences may be considered.

The first type of evidence is provided by nuclear transplantation experiments mainly performed in amphibian species. When nuclei from amphibian blastulae, gastrulae, neurulae or tadpoles were injected into enucleated eggs, they supported the development of the recipient egg to tadpole or even to adult stages (reviews in Gurdon (31), Mc Kinnel (44)). It was observed that the most advanced developmental stage reached by the recipient egg was dependent on the developmental stage of the donor cell. The more advanced the developmental stage of the donor cell, the less advanced the developmental stage that could be reached by the recipient egg. Nuclei from adult tissues never allowed the recipient egg to develop further than the young tadpole stage. As a rule, serial transplantations improved the results (percentages of successful development) but did not basically change the general conclusion. The results of these experiments have been understood as a demonstration that nuclei of advanced embryos and tadpoles still have the complete undisturbed genetic information normally present in the zygote. Failures were explained by the disparity between the programmed cell cycle of the cytoplasm of the recipient egg and the phase and pace of the cell cycle programmed in the donor nucleus. The disparity would generate abnormalities during the first few S and M phases and the resulting chromosomal aberrations would be incompatible with normal development. The more advanced the developmental stage of the donor nucleus the more important would be the disparity in the cell cycle. When nuclei of differentiated cells from the gut (29) or epidermis (11) of advanced tadpoles or from the adult skin (30) were injected into enucleated eggs a small percentage (2-8%) of the recipient eggs developed into advanced tadpoles. The differentiation of the donor cell was ascertained by morphological criteria. The argument says that the successful cases demonstrate that the differentiated cells still possess the unaltered genetic information for all other cell types. However, it could be objected that undifferentiated stem cells could have been erroneously used in a few cases. Errors would be rare but the success was also a rare event. It may be concluded that the results of nuclear transplatations in Amphibians suggest that embryogenesis is not associated with genetic alterations but that the evidence is not conclusive.

Nuclear transplantations performed on mammalian eggs have given very different results than those performed on amphibian eggs. When the two pronuclei of a mouse donor egg are injected into an enucleated egg, 90% of the recipient eggs develop until the blastula stage. When the donor nucleus is taken from a 2 cell stage embryo, only 20% of the recipients reach the blastula stage. When the donor nucleus is taken from a 4 or 8 cell stage embryo, only 5% and 0%, respectively, of the recipients reach the morula stage (43).

These and other results indicate that the capacity of nuclei from embryonic stages to support a normal development is much more restricted in Mammals than in Amphibians. The difference does not seem to be attributable to a greater disparity in the cell cycle of the donor and recipient cell. The failure to obtain a normal development by nuclear transplantation in Mammals is not a proof that the genetic material is irreversibly changed during early embryogenesis. Indeed, eggs possessing two paternal or two maternal genomes are lethal (69). A specific imprinting of the genomic material during gametogenesis is required for a normal development. The imprinting affects specific chromosomes and chromosome regions (42,12). Similar imprinting mechanisms could be at work during embryogenesis and explain the failure of nuclear transplantations in both mammalian and amphibian species when cells from late developmental stages are used. Imprinting would merely happen earlier in Mammals than in Amphibians. However, it remains that nuclear transplantations in both Amphibians and Mammals have not provided the convincing evidence that embryogenesis is not controlled by specific and orderly alterations in the genomic material.

The second main set of evidence for an epigenetic control of developmental processes comes from the detailed analysis of the DNA structure in differentiated adult tissues. An extensive variety of studies indicates that, as a rule, differentiated cells are not characterized by selective amplifications or selective losses of DNA sequences (15). Recent studies using cDNA recombinant techniques (39,50) have demonstrated that DNA sequences involved in the development of the Drosophila and Xenopus embryo do not undergo major deletions, amplifications or rearrangements. However, minor modifications such as base substitutions or small deletions or insertions would admittedly not be detected by these techniques and could possibly be of regulatory importance. In addition, an increasing number of examples of modifications of the genetic content of eukaryotic cells during differentiation or embryogenesis has been well documented in recent years: an important proportion of DNA and chromosomes are eliminated during the development of some insect (6) and worm (70) species; some genes are amplified during oogenesis in Drosophila (68) and Xenopus (10); immunoglobulin genes undergo rearrangements during development (8,60); genetic re-arrangments are observed in the switch of mating types in yeast (33) and in the modification of surface antigens in trypanosomes (48). It is still difficult to decide whether these observations correspond to very special mechanisms that bear little on the processes involved in embryogenesis.

It may be concluded that there is no convincing evidence against the hypothesis that embryogenesis is primarily controlled by epigenetic mechanisms which regulate the genetic expression in a coordinated way. However, a direct demonstration of the hypothesis is still lacking.

ONCOGENESIS IS THE RESULT OF A GENETIC ALTERATION AND NOT THE RESULT OF AN ALTERATION IN THE GENETIC REGULATION.

The discovery of oncogenes and protooncogenes and the analysis of their expression in normal and cancer cells has lead to significant progress in the understanding of oncogenesis. It is now broadly assumed that genetic alterations are always at the origin of the oncogenic transformation. In contrast, epigenetic theories such as those relating the origin of neoplasia to some failure in embryogenesis or differentiation, have so far failed to provide a decisive insight into the oncogenic process. However, two main evidences seem to favor the possibility that epigenetic mechanisms could also be at the origin of the oncogenic transformation and should be analyzed in detail: the first one is related to the experimental reversion of the malignant phenotype and the second one is based on the experimental induction of teratocarcinomas.

Reversion of the malignant phenotype to a normal phenotype under the influence of an embryonic environment has been considered as evidence that the initial step of the oncogenic transformation was not a genetic alteration in these tumor cells. When some types of malignant cells were inserted into mouse embryos at the appropriate stage, tumor-derived cells participated in the normal development. Adult animals, derived from the host embryos after transfer to a forster mother, did not develop tumors although they were proven to be mosaics containing many normally differentiated tumor-derived cells in a few or in a majority of the organs. The same result was also observed after the injection of cloned malignant cells. In some instances, even germ cells were proven to be tumor-derived cells (reviewed in Mintz and Fleischman (45)). Reversion of the neoplastic phenotype under the influence of embryonic tissues was demonstrated for teratocarcinoma cells by Brinster (9) and by well known experiments performed by Mintz and collaborators (48,45). Similar reversions were also observed for neuroblastoma (55,56), mammary carcinoma (17) and myeloid leukemic cells (27). The ability of these malignant cells to loose their abnormal phenotype under the influence of embryonic cells and to form normally functioning differentiated adult cells has been understood by several authors as clear evidence that the primary event leading to the malignant transformation in these cells was not a structural genetic alteration. Mintz and collaborators (48,45) concluded that malignancy in the stem cells of these tumors had been caused by a disorganized cellular environment rather than by mutation. It had already been similarly proposed by Pierce (54) that carcinogenesis may result from altered developmental influences rather than from alterations of the genome.

Several arguments against a mutational origin of the neoplastic phenotype in these particular cells have been pointed out by these authors (45). First a progeny was obtained from the tumor-lineage germ cells of some mosaic animals. In this progeny, no impairment of development and survival and no increased incidence of tumors was observed. Second, reversal of the malignant phenotype was permanent. Tissues obtained from mosaic animals and containing tumor-derived cells were grafted on histocompatible animals and no tumors ever grew. Thirdly, the appearance of tumors in a small proportion of adult mosaic animals can be explained by the failure of some of the injected cells to be incorporated into the inner cell mass of the embryo. The conclusion was that, in addition to mutational causes, epigenetic mechanisms may also induce abnormal expression leading to the malignant phenotype.

However, these and other arguments admittedly point to indirect evidence. One could also argue that a mutation would not be incompatible with reversal of the malignant phenotype by the embryonic environment. For example, a genetic alteration leading to an overexpression of some oncogene or to the expression of an abnormal form of a protooncogene would result in a transformed phenotype in the adult environment because the abnormality would result in an increased proliferative response to specific growth factors present in the adult environment. When the same cell is placed into the embryo, the abnormal expression of the oncogene would not result in a transformed phenotype because the growth factors would not be present in the embryo or would have another specificity. Later in development, the abnormal gene would be permanently repressed at some time during this second run through developmental processes.

The second main evidence in favor of epigenetic mechanisms is related to experimentally induced teratocarcinomas. When embryonic germinal cells or early embryos are grafted into adults at ectopic places, tumors will often arise from the grafted cells. In many strains of mice, the grafted embryo will generate a tumor in almost all experimental animals. A majority of these tumors are malignant teratocarcinomas (64). It has been pointed out that the mutational rate in the small population of grafted cells should be exceedingly high to explain the observed frequency of malignant tumors (45). However, in some strains of mice the same experiment will not induce the development of teratocarcinomas (65). In addition, rats and other mammalian species are also insensitive to experimental teratocarcinogenesis (66). The reason for this discrepancy is not known.

In the author's laboratory, experiments have been performed on an amphibian species, <u>Xenopus borealis</u>, in order to verify if the experimental teratocarcinogenesis observed in mice can be extended to non mammalian species. It has been demonstrated in the author's laboratory and by other authors that amphibian species are susceptible to viral (28) and chemical (5,35,52) carcinogenesis.

Rare cases of spontaneous teratomas and teracarcinomas have been reported in Amphibians (4,5). The implantation of embryos into adult amphibians has been performed by several workers (3,37,2,24,59,18,62). Most of these authors concluded that benign teratomas evolved from the implanted embryos. One of the main difficulties in these experiments is the lack of histocompatible strains in most amphibian species.

In a first series of experiments (57), random bred _Xenopus borealis_ from a small colony in the author's laboratory were used for embryo transplantations. Sibling embryos were grafted under the dorsal skin of sibling adult hosts obtained from another couple. Tumor induction was more successful with tailbud embryos (stage 28) than with gastrulae (stage 10) (Fig. 1 and Table 1). When tailbud stage embryos were implanted either into premetamorphic tadpoles (stage 56) or into young adults, the development of tumors was higher in adults than in tadpoles (Table 1). When grafted embryos (tailbud stage) and young adult hosts were all siblings, all hosts carried a tumor during the 20 weeks of observation (Fig. 2).

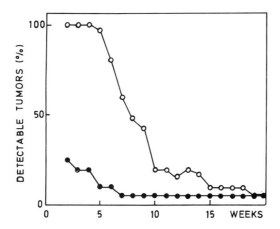

Fig. 1. Influence of the age of the implanted embryo on the development of teratomas. Sibling tailbud stage (Stage 26-28)(0-0) and gastrulae (stage 10)(●-●) from the _Xenopus borealis_ species were implanted under the dorsal skin of young sibling adults derived from another couple. Tumors were detected by manual palpation.

TABLE I

INFLUENCE OF THE AGE OF THE EMBRYO AND THE HOST ON THE DEVELOPMENT
OF TERATOMAS

Age		Tumor-bearing animals (%)	
Embryo	Host	2 weeks	12 weeks
st. 10	toadlet	26	5
st. 28	toadlet	100	15
st. 28	st. 56	80	6
st. 28	toadlet	100	15

Influence of the age of the embryo and the host on the development
of teratomas in <u>Xenopus borealis</u>. Twenty sibling embryos of the
developmental age indicated in the table were implanted each under
the dorsal skin of genetically unrelated sibling hosts (young adults
or late tadpoles). Tumors were recorded by manual palpation at 2 and
12 weeks after implantation.

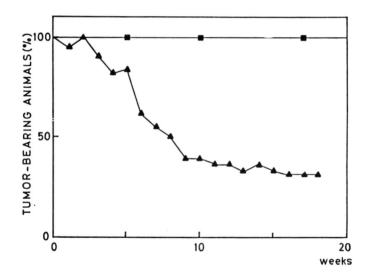

Fig. 2. Influence of the genomic relationship between embryos and
hosts on the evolution of teratomas. Sibling tailbud stage <u>Xenopus
borealis</u> embryos were implanted under the dorsal skin either into
sibling genetically unrelated adults (▲-▲) or into adults generated
by the parents of the embryos (■-■). Tumors were recorded by manual
palpation.

Histologically, all tumors were benign teratomas. Metastases
were never observed. In an attempt to increase the
probability of teratocarcinogenesis, embryos were first incubated

for 24 hrs at 23^b in a physiological salt solution containing
N-methyl-N'-nitro- N-nitrosoguanidine (MNNG). Embryos were cut into
three pieces to allow proper diffusion of the chemical into the
tissues. No toxic effects were observed at concentrations
below 0.3 x 10^{-3}M. Embryos were incubated in 10^{-4}M MNNG and the
three pieces were implanted into young adult hosts. Control embryos
were incubated in the physiological salt solution. Embryos and hosts
were all siblings. The evolution of the weight of the tumors was
significantly different in the two groups of animals (Fig. 3). The
mean weight of the tumors from the control group increased markedly
during the 25 weeks of observation. All animals developed tumors.
Some tumors reached huge volumes and the animals were unable to
survive due to mechanical problems (impairment of feeding or
breathing). In the experimental animals, the mean weight of the
tumors increased slowly during the 52 weeks of observation (Fig. 3).
Tumors in both groups were histologically classified as benign
teratomas. They contained the usual mixture of many different well
differentiated tissues belonging to the three embryonic layers. Most
tumors had one or several cysts filled with a mucous liquid. The
tumors were surrounded by a fibrous capsule and were irrigated by
one or two vascular pedicles. Neighbouring tissues were never
invaded by the tumors. No metastases were ever detected. No
qualitative differences were observed between the control and
experimental groups. When teratomas from both groups were
transplanted, they slowly regressed and no teratocarcinomas were
observed (57).

The failure to induce teratocarcinomas in these experiments may
be due to several reasons already discussed by other authors
(41,64,45). The recent development in the author's laboratory of an
histocompatible strain of <u>Xenopus borealis</u> (1) could make it
possible to improve the experimental design. Finally, Amphibians
develop more slowly and survive for much longer periods than rats
and mice and the observation should possibly be extended over longer
periods than in the present experiment.

Let us return to the argument in favor of the epigenetic
mechanism developed by Mintz and Fleichman (45). The very high
percentage of success in experimental teratocarcinogenesis observed

144

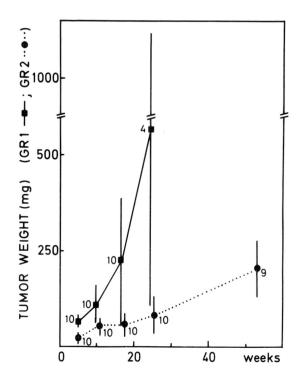

Fig. 3. Growth of teratomas generated by tailbud stage <u>Xenopus</u> <u>borealis</u> embryos in sibling adults. The mean weight of the tumor was recorded as a function of time after the graft. Embryos were cut into three pieces and incubated for 24 hrs either in a physiological salt solution (■-■) or in the same solution containing MNNG (10^{-4}M) (●-●). After incubation, the three pieces of each embryo were implanted under the dorsal skin of each host.

in the mouse does not seem to be convincing evidence. Sensitive strains of mice could have viral sequences integrated in their genome and the unusual environment of the ectopic embryo would result in the expression of these sequences with a high frequency. In these cases, experimental induction of teratocarcinomas would not be different from other inductions of tumors that result both from a structural alteration of the genome and from some associated epigenetic stimuli.

We may conclude that neither the reversion of the malignant phenotype by embryonic tissues nor the high frequency of teratocarcinomas developing from ectopic mouse embryos give convincing evidence that epigenetic mechanisms without genomic alteration can induce the oncogenic transformation.

IS EXPRESSION OF EMBRYONIC GENES ASSOCIATED WITH OR INVOLVED IN THE ONCOGENIC TRANSFORMATION ?

Many authors have long been impressed by similarities between embryonic and tumor cells, in growth properties, in differentiation and in ability to invade the neighbouring tissues and to migrate at long distances (reviewed in Sherbert (61)). The synthesis in numerous cancer cells of ectopic peptides, normally observed in embryos or fetuses, such as the alpha-fetoprotein, the carcinoembryonic antigen and several others, or of cell surface markers and isozymes seemed to some authors to indicate that some mechanisms active in embryogenesis are also active in oncogenesis (71). In addition, associations between teratogenesis and oncogenesis appeared to some authors to imply that the two processes are intimately related at the genetic or epigenetic level (7,26).

Embryonic genes may be defined as genes expressed in some or all cells during embryogenesis and inactive or active at low levels in adult tissues. Due to the small size of most embryos, extensive studies of specific gene activity during embryogenesis has long been very difficult. Studies on the control of the synthesis of RNAs and proteins corresponding to defined embryonic genes have been even scarcer until recently. Among an increasing number of pertinent studies using recombinant cDNA techniques, one may mention the homeotic genes that control embryonic segmentation in Drosophila and other organisms (40,32). Another example, are the several DG genes (differentially expressed in gastrula) analyzed in Xenopus embryos by Dawid and coworkers (16). These genes have a specific spatial and temporal expression in the embryo and are all repressed in the adult tissues. Most of them have still unknown functions.

In the context of the present review, one would expect to find a few embryonic genes expressed in some malignant tumors if some abnormality in the genetic expression that controls embryogenesis is primarily involved in some cases of oncogenesis. Alterations of the genome could also induce an abnormal expression of these embryonic genes or an expression of abnormal embryonic genes. It has been observed that some embryonic or fetal antigens as well as fetal isozymes and other markers are expressed in some cancer cells (71,34). Among other examples , it may be mentioned that a 55-kdalton phosphoprotein, induced in mouse cells after SV40 transformation is also expressed in embryos in a stage-specific way (13). Using monoclonal antibodies, it has been shown that some glycoproteins and glycolipids have antigenic domains that are expressed only in embryos and cancer cells (23). Finally, it has been demonstrated that some protooncogenes are expressed in embryonic tissues: c-src is expressed during organogenesis of the neural tissue (67,25); high levels of c-fos products are observed in fetal membranes (14,59); c-myc has specific patterns of expression in human embryos (51).

In the author's laboratory, Lempereur et al. (38) have shown that _Xenopus_ embryos and a tumorigenic _Xenopus_ cell line express at least four common antigens at a much higher level than adult liver cells and non transformed cells. A rabbit antiserum was prepared by immunization with extracts from a tumorigenic cell line, XB693T. This cell line induces malignant adenocarcinomas when injected into histocompatible _Xenopus_ hosts (52). Cellular extracts from the tumorigenic cells (XB693T cell strain), from the XB693 cell strain (the non transformed cell strain from which XB693T cells were derived by _in vitro_ chemical mutagenesis), from embryos (neurula stage) and from adult _Xenopus_ liver were analyzed with the antiserum. All cellular extracts were prepared in the same buffer. Extracts from the two cell strains were obtained from cells at confluence. One example of such an analysis is shown in Fig 4. Two antigens of about 19 and 46 kdalton are detected in the tumorigenic cell line and in the embryos and are absent or present at low levels in both the non transformed cells and the adult liver. Similar analyses showed that two additional antigens of about 78 and 36 kdalton are observed in embryos and transformed cells and absent or less abundant in untransformed cells and adult liver (37). These experiments demonstrate that the expression of a few antigens is probably restricted to embryos and malignant cells. The nature and function of these antigens is unknown.

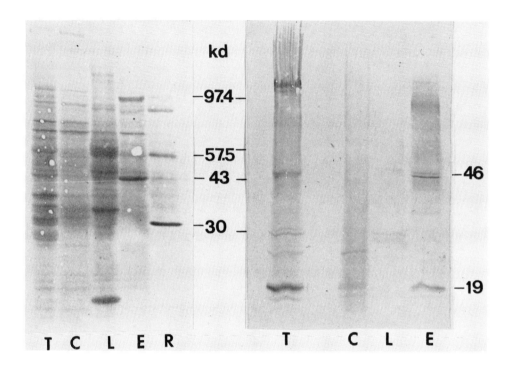

Fig. 4. Immunoblot analysis of cellular extracts from <u>Xenopus</u> <u>borealis</u>. T, extract from XB693T cell strain (tumorigenic); C, extract from XB693 cell strain (non-transformed); L, extract from adult liver; E, extract from neurula (stage 17) embryos; R, molecular weight protein markers. Each track was loaded with 40 µg protein. The proteins were separated by electrophoresis on a 5 to 25 % acrylamide gradient SDS-polyacrylamide gel. <u>Left</u>: Amido black 10B staining of a nitrocellulose transfer. <u>Right</u>: nitrocellulose transfer and immunoblotting with a rabbit anti-XB693T cells (diluted 1/100) revealed with a swine HRP- conjugated anti-rabbit IgG (Dako; 1/1000). The two antigens of about 19 and 46 kdalton are present in T and E and absent or at very low concentration in C and L.

Using a different approach, we have recently shown that the same tumorigenic <u>Xenopus</u> cell line expresses several maternal and early embryonic mRNAs (i.e. mRNAs present in oocytes and embryos) (53). RNAs were prepared from <u>Xenopus</u> oocytes, gastrulae and tadpoles and used by Dworkin and collaborators to construct cDNA libraries in pBR322 or PBR322-derived vectors (19,21). About 550 clones were found to give an hybridization signal with ^{32}P-cDNA probes prepared from RNAs isolated from develomental stages (20). These clones were first screened by colony hybridization with ^{32}P-cDNA probes from RNAs isolated from <u>Xenopus</u> adult liver, XB693

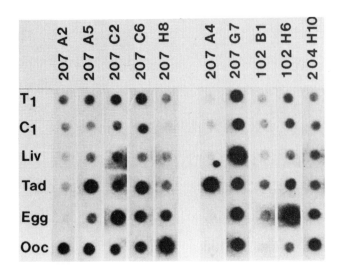

Fig. 5. DNA dot hybridizations.
[32]P-cDNA probes were prepared from poly(A)$^+$RNA isolated from Xenopus
borealis XB693 Tcells (T1) (tumorigenic cells), XB693 cells (C1)
(untransformed cells), adult liver (Liv), stage 41 tadpoles (Tad),
eggs (Egg) and a mixture of stage I to V oocytes (Ooc). The two cell
lines were at confluence (T1 and C1). The left half of the figure
shows data from five of the selected sequences. The right half of
the figure shows data from five control sequences as defined in the
text. All data are taken from the same experiment.

cells (the non transformed cell line) and XB693T cells (the

tumorigenic substrains of XB693). Clones were selected when they

gave a signal with probes from transformed cells and no signal with

the two other probes. The selected clones were again screened using

DNA dot hybridizations with the same three probes as well as with

probes prepared from developmental stages. An example of DNA

hybridization is given in Fig. 5. In this experiment five sequences

were selected for a higher expression in the tumorigenic cell line

than in the non transformed cell line (53). Southern gel transfer

experiments allowed to discard sequences homologous to rRNA and to

verify that the selected sequences were unrelated to each other.

Several plasmids contained sequences expressed at equal titer in the

two cell lines. These sequences were called control sequences. They

were used to adjust RNA concentrations in RNA dot blot

hybridizations. Finally, probes were synthesized by nick translation

of the selected clones and hybridized to RNA dots prepared from the

three types of cells.

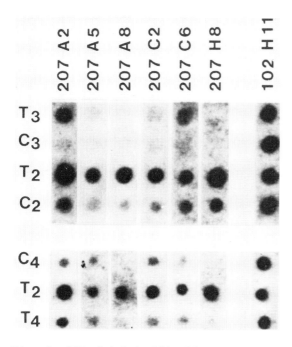

Fig. 6. RNA dot hybridizations.
^{32}P-probes were synthesized by nick translation of six selected sequences and one of the control sequences and were hybridized to RNA dots. Total RNA was extracted from unfractionated XB693 cells at confluence (C2;C4), XB693T cells at confluence (T2;T4), Xb693 cells during exponential growth (C3) and XB693T cells during exponential growth (T3). The top four rows and the bottom three rows are taken from two different experiments. The names of the probes are indicated above.

An example of this type of analysis is shown in Fig. 6. In many experiments, the selected sequence hybridized more strongly with RNA samples from XB693T cells than with RNA samples from XB693 cells, when both cell types were at confluence (Fig. 6: C2/T2 and C4/T2). However, variations in the level of the sequences were observed in similar RNA preparations (Fig. 6: C2/C4 and T2/T4, at confluence). In addition, when compared to cells at confluence, the levels of the selected sequences were reduced in both XB693 and XB693T cells in the exponentially growing phase (Fig. 6: C3/T3). This variation was not seen with control sequences such as 102H11 and is therefore probably not due to experimental artifacts. As a whole, six sequences were selected that were expressed at a higher titer in RNA samples from the tumorigenic cell line than in RNA samples from the non transformed cell line. All these sequences are expressed in significant amounts in early oogenesis. Sequences corresponding to 207H8 and 207A2 decrease during oogenesis and embryogenesis. The RNA corresponding to 207A5 decreases during oogenesis and persists during embryogenesis (22). Three of the sequences, 207A2, 207A5 and 207H8 were identified by DNA sequencing followed by a computer search of protein data banks as coding for, respectively, the glycolytic enzyme enolase, the ATP-ADP binding protein and alpha-tubulin. In vitro experimental conditions that may influence the expression of the six sequences are currently investigated.

The results obtained in the author's laboratory on the level of mRNAs and of antigens are in accordance with the literature summarized above. They point to the conclusion that some embryonic genes are expressed at least in some malignant cells while they are repressed or expressed at low titer in normal adult cells; they are no proof that the expression of embryonic genes in tumor cells is a rule nor that the inappropriate expression of embryonic genes in adult cells is required in the oncogenic process. These observations could be circumstantial and should be confirmed by similar analyses on other species and tumors. They could be linked to cellular proliferation. They could also be more or less remote effects of the oncogenic process or of the successive adaptations of the transformed cell to the expression of oncogenes. However, the accumulation in recent years of similar observations suggests that some embryonic genes could play some crucial but still unknown role in oncogenesis.

CONCLUSIONS

It may be concluded that there is so far no convincing evidence that neoplasia may be initiated by epigenetic mechanisms. There are well established data indicating that several malignant tumors express embryonic genes. Due to our still very limited knowledge of gene expression in embryos it can be expected that more examples will be discovered in the near future. The significance of these observations is unknown. The abnormal expression could be due to alterations in the genome as well as to a cellular adaptation to the oncogenic transformation.

Expression of one or two abnormal oncogenes or a qualitatively abnormal expression of oncogenes has been demonstrated to be sufficient for the induction of uncontrolled growth. However, development of a clinical cancer is admittedly a multistep process and requires more than the loss of control on proliferation. It has been recently pointed out by several authors (36,49,63,51) that a high level of expression of cellular or viral oncogenes or the expression of mutated oncogenes is not sufficient to achieve the full conversion of normal cells to tumorigenic cells. It remains difficult to explain how the known oncogenes would induce the profound metabolic changes, the invasive properties and the ability to metastasize. Successive alterations and a cascade of regulatory adaptations are probably required for the tumorigenic conversion. Some embryonic genes could possibly be involved in these alterations.

REFERENCES

1. Afifi A, Picard JJ, Querinjean P (1985) Lab Anim Sci 35: 139-141

2. Allison JE (1955) Anat Rec 122: 561

3. Andres G (1950) Rev Suisse Zool 57: 1-12

4. Balls M, Clothier RH (1974) Oncology 29:501-519

5. Balls, Clothier RH, Ruben L (1978) In: Animal models of comparative and developmental aspects of immunity and disease, Gershwin ME, Cooper EL (eds), Pergamon Press, New York, pp 48-62

6. Bantock CR (1970) J Embryol exp Morph 24: 257-286

7. Bolande RP (1984) J Histochem Cytochem 32: 878-884

8. Brack C, Hirama M, Lenhard-Schuller R et al. (1978) Cell 15: 1-14

9. Brinster RL (1974) J Exp Med 140:1049-1056

10. Brown DD, Dawid IB (1968) Science 160: 272-280

11. Brun RB, Kobel HR (1972) Rev Suisse Zool 79: 961-965

12. Cattanach BM, Kirk M (1985) Nature 315: 496-498

13. Chandrasekaran K, McFarland VW, Simmons DT et al. (1981), Proc Natl Acad Sci, USA 78: 6953-6957

14. Curran T, Miller AD, Zokas L et al. (1984) Cell 136: 259-268

15. Davidson EH, Britten RJ (1973) Quart Rev Biol 48: 565-613

16. Dawid IB, Sargent TD (1986) Trends Genet 2:47-50

17. Decosse JJ, Gossens CL, Kuzma JF et al. (1973) Science 181: 1057-1058

18. Dent JN, Benson DG (1966) Anat Rec 155: 315

19. Dworkin MB, Dawid IB (1980a) Develop Biol 76: 435-448

20. Dworkin MB, Dawid IB (1980b) Develop Biol 76: 449-464

21. Dworkin MB, Dworkin-Rastl E, (1985) Develop Biol 112: 451-457

22. Dworkin MB, Shrutkowski A, Dworkin-Rastl E (1985) Proc Natl Acad Sci, U.S. 82: 7636-7640

23. Feizi T (1985) Nature 314: 53-57

24. Frankhauser G, Stonesifer GL (1956) J exp Zool 132: 85-103

25. Fults DW, Towle AC, Lauder JM et al. (1985) Molec cell Biol 5: 27-32

26. Gill TJ (1984) Biochim Biophys Acta 738: 93-102

27. Gootwine E, Webb CG, Sachs L (1982) Nature 299: 63-65

28. Granoff A, Gravell M, Darlingrton RW (1969) In : Biology of amphibian tumors, Mizell M (ed), Springler-Verlag,NY pp 279-295

29. Gurdon JB (1968) Scient Amer 219: 24-35

30. Gurdon JB, Laskey RA (1970) J Embryol exp Morph 24: 227-248

31. Gurdon JB (1974) The control of gene expression in animal development, Clarendon Press, Oxford

32. Harding K, Wedeen C, McGinnis W et al. (1985) Science 229: 1236-1242

33. Hicks J, Strathern JN and Klar AJS (1979) Nature 282: 478-483

34. Ibsen KH, Fishman WH (1979) Biochim Biophys Acta 560: 243-280

35. Khudoley VV, Picard JJ (1980) Int J Cancer 25: 679-683

36. Land H, Parada LF, Weinberg RA (1983) Science 222: 771-778

37. Lehman FE (1950) Rev Suisse Zool 57: 13-24

38. Lempereur P, Querinjean P, Picard JJ Arch Intern Biochim. In press

39. Levine M, Garen A, Lepesant J et al. (1981) Proc Natl Acad Sci, USA, 78: 2417-2421

40. Lewis EB (1978) Nature 276: 565-570

41. Martin GR (1982) In: Teratocarcinoma and embryonic interactions, Muramatsu T, Gachelin G et al. (eds) Academic Press, New York, pp 3-17

42. McGrath J, Solter D (1984) Nature 308: 550-551

43. McGrath J (1986) Nuclear transfer in mouse embryos, Comm. at the B.S.D.B. Symposium on Determinative Mechanisms in Early Development. Univers. East Anglia, Norwich, 6-9 April

44. McKinnel RG (1978), Cloning. Nuclear transplatation in Amphibia, Univ Minnesota Press, Oxford

45. Mintz B, Fleischman RA (1981) Adv Cancer Res 34: 211-278

46. Mintz B, Illmensee K (1975) Proc Natl Sci, USA, 72: 3585-3589

47. Mintz B, Illmensee K, Gearhart JD (1975) In: Teratomas and Differentiation,Sherman MJ,Solter D (eds),Acad Press,NY,pp 59-82

48. Moeijmakers JHJ, Frasch ACC, Bernards A et al. (1980) Nature, 284:78-80

49. Muller R, Verma IM (1984)   Curr Topics Microbiol Immunol 112: 73-115

50. Okada A, Shin T, Dworkin-Rastl E et al. (1985) Differentiation 29: 14-19

51. Pfeifer-Ohlsson S, Rydnert J, Goustin AS et al. (1985) Proc Natl Acad Sci, USA, 82: 5050-5054

52. Picard JJ, Afifi A, Pays A (1983) Carcinogenesis 4: 739-742

53. Picard JJ, Pelle R, Schonne E et al. (1986) Exptl Cell Res ,in press

54. Pierce GB (1967) In: Current Topics in Developmental Biology, Moscona AA, Monroy A (eds), Vol 2, Acad Press, NY, pp 223-246

55. Pierce GB, Pantazis CG, Caldwell JE et al. (1982) Cancer Res 42: 1082-1087

56. Podesta AH, Mullins J, Pierce GB et al. (1984)   Proc Natl Acad Sci, USA, 81: 7608-7611

57. Querinjean PJ, Picard JJ (1980) Fed Proc 39: 884

58. Rafferty NS (1961) J exp Zool 147: 33-41

59. Ruther U, Wagner EF, Muller R (1985) EMBO J 4: 1775-1781

60. Seidman JG, Max EE, Leder P (1979) Nature 280: 370-375

61. Sherbert GV (1982) The Biology of tumour malignancy, Acad Press, London

62. Simnett DJ (1966) Develop Biol 13: 112-143

63. Slamon DJ, Cline MJ (1984) Proc Natl Acad Sci USA 81:7141-7145

64. Solter D, Damjanov I (1982) In: Teratocarcinoma and embryonic cell interaction, Muramatsu T, Gachelin G, Moscona AA, Ikawa Y (eds), Acad Press, NY, pp 31-40

65. Solter D, Dominis M, Damjanov I (1979) Int J Cancer 24: 770-772

66. Solter D, Skreb N, Damjanov I (1970) Nature 227: 503-504

67. Sorge IK, Levy BT, Maness PF (1984) Cell 36: 249-257

68. Spralding AC, Mahowald PA (1980) Proc Natl Acad Sci, USA, 77: 1096-1100

69. Surani MAH, Barton SC, Norris ML (1984) Nature 308: 548-550

70. Tobler H, Smith KD, Ursprung H (1972) Develop Biol 27: 190-203

71. Uriel J (1979) Adv Cancer Res 29: 127-174

THE TISSUE LEVEL:
MULTISTEP CARCINOGENESIS

FROM NORMAL CELL TO CANCER : AN OVERVIEW INTRODUCING THE CONCEPT OF MODULATION OF CARCINOGENESIS

MB ROBERFROID

Unité de Biochimie Toxicologique et Cancérologique, Université Catholique de Louvain, U.C.L. 73.69, B - 1200 Brussels, Belgium

FOREWORD

This paper has been written as a controversial paper. To stimulate debate it is presented provocatively. It has been written to be presented during a symposium on "Concepts and Theories in Carcinogenesis".

INTRODUCTION

Most scientific reports on (chemical) carcinogenesis begin with the statement "that carcinogenesis is a long lasting multistage, multiphase or multistep process". It means that cancer is regarded as the end-point of a connected series of changes and/or actions. The changes are assumed to follow stages (in other words "several definite periods"), or phases (in other words " characteristic or decisive distinct stages or periods"). Moreover, they are assumed to require steps (in other words "single actions or proceedings regarded as leading to..") in order to take place or in order to be completed.

That carcinogenesis may be a long lasting process characterized by a latency period between the carcinogenic insult and the appearance of malignant neoplasms is known since the description by Pott of soot cancers in chimney sweeps.

That, preneoplastic and premalignant lesions often, but not always, preceed the appearance of cancer is known since the last century from the works of pathologists, studying human cancer, who made extensive descriptions of the natural history of neoplastic development.

That, in humans, such early lesions may play a role in the development of malignant neoplasia came from epidemiological studies of carcinoma in situ of the human cervix in relation to the occurrence of invasive carcinoma .

For human pathologists, a long lasting period exists between the "carcinogenic insult" and the appearance of cancer. During that period preneoplastic lesions appear that could, in some way or the other, play a role in the development of malignant neoplasia. Such a descriptive statement does imply neither that definite steps periods (stages) or characteristic/decisive distinct periods (phases) do exist during that long lasting process nor that the morphological changes leading to preneoplasia or neoplasia require single actions or proceedings (steps) to take place or to be completed.

During the last 40-45 years, experimental carcinogenesis has developed with the aim to give scientific bases to the experimental dissection of the history of neoplastic development (19). It remains however to be known whether such an approach has only dissected the "natural history" of neoplastic development or whether it has artificially manipulated it in such a way that its conclusions no longer concerns that "natural history" alone.

The multistage, multiphase or multistep nature of carcinogenesis has first been demonstrated on mouse skin and more recently for other tissues like the liver, the urinary bladder, the thyroid, the mammary glands, the lungs... The concept that cancer is the end point of a long lasting process during which stages/phases do arise that require steps to take place or to be completed relies most exclusively on operational rather than on biological evidences. It means that each "stage or phase" has been identified as resulting from the effect(s) of specific chemical, nutritional or surgical treatments considered as step(s). No one has been clearly defined by its biological nature. "The concept that carcinogenesis is a two-or a multistage process has developped mainly by indirect ways from experiments in which certain operational steps were used" (1).

1. THE MOUSE SKIN CARCINOGENIC PROCESSES

The efficiency of the two-stage protocol for rapid production of skin tumors (papillomas and squamous cells carcinomas) in mice is obvious.

Rous and Kidd (23) were the first to demonstrate that wounding of the skin of the rabbit's ear previously treated with a

carcinogenic polycyclic aromatic hydrocarbon resulted in the rapid
appearance of neoplastic growth compared with that on the ears of
animals treated only with the hydrocarbon. These experiments
suggested to the authors that the application of a polycyclic
aromatic hydrocarbon to mouse skin had begun a process in skin cells
that they termed initiation whereas the wounding had begun a second
process which they termed promotion (in other words an action or a
proceeding contributing to or helping the progress, development or
growth of "initiated cells or tissue").

A few years later Mottram (15), using mice, demonstrated
similarly that the application of a polycyclic aromatic hydrocarbon
on the shaved skin resulted in the rapid appearance of neoplasms
only in those animals subsequently treated with another agent, the
vesicant croton oil.

In 1947, Berenblum and Shubik (3) extended the Mottram's study
and demonstrated that two distinct stages analogous if not identical
with those of initiation and promotion could be shown in mouse skin
carcinogenesis. Furthermore they reported that the administration
of the promoting treatment must follow the application of the
initiating agent. Moreover the application of croton oil could be
delayed for many months after the application of the polycyclic
aromatic hydrocarbon without significantly affecting the yield of
neoplasms at the end of the experiment.

For the next four decades following these pioneering
experiments, numerous studies based on the mouse skin system
confirmed but also extended these observations demonstrating the
reversibility of promotion (4) as opposed to the irreversibility of
initiation, the non additivity of the effect of a promoting agent
(4) and the subdivision of tumor promotion into stage I and stage II
(4,26,9,27).

All these data are used to support the two-stage theory of skin
carcinogenesis "that over the years has taken on all the qualities
of what is traditionally called a paradigm. For the adherents it
represents the undisputed truth"..."The beneficial effects of
paradigm are that they make good, detailed research possible, and
the two-stage theory has certainly served extremely well in this
capacity. It has given us an overhelming mass of particular

information on cell biology and on the cellular effects of a few selected substances, <u>but until now it has not really helped us to understand carcinogenesis, the basic mechanisms of which still remain unexplained...</u>"We certainly do not object to the two-stage protocol as a good method for the rapid experimental production of skin cancer, we only disagree with some of the highly speculative and sweeping interpretations of the experimental results, which have led too many scientists to believe too strongly that <u>carcinogenesis</u> is already essentially explained : i.e. that it <u>really is a two-step process...</u>" (sentences taken from Iversen and Astrup (11)).

Indeed many experimental evidences that have been repeteadly reported are not at all integrated by the two-stage theory. They give rise to interpretations that are outside the paradigm. Thus they are not easily accepted.

Among these experimental evidences are the following facts :
- a single application of a skin carcinogen is enough to provoke both benign and malignant tumors (26,30);
- repeated doses of the same compound applied on the skin at regular intervals (weekly) induce both benign and malignant tumors. The repeated treatment with initiating doses of 7,12 dimethylbenz(a)anthracene produces fewer papillomas but many more carcinomas than the two-step protocol (26);
- treatment with a "promotor" before initiation, can in some experimental conditions, increase the tumor yield the way it does when given after (12);
- felt wheel abrasion alone works as a good tumor promotion treatment. It even produces malignant tumors in mice pretreated with a small dose of 7,12 dimethylbenz(a)anthracene (23);
- all chemicals with skin cancer promoting activity that have been tested induce papillomas and/or carcinomas when applied chronically to mouse skin not previously "initiated" (11);
- a pure "initiating treatment" given repeatedly after initiation and short term promotion is an excellent promoting treatment (10).

Even though a <u>two-step protocol</u> for skin carcinogenesis may be useful for the <u>rapid experimental production</u> of skin tumors and skin cancers mostly in mouse, the <u>two-stage/two phase/multistage/multiphase theory of skin carcinogenesis</u> to which that protocol gives support, has not all the qualities of a paradigm.

2. THE RODENT LIVER CARCINOGENIC PROCESSES

The second most frequently used target for experimental cancer research is the rodent liver (mainly the rat sometimes the mouse). (For review see Farber and Sarma, this book).

That hepatocarcinogenesis may occur in distinct stages equivalent to those seen in skin was first suspected by the demonstration of Farber (6) that the hyperplastic nodule may, in some instances, be a potential precursor to hepatocellular carcinoma. The studies of Teebor and Becker (29) lessened the impact of this concept by demonstrating that such nodules induced by the intermittent feeding of 2-acetylaminofluorene were reversible and disappeared after stopping the treatment.

The first two-step protocol for hepatocarcinogenesis has been described by Peraino et al. (16), who demonstrated that chronic phenobarbital feeding "markedly enhanced" the hepatocarcinogenic action of 2-acetylaminofluorene. During the last fifteen years, other protocols for the production of hepatic cancer have been reported by Scherer and Emmelot (24), Solt and Farber (28), Pitot (17), Lans et al. (13), Préat et al. (20,21) and Shivapurkar et al. (25). The protocol proposed by Scherer and Emmelot is not a two-step protocol but it has been modified by Pitot to become such. Except that proposed by Peraino, all these protocols use the same chemical as the initiating treatment i.e. diethylnitrosamine.

Given as a single dose treatment either alone (high dose) (25) or in combination with partial hepatectomy (low dose) (24) diethylnitrosamine is by itself fully carcinogenic if the rats are allowed to survive for up to 2 years.

Feeding rats chronically with PB after such a single dose treatment with either diethylnitrosamine (high dose) alone (25) or feeding them chronically with a peroxysome proliferator (Nafenopin) after a single high dose of diethylnitrosamine (21) increases tumor yield and shortens the latency period between the initiating treatment and the appearance of first tumors.

A 2 week treatment with 2-acetylaminofluorene combined with a stimulus of proliferation in the middle of that treatment results in essentially the same effects (28). According to the authors of that report, that treatment is a "short term promoting treatment ". Feeding rats chronically with PB after they had been submitted to a Solt and Farber recipe further increases tumor yield and further reduces the latency period for the appearance of the first cancer (5,13). In such a three-step protocol, the chronic administration of PB can be replaced by a porto-cava anastomosis to give essentially the same results (20).

The chronic administration of 2-acetylaminofluorene, (29) diethylnitrosamine (2) (as well as other nitrosamines), PB or Nafenopin is carcinogenic for rats.

In the liver of the rats treated according to either one of these protocols, whenever it has been analyzed, enzyme altered foci, preneoplastic lesions and/or hyperplastic nodules have been identified and characterized histologically, histochemically or even biochemically (for a review see Farber and Sarma, this book). One major exception has however been reported by Préat et al. (21) using the "promoting effect" of Nafenopin. Indeed the livers of the rats submitted to that two-step protocol have very rare preneoplastic lesions which furthermore show unusual patterns of morphologic alterations (Preat et al. manuscript in preparation).

At least 5 studies with different models (see 8 for references) have given support to the hypothesis that cancer can but do not necessarily arise inside hepatocytes nodules. However not all nodules are precursor of cancer. Indeed it has been shown that most of the early hepatocyte nodules disappear most probably through a remodelling process (21).

Based on these results it has been concluded that "the two-stage mechanism of initiation and promotion as first described for skin carcinogenesis is not a unique feature of this system, and that entirely comparable stages have now been demonstrated for the carcinogenic process in the liver"...(Pitot, 15).

However, such a conclusion is rather surprising because, once again, many experimental evidences are not integrated by the two-stage theory.

Among these experimental evidences are the following facts:

- a single application of an hepatocarcinogen to young rats or to previously hepatectomized adult rats is enough to provoke both benign and malignant tumors (24,25);

- intermittent feeding of the same compound i.e. 2-acetyl amino-fluorene (29) or diethylnitrosamine (2) or continuous feeding of nitrosomorpholine (1) induces both benign and malignant tumors. The chronic treatment with 2-acetylaminofluorene produces in a much shorter time more tumors and more hepatocellular carcinomas than the Peraino's two-step protocol (28);

- porto cava anastomosis works as well as PB, as a promoting treatment (20);

- all chemicals with liver cancer promoting activity that have been tested induce preneoplastic lesions and/or carcinomas when given chronically to rats not previously "initiated";

- a pure initiating treatment (dialkynitrosamine) administred repeatedly after initiation and short term promotion is an excellent promoting treatment (J. de Gerlache, personal communication);

- depending upon either the protocol used (single step, two-step , three-step) or the promoting treatment (PB or Nafenopin or porto cava anastomosis) the pathway from "initiated cells" to "cancer" may vary as well as the nature, the homogeneity or the diversity of the malignant tumors (5,21).

Even though a <u>two- or a three-step protocol</u> for hepatocarcinogenesis may be useful for the <u>rapid experimental production</u> of tumors and cancers mostly in rats, the <u>two-stage/two-phase/multistage/multiphase theory of hepato-carcinogenesis</u> to which these protocols give support, has not yet the qualities of a paradigm.

CONCLUSIONS

Experimental evidences accumulated over the recent years on mouse skin and rat liver carcinogenesis support the following conclusions which still need to be put together in A THEORY OF CARCINOGENESIS :

1. an <u>initiating treatment</u> is <u>necessary</u> to begin the process;

2. even <u>a single initiating dose</u> of a chemical is <u>a carcinogenic</u>

treatment (26,30);

3. sequential administration of chemicals with initiating or "promoting" activity (wathever the sequence may be, shows synergy between the two (three) classes of chemicals (11);

4. the consequence of that synergism is a reduction of the latency period between the initiating treatment and the appearance of tumors (5);

5. often that consequence is also a modification of the pathway from initiated cells to cancers (21);

6. the long term chronic administration of an initiating treatment is more carcinogenic than a two (three) step protocol (29);

7. even the repeated administration of an initiating treatment has the effects of a promoting treatment (10).

Beyond the initiating treatment for which, in some cases, a single dose is enough, the tissue/the cells slowly become malignant. In most cases the appearance of malignancy is preceded by premalignant lesions from which cancers seem to arise.

Additional exogenous treatments can be used to modify and accelerate that history.

A single step protocol begins a "natural" carcinogenic process. We do not know yet how multiphase/multistage that process is.

A multi-step protocol induces a modified carcinogenic process which has the characteristic of a multiphase/multistage process. We do not know for sure if that modified process simply mimics the "natural process". We do not know whether what we learn from the former can simply be transposed to the later.

Carcinogenesis is a long lasting process during which, in many but not all cases (cfr for example colonic carcinogenesis in rat) (14), preneoplastic lesions can be morphologically identified which preceed the appearance and/or which could be the precursor of malignant lesions. An initiating treatment (sometimes a single dose of chemical) is the only necessary treatment that, in adequate experimental conditions may be sufficient.

In experimental animals, various experimental means have been discovered which applied after such an initiating treatment (single fully, weakly or sub-carcinogenic dose; repeated fully, weakly or sub-carcinogenic doses) may :

- shorten the duration, (shorter latency period);
- amplify the intensity (increased number of tumors or cancers);
- potentiate a sub... treatment to make it able to induce a full
  carcinogenic process.

Such an experimental mean has been called a promoting treatment that, by definition, is thought to complete, contribute to, help, but not "induce" the neoplastic transformation.

However any time they have been tested, chemicals that have such a promoting activity have also been shown to be carcinogenic by themselves. Moreover chemicals with recognized initiating activity have been shown to have also promoting effects. With regards to the sequence of administration of the treatments, repeated experiments have similarly questionned the dogma of the Initiation before Promotion sequence by showing that, even though such a protocol may be less effective than the preceeding one, to reverse the sequence promotion followed by Initiation is also more carcinogenic than the initiating treatment alone.

Finally, repeated administration of an initiating treatment is always more efficient than the sequential administration of initiating and promoting treatments. Moreover the pathway to malignancy as well as the nature of malignancy induced by these two protocols may be different.

Besides these experimental evidences, Initiation is still defined as the production of potentially tumorigenic cells by limited exposure to carcinogen that induces neither a cancer cell nor a neoplastic cell (i.e cell that can proliferate without the need of a stimulus) but rather that produces some cell that can be differentially stimulated to produce a focal proliferation (7).

Such a definition strongly binds the initiated state to the promotion step because it says that : an initiated state cannot be detected per se but can only make itself evident only when promoting or selecting environment is created.

The further history of initiated-potentially tumorigenic cells is closely dependent upon the imposition of a suitable promoting environment.

Based on such assertions which however do not take into account all experimental evidences, it became self evident that PROMOTION is a biological process which is PART of carcinogenesis. In order to avoid such a confusion my suggestion is that any type of treatment given either before or after an initiating treatment should be called MODULATING TREATMENT, Modulation being defined as the process of varying the frequency, the amplitude, the intensity of ...

The "natural"history of cancer development is the one which starts after a single dose initiating treatment. It is a long story which probably goes through various stages/phases. We have discovered means to modulate it positively (acceleration increase in intensity...) or negatively (inhibition-slowing down....) We do not know yet if the modulated story is equivalent to the natural one. Perhaps something equivalent to promotion (endogenously mediated?) takes place during that long lasting natural history. Before making a paradigmatic theory out of still partial knowledges we have to be very careful. Let us be more modest.

We know a little bit about "initiating treatments";

We know they may be carcinogenic;

We know we can modulate that carcinogenic process;

We do not know yet how different are the effects of the various modulating treatments;

We do not know whether the process we described after modulation is similar, equivalent or different from the one we would see after pure initiation.

REFERENCES

1. Bannasch P (1984) J Cancer Res Clin Oncol 108: 11-22

2. Barbason H, Fridman-Manduzo A, Lelievre P et al. (1977) Eur J Cancer 13: 13-18

3. Berenblum I, Shubik P (1947) Brit J Cancer 1: 383-391

4. Boutwell RK (1964) Prog Exp Tumor Res 4: 207-250

5. de Gerlache J, Lans M, Preat V et al. (1984) Toxicol Pathol 12: 374-382

6. Farber E (1973) Cancer Res 33: 2537-2550

7. Farber E (1982) In: Sequential Events in Chemical Carcinogenesis in Cancer: a Comprehensive Treatise, Becker FF (ed) Vol 1, 2nd Ed, Plenum Publ Corp, NY, pp 485-506

8. Farber E (1984) Cancer Res 44: 5463-5474

9. Furstenberger G, Berry DL, Sory B et al. (1982) Proc Natl Acad

Sci USA 78: 7722-7726

10. Hennings H, Shores R, Wenk ML et al. (1983) Nature 304: 67-69

11. Iverson OH and Astrup EG (1984) Cancer Investig 2: 51-60

12. Iversen OH and Iversen U (1982) Brit J Cancer 45: 912-920

13. Lans M, de Gerlache J, Taper HS et al. (1983) Carcinogenesis 4: 141-144

14. Maskens AP (1983) In: Precancerous Lesions of the Gastrointestinal Tract, Sherlock P, Morson BC, Barbara S and Veronesi V (eds), Raven Press, NY, pp 223-240

15. Mottram JC, (1944) J Pathol Bacteriol 56: 181-187

16. Peraino C, Fry RJM and Staffeldt E (1971) Cancer Res 31: 1506-1512

17. Pitot HC, Barsness L, Goldsworthy, T et al. (1978) Nature 271: 456-458

18. Pitot HC and Sirica AE (1980) Biochim Biophys Acta 605: 191-215

19. Pitot HC (1983) Cancer Surveys 2: 519-538

20. Preat V, Pector JC, Taper H et al. (1984) Carcinogenesis, 5: 1151-1154

21. Preat V, Lans M, de Gerlache J et al. (1986) Jpn J Cancer Res (GANN) 77, In Press

22. Roomi MW, Ho RK, Sarma DSR et al. (1985) Cancer Res 45: 564-571

23. Rous P and Kidd JG (1941) J Exp Med 73: 365-384

24. Scherer E and Emmelot P (1975) Eur J Cancer 11: 145-154

25. Shivapurkar N, Hoover KL and Poirier LA (1986) Carcinogenesis 7: 547-550

26. Shubik P (1977) Cancer 40: 1821-1824

27. Slaga JT, Fischer SM, Nelson K et al. (1980) Proc Natl Acad Sci USA, 77: 3659-3663

28. Solt DB and Farber E (1976) Nature 263: 702-703

29. Teebor GW and Becker FF (1971) Cancer Res 31: 1-3

30. Terracini B, Schubik P and Della Porta G (1960) Cancer Res 20: 1538-1542

FROM THE NORMAL CELL TO CANCER: THE MULTISTEP PROCESS OF EXPERIMENTAL SKIN CARCINOGENESIS

F. MARKS and G. FÜRSTENBERGER
Deutsches Krebsforschungszentrum, Institut für Biochemie, Im Neuenheimer Feld 280, 6900 Heidelberg, F.R.G.

Cancer is generally assumed to be the result of genotoxic effects leading to a somatic mutation or to an improper gene activation. The complex pattern of tumor development indicates, however, that such a genetic alteration can only be regarded as the very beginning of the neoplastic process. Especially the development of human cancer is characterized by long latency periods and the existence of different precancerous stages which frequently appear to be reversible.

To deal with a carcinogenic mutation, the organism seems to possess, therefore, an arsenal of defense systems which have to be overrun step by step before a malignant tumor becomes clinically manifest.

If step-wise tumor development generally occurs it would provide the chance to interfere with the neoplastic process not only at its starting point but also at later stages. The purpose of such therapeutic approaches would be to allow the patient to live with his cancer cells. Consequently, it is highly desirable to imitate the step-wise development of tumors under experimental conditions and, in this way, to study the different stages in detail.

THE CLASSICAL APPROACH OF 2-STAGE SKIN CARCINOGENESIS

Skin has to be considered as the classical target organ of chemical carcinogenesis in animal experiments. In 1914 Yamagiwa's and Ichikawa's approach to induction of skin cancer in rabbits by prolonged application of coal tar (1) opened an era of experimental carcinogenesis characterized by painting animal skin with tar, or later with polycyclic aromatic hydrocarbons. It was observed that carcinoma development thus induced always followed a step-wise scheme, starting with an early inflammatory reaction and the development of epidermal hyperplasia. Repeated application of the carcinogenic agent for many weeks resulted in the formation of benign papillomas, a few of which finally developed into malignant carcinomas. Originally, the inflammatory response was regarded as providing an important condition for tumorigenesis, especially since irritating manipulations such as application of unsaturated fatty acids, turpentine or wounding could accelerate tumor development in coal tar-treated skin. However, it turned out later that irritation alone was insufficient to induce neoplastic growth.

In 1941 Rous et al. (2) succeeded in dissecting the process of experimental skin tumorigenesis into two stages. In the first stage, called "initiation", a limited treatment of animal skin with coal tar or benzopyrene was carried out. The papillomas thus elicited generally disappeared when the treatment was stopped, but could be elicited again at the same sites by a subsequent treatment with a non-tumorigenic skin irritant or by wounding. This second treatment was called "promotion". Promotion did not exhibit a carcinogenic effect without prior initiation, at least within the limits of the experiment. This result could be only explained by the assumption that despite a complete regression of the visible papilloma one or a few initiated cells irreversibly remained in the epidermis, which, when promoted, gave rise to new tumor formation.

At about the same time, croton oil, the seed oil of the Euphorbiacea Croton tiglium, was found to contain extremely potent skin tumor promoters which were later identified as phorbol esters such as TPA (3-5). Recently, other types of skin tumor promoters have been identified in different natural sources (6). Based on the work of Rous et al., Mottram (7) and Berenblum (8) introduced a standard approach of two-stage carcinogenesis in mouse skin which is still in use. It consists of a single application of an initiator, usually a polycyclic aromatic hydrocarbon such as DMBA, followed by chronic promoter treatment, for instance, phorbol ester application twice a week over a period of about 18 to 20 weeks. In order to obtain clear-cut experimental conditions, the dose of the initiator chosen is so low that, without subsequent promotion, no tumors become visible ("subthreshold dose").

Fundamental observations made by applying the Berenblum-Mottram scheme may be summarized as follows (8,9). Under the described conditions initiation led to invisible alterations in epidermal cells. These alterations were virtually irreversible, since between initiation and promotion the experiment could be interrupted for more than a year without a considerable decrease in tumor incidence. Such irreversibility is consistent with the generally accepted theory that the initiating effect of a carcinogenic agent is due to a genetic alteration. Recently, this concept has gained additional support by the demonstration of an overexpressed and point-mutated H-ras protooncogene in skin tumors generated along the two-stage approach (10). In contrast to initiation, promotion was found to be a reversible process. That is, when the time interval between two subsequent promoter applications was increased from 3 days up to about 1-2 weeks tumor development was drastically impaired. The recent finding that a more persistent component is included in the effect of the tumor promoter TPA on initiated skin, has prompted, however, a modification of the concept of reversibility (see below). Contrary to the effect of an initiator, the effect of repeated promoter treatments was observed to be not additive. When the overall dose of a promoter was splitted into smaller doses given in shorter time intervals, the tumor incidence dropped considerably. Tumors were found to develop only when the initiating carcinogen was applied prior to the promoter but not vice versa, i.e. a promoter did not act additively with the initiator but completed a process started with initiation (11). According to Berenblum this indicates that the mechanism of promotion must be different from that of initiation.

It should be emphasized that initiation and promotion are first of all operationally defined terms; their definition is based on a distinct experimental approach designed in such a way that both processes can be clearly distinguished and experimentally characterized. Outside of these experimental conditions, the situation becomes less clear for two reasons:

1) Practically all initiating agents are "complete carcinogens", which produce tumors in the absence of promotion, provided they are applied in a sufficient dose over a long enough period of time; one wonders if a promoting component is included in this carcinogenic activity and, if so, if it follows the same mechanistic pathways as

in the two-stage experiment.

2) Every promoting agent induces a few tumors if applied long enough. Therefore, promoters have to be classified, in the strict sense of the word, as carcinogens, albeit weak ones. But does the carcinogenic effect of promoters come about by the same mechanism as that of initiation? Or is it due to the existence of "spontaneously" initiated cells in the tissue?

If a two-stage carcinogenesis experiment is carried out in the correct way, both the complete carcinogenic activity of the initiating agent and the carcinogenic effect of the promoter do not significantly contribute to the final result and may thus be neglected. It has to be emphasized that this is a model situation designed to study processes in carcinogenesis rather than agents with the ultimate goal to arrive at an understanding of the mechanisms involved. Therefore, whether or not the observations thus made are relevant for an understanding of neoplastic processes in humans is another question which will be discussed below.

The sequence of events observed in the course of skin tumor promotion resembles that observed in coal tar carcinogenesis, including initial inflammatory and hyperplasic events, the appearance of benign papillomas after several weeks and of a few malignant carcinomas after prolonged treatment (12). Under the experimental conditions described above, the rate of progression from the papilloma to the carcinoma stage is rather low (less than 10%) but can be increased by a second treatment with initiating agents following promoter treatment (13). This indicates that an additional attack on the cellular genome might be required to achieve malignancy. The dose of the promoter and the duration of promoter treatment has no effect on the rate of malignant progression (13). On the other hand, carcinoma development does practically not occur in initiated skin without promotion. This indicates that promotion has to be regarded as a prerequisite for malignant progression, probably because the carcinomas develop from papillomas, the development of which, in turn, depends on promotion. It is easily conceivable that, if malignant progression is the result of a second genotoxic effect the probability of this effect to occur will be much higher in papillomas (being the result of a clonal expansion of tumor cells) than in single initiated cells. If promoter treatment is stopped before malignant carcinomas appear, the whole process of skin tumorigenesis exhibits a high degree of remission, i.e. most of the papillomas disappear. A prevention or inhibition of promotion thus brings cancer development to a halt.

The investigation of the mechanism of tumor promotion and the identification of tumor promoters in the environment may, therefore, provide a possibility of cancer prevention.

INITIATION, CONVERSION AND PROMOTION: THE THREE-STAGE APPROACH OF SKIN TUMORIGENESIS

Considering the fact that under the conditions of an initiation-promotion experiment predominantly reversibly growing, non-autonomous papillomas appear in mouse skin (12) one may arrive at the conclusion that promotion is simply due to the generation of a chronic hyperproliferative status in epidermis required to make these papillomas grow to a visible size. An initiated cell would then be a single papilloma cell which by local growth restraints is prevented from forming a clone and a tumor. These local growth restraints are thought to be overcome by the tumor promoter. As a result conditions for a clonal expansion of initiated cells are provided (14).

At a first glance, such a hypothesis seems to be highly consistent with the fact that all skin tumor promoters are strong hyperplasia-inducing mitogens. On the other hand, mouse epidermis responds to all kinds of chemical irritation or mechanical injury by a hyperplastic reaction, regardless whether the stimulus exhibits tumor-promoting potency or not. To deal with this discrepancy an additional postulate was included into the hypothesis mentioned above. According to this postulate a selective advantage has to be provided for initiated cells in addition to growth stimulation. Such a selective advantage is thought to be achieved by a stimulatory effect of tumor promoters on terminal differentiation of non-initiated epidermal cells (14). Recent observations seem to support this assumption (15).

Another explanation of the fact that not every

hyperplasia-inducing agent is a good tumor promoter is provided by
the assumption that an initiated cell, - albeit genetically
transformed - represents some kind of a recessive mutant being
unable to express its neoplastic phenotype. Such a cell would behave
like a normal epidermal stem cell except it comes under the
influence of a tumor promoter, which first induces the expression of
the neoplastic phenotype, i.e. "converts" the initiated cell into a
papilloma cell, and then "propagates" the clonal expansion of this
papilloma cell. According to this hypothesis tumor promotion would
be the result of two mechanistically quite different processes, i.e.
"conversion" and "propagation" which may be defined as stages of
promotion (9). A tumor-promoting agent could be distinguished from a
non-promoting mitogen by its "convertogenic" efficacy which it
exhibits in addition to its growth-stimulatory or "propagating"
effect. This hypothesis has been put forward initially by Boutwell
(9) in order to explain the following observation: when initiated
mouse skin was treated with croton oil only for a short period of
time, no tumor development was observed. But when this treatment
(conversion) was followed by a subsequent chronic application of the
mitogenic turpentine (propagation) many tumors appeared. Later on,
this experiment was repeated by using TPA to induce conversion or
"stage 1 of promotion" and the diterpene ester mezerein (the toxic
principle of Daphne mezereum) as a propagating agent or "stage 2
promoter" (16). Without prior croton oil or TPA treatment, neither
turpentine nor mezerein could significantly promote tumor growth in
initiated skin. Thus, it appeared that these "incomplete" promoters
acted as propagating agents only, whereas a "complete" promoter such
as TPA or croton oil exhibited additional convertogenic efficacity.
Then it should perhaps be possible to abolish one of these
efficacies of TPA by a chemical alteration of the molecule. Indeed,
a phorbol ester (called "Ti8" and isolated from certain plant
species, ref. 17) differring from TPA by 4 conjugated double bonds
in the C_{14} fatty acid side chain (Fig. 1) turned out to be a strong
irritant skin mitogen but almost completely devoid of tumor
promoting potency (18). Based on this finding, a "disarmament" of
the promoter TPA was tried by replacing its satured tetradecanoyl
residue by a highly unsaturated residue such as retinoic acid (19).

The resulting phorbol ester 12-retinoylphorbol-14-acetate (RPA, Fig. 1) exhibited properties similar to that of Ti8, i.e. it was a strong irritant skin mitogen, but almost unable to promote tumor development after initiation (20). "Disarmed" tumor promoters such

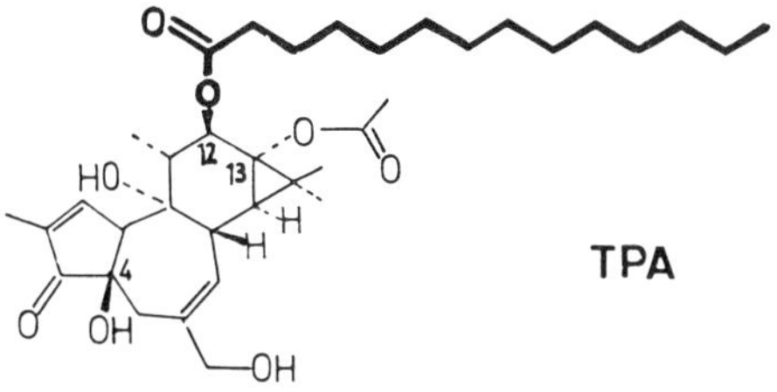

TPA

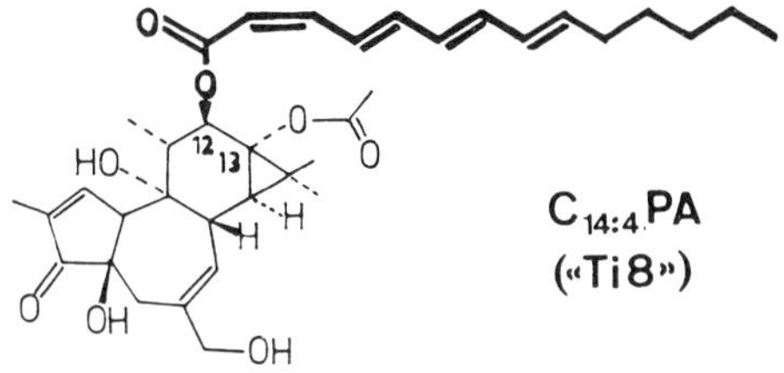

C$_{14:4}$PA
("Ti8")

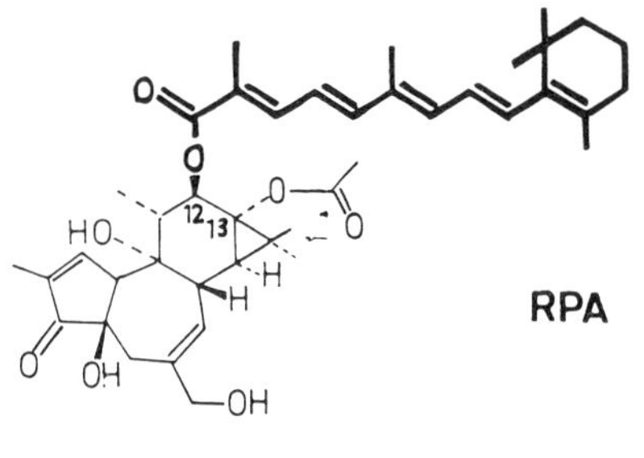

RPA

Fig.1. Phorbol esters with different effects in skin carcinogenesis. 12-0-tetradecanoylphorbol-13-acetate (TPA) exhibits both convertogenic and promoting efficacy. The replacement of the tetradecanoyl residue by an unsaturated side chain yields two phorbol esters, the naturally occuring "Ti8" and the semisynthetic 12-0-retinoylphorbol-13-acetate (RPA), the convertogenic efficacy of which is drastically diminished. Under certain experimental conditions (controlled dosage and time-schedule of treatment) they exhibit a "pure" tumor-promoting effect on initiated and converted mouse skin (strain NMRI).

as Ti8 (21) or RPA (20) turned out to be very efficient propagating agents, i.e. they could elicit papilloma growth when applied after one single application of TPA onto initiated mouse skin. It was observed that in the course of conversion, TPA induced in initiated skin rather persistant alterations (22). That is, the converted state as measured by the tumorigenic effect of subsequent RPA treatment disappeared only gradually, with a half-life of 10-12 weeks (at least as far as the back skin of the NMRI mouse strain is concerned).

Conversion was thought to be a first stage of promotion until it was found that it could occur also several weeks _prior_ to initiation (22), whereas promotion is strictly defined as completing the tumorigenic process started with initiation. This prompted us to reconsider conversion as a discrete element of multistage carcinogenesis in mouse skin rather than as a component of promotion (22). Consequently, we proposed to restrict the term promotion to those events occurring _after_ carcinogen treatment which have been called stage II of promotion or propagation. According to this new scheme, a "disarmed" phorbol ester, such as Ti8 or RPA, is a true promoting agent rather than an incomplete promoter, whereas TPA is a promoter with additional convertogenic potency. It may be emphasized that such a re-evaluation of the nomenclature is more than a matter of semantics since it may help to overcome the discrepancy that no differences between the biological effects of RPA, Ti8, mezerein or TPA could be found in systems other than the skin of the living mouse. Since the other systems are mainly _in vitro_ models, the question that arises is whether or not conversion is restricted to the _in vivo_ situation, and perhaps only valid for the skin model.

MECHANISTIC ASPECTS OF CONVERSION AND TUMOR PROMOTION IN SKIN

The terms conversion and promotion are first of all operationally defined as discrete stages of carcinogenesis observed under the special experimental conditions described above (Fig 2). Conversion may be described as a manipulation required to make the tissue sensitive for promotion (induction of promotability), whereas promotion describes a manipulation necessary to elicit papilloma development in initiated and converted skin. Considerable efforts have been made to replace these operational definitions by mechanistic ones. The results of this task are still fragmentary.

As yet, there is every reason to assume that promotion is the

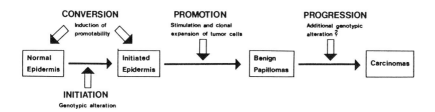

Fig. 2. Schematic representation of experimental multistage carcinogenesis in mouse skin.

result of a chronic hyperproliferative process which allows the clonal expansion of tumor cells. This means that the mechanisms involved in the hyperplastic response of epidermis to external injury have to be regarded as important or even essential parameters of the promoting process. The development of a hyperplastic condition in epidermis is a rather dramatic event proceeding within 1-2 days and being accompanied by strong symptoms of inflammation. This so-called hyperplastic transformation (23,24) is not simply the result of overshooting cellular proliferation, but due to distinct cellular and molecular events which result in a temporary disturbance of tissue homeostasis, i.e. in a disequilibrium between the rates of cell gain and cell loss. This idea is strongly supported by the fact that, under certain conditions (such as skin massage or application of the phorbol ester 4-0-methyl-TPA), a strong hyperproliferative response can be evoked in epidermis which does not result in hyperplasia at all. One cannot escape the conclusion that, in this case, the endogenous devices for steady state control remain intact, providing an exact matching of the rate of cell gain by the rate of cell loss ("balanced hyperproliferation").

Since all skin tumor promoters induce hyperplastic transformation, this special response seems to be a condition of promotion. This conclusion is consistent with the observation that sustained epidermal hyperplasia is essential for promotion (25). Hyperplastic transformation of skin is characterized by chemical and cellular events which are not observed in the case of balanced hyperproliferation (23,24).

Two prominent events occur in mouse skin almost immediately after hyperplasiogenic stimulation: an induction of the arachidonic acid cascade resulting in the production of prostaglandins and metabolites produced along the lipoxygenase pathway (26), and an activation of the enzyme protein kinase C. The latter response is especially seen after application of phorbol esters, which have been found to be specific stimulators of protein kinase C (27,28) by mimicking the effect of the physiological activator of the enzyme, diacylglycerol, which is a second messenger of certain hormones. Within the phorbol ester series, a good correlation exists between the degree of protein kinase C stimulation and the evocation of the hyperplastic response in epidermis. Whereas the function of proteinkinase C activation in the hyperproliferative process is still not entirely clear, the role of arachidonic acid metabolites is much better understood. The initial hyperplastic response depends critically on the accumulation of prostaglandin E_2 in epidermis, whereas, after repeated stimulation, this role seems to be taken over by prostaglandin F_2 alpha (26). By itself, prostaglandins are unable to evoke epidermal hyperproliferation; they act synergistically with the exogenous stimulus. In mouse skin, prostaglandins are exclusively involved in the induction of epidermal hyperproliferation, whereas the inflammatory response is probably mediated by arachidonic acid metabolites of the lipoxygenase pathway.

Later events in the course of hyperplastic transformation, not seen during balanced hyperproliferation, include an increase of polyamine biosynthesis caused by an induction of the enzyme ornithine decarboxylase, desensitization of epidermal cells for antiproliferative endogenous signals such as catecholamine and chalone and an impairment of intercellular communication (23,24).

As expected from the prostaglandin requirement of hyperplastic transformation, tumor promotion, achieved for instance by repeated RPA treatment, is depressed by the cyclooxygenase inhibitor indomethacin (25). Other inhibitors include corticosteroids, retinoic acid, antioxidants and cyclosporin A (29-33). Most symptoms of hyperplastic transformation induced by a single stimulation cease within one to two weeks. It appears as if the reversibility of promotion, as demonstrated by the decrease of tumor incidence upon prolongation of the time interval between subsequent promoter treatments, is closely related to the remission rate of epidermal hyperplasia. Being a general response of skin to all kinds of chemical irritation and mechanical injury, hyperplastic transformation provides an important physiological defense mechanism. Bearing this in mind, one hesitates to describe tumor promotion as the result of a special cytotoxic event, for instance comparable to the "genotoxic" effect of an initiator. Instead, one could understand promotion as an over-activation of a normal physiological process. The fact that protein kinase C plays a critical role in this response makes the phorbol esters and other C kinase-activating agents extremely potent hyperplasiogenic agents and skin tumor promoters. In other tissues the induction of hyperproliferative processes may proceed along quite different biochemical pathways. This means that the mechanistic parameters of promoter action as delineated from experiments with the skin model cannot be generalized. Instead, the molecular mechanisms of growth control, hyperproliferative responses and tumor promotion have to be determined specifically for every tissue.

While tumor promotion seems to be deeply linked to the process of hyperplastic transformation of skin, much less is known about the molecular events involved in the conversion-stage of tumorigenesis. Conversion has been shown to depend on an induction of epidermal DNA-synthesis by the convertogenic agent such as TPA (34,35) and to be subject to inhibition by retinoic acid and inhibitors of the arachidonic acid cascade (30). Thus, conversion seems to be closely related to promotion and hyperplastic transformation. On the other hand, the alteration induced by the convertogenic agent (i.e. promotability of skin) exhibits a much longer half-life (10-12 weeks) than the events occurring in the course of hyperplastic transformation (2 weeks). Furthermore, reactions probably involved in hyperplasia and promotion such as an activation of the C kinase are apparently not critical for conversion (30).

The three-stage experiment as described above demonstrates that conversion - either before or after initiation - is required for initiated skin to respond to promoter application by tumor development. Providing that our assumption is correct that promotion is explainable by clonal expansion of tumor cells in the course of a chronic hyperproliferative reaction, this would mean that in the absence of conversion an initiated cell is unable to respond to the mitogenic effect of the promoter. If initiation occurs in a rather undifferentiated stem cell population of the epidermis (as indicated by Rous' classical experiment on the irreversible character of initiation, see above) it may be speculated that such stem cells lack expression of perhaps one or another constituent (enzyme?) required for the hyperplastic response and that the formation of this constituent would be induced by the convertogenic agent. On the other hand, an initiated cell may well respond to the mitogenic effect of a promoter, but - as already proposed by Boutwell (9) - may be unable to express its neoplastic phenotype in the absence of conversion. Such a hypothesis seems to be in conflict with the observation that conversion can be carried out prior to initiation (22). It could well be, however, that the convertogenic agent creates a rather persistent situation in the tissue which allows spontaneous phenotypic expression of initiated cells, provided that initiation occurs within the time interval when the tissue is in the converted state.

At present, our knowledge is not sufficient for a final decision between these two hypotheses, which are not necessarily mutually exclusive. Moreover, we do not know whether conversion is a general phenomenon of neoplastic development or whether it is restricted to the mouse skin model in vivo. It must be emphasized, however, that convertogenic potency is not a speciality of exotic chemical compounds such as the phorbol esters, but that skin wounding exhibits a strong convertogenic effect (21). This indicates that a convertogenic agent induces pathways or mimicks factors which are normally involved in the wound response. It appears as if a convertogenic agent such as TPA makes the tissue "believe" that it is wounded. For conversion the wound must be deep, i.e. include dermis and blood vessels. Superficial wounding such as a removal of the horny layer of epidermis induces hyperplastic transformation but does not exhibit convertogenic efficacy. This indicates a difference in the response of skin to superficial versus more extended wounding which may reflect the difference between promotion and conversion.

Initiation is carried out by a single local treatment with a carcinogenic agent, promotion by chronical application (once or twice a week) of a promoter such as the phorbol ester RPA. For conversion, i.e. induction of promotability, a single topical application of a convertogenic agent (for instance TPA) or single skin wounding either before or after initiation is sufficient. Between conversion and promotion the experiment can be interrupted for several months (NMRI mice), whereas an increase of the time interval between two subsequent promoter treatments (from 3-6 days up to 2 weeks) results in a pronounced drop of tumor yield. The progression from the benign to the malignant state can be augmented by an additional treatment of papilloma-bearing skin with an initiating agent.

THE POTENTIAL IMPORTANCE OF THE MULTISTAGE APPROACH OF SKIN CARCINOGENESIS FOR A PREVENTION OF HUMAN CANCER

The multistage model of skin carcinogenesis is a highly artificial approach which allows the investigator to dissect the complex pattern of tumor development so that the process can be analyzed stage by stage. There is no other possibility to acquire an understanding of the mechanisms involved. The argument that such a situation never occurs in daily life and the model, therefore, is irrelevant for the human situation is frequently raised, but nevertheless trivial. From our animal model one should not demand more than it can provide, i.e. an insight into biological pathways along which tumors may develop. The most important results which have emerged from the skin model are:

1) the initiating effect of a carcinogenic agent on the tissue is irreversible but remains silent provided the dose of the agent is low; it is most probably due to an alteration at the level of the cellular genome which occurs with a low degree of probability;

2) the post-initiation stages of skin carcinogensis, i.e. conversion and promotion, proceed along physiological pathways normally involved in wound response and tissue regeneration; they

facilitate the formation of papillomas from initiated cells;

3) the progression from the benign to the malignant state requires most probably an additional effect on the cellular genome of a papilloma cell; the preceeding clonal expansion of papilloma cells due to promotion greatly increases the probability of such a genetic alteration.

The close relationship of conversion and promotion to physiological processes allows the proposal that the development of tumors from initiated cells could be induced not only by exogenous (environmental) influences but, perhaps with a lower frequency, also by endogenous factors. This may help to explain the well known effect of certain hormones on human cancer development.

Epidemiological studies indicate that promoting influences may be important, or even critical, in the development of certain human cancers. The most striking evidence for this is the rather long latency period of most malignant diseases. In addition, risk reversibility and the synergistic effect of many carcinogenic agents show a striking parallelism to the situation in the skin model. For example, the carcinogenic effects of tobacco smoke and asbestos or ionizing radiation potentiate each other (31), as do the carcinogenic effects of initiators and promoters in the animal model. The risk of getting lung cancer decreases once smoking is stopped showing that the process has a reversible component (36,37). In fact this is exactly what one would predict from the animal model, where the risk of getting skin carcinomas is drastically reduced when promoter treatment is stopped before the endpoint of papilloma development is reached. Another practical impact of the multistage model is that it may help to develop measures of cancer chemoprevention, i.e. it may provide the opportunity for a patient to live with initiated or even fully transformed cells provided one would be able to inhibit the post-initiation stages of carcinogenesis. As mentioned above, conversion and promotion in mouse skin can be effectively suppressed by local treatment with vitamin A acid and its derivatives, by glucocorticosteroids, non-steroidal antiphlogistica, antioxidants, and, at least in the case of promotion, by the immunodepressive drug cyclosporin A. It must be emphasized, however, that in other organs multistage carcinogenesis may proceed along other cellular pathways and may, therefore, be sensitive to other types of inhibitors. It may thus be impossible to design a generalized scheme for the chemoprevention of the post-initiation stages of tumor development. Rather, preventive measures have to be determined specifically for every tissue and tumor type.

REFERENCES

1. Yamagiwa K, Ichikawa K (1914) Gann 8: 11-15

2. Rous P, Kidd JG (1941) J Exp Med 73: 365-389
   Friedwald WF, Rous P (1944) J Exp Med 80: 101-125

3. Berenblum I (1941) Cancer Res 1: 44-48

4. Van Duuren BL (1969) Progr Exp Tumor Res 11: 31-68

5. Hecker E, Schmidt R (1974) Progr Chem Org Natur Prod 31: 378-467

6. Fujiki H, Suganuma M, Tahira T et al. (1984) In: Cellular Interactions by Environmental Tumor Promoters. Fujiki et al. (eds), pp 37-48, Japan Sc Soc Press, Tokyo; VNU Science Press, Utrecht

7. Mottram JC (1944) Pathol Bact 56: 181-187

8. Berenblum I (1954) Adv Cancer Res 2: 129-175 – Berenblum I (1975) In: Cancer, a Comprehensive Treatise, Vol 1, Becker FF (ed) pp 323-244, Plenum Press, New York

9. Boutwell RK (1964) Progr Exp Tumor Res 4: 207-250

10. Quintanilla M, Brown K, Ramsden M et al. (1986) Nature 322: 78-80

11. Berenblum I, Haran N (1955) Brit J Cancer 9: 268-271

12. Burns FJ, Vanderlaan M, Snyder E et al. (1978) In: Mechanisms of Tumor Promotion and Cocarcinogenesis. Slaga TJ et al. (eds), pp 91-96, Raven Press, New York

13. Hennings H, Shores R, Wenk ML et al. (1983) Nature 304: 67-69

14. Yuspa SH (1984) In: Cellular Interactions by Environmental Tumor Promoters. Fujiki H et al. (eds), pp 315-326, Japan Sc Soc Press, Tokyo; VNU Science Press, Utrecht

15. Parkinson EK (1985) Brit J Cancer 52: 479-493

16. Slaga TJ, Fischer SM, Nelson K et al. (1980) Proc Natl Acad Sci USA 77: 3659-3663

17. Fürstenberger G, Hecker E (1986) J Natural Products (Lloydia), in Press

18. Marks F, Bertsch, Fürstenberger G (1979) Cancer Res. 39: 4183-4188

19. Sorg B, Fürstenberger G, Berry DL et al. (1982) J Lipid Res 23: 443-447

20. Fürstenberger G, Berry DL, Sorg B et al. (1981) Proc Natl Acad Sci USA 78: 7722-7726

21. Fürstenberger G, Marks F (1983) J Invest Dermatol 81: 157s-161s

22. Fürstenberger G, Kinzel V, Schwarz M et al. (1985) Science 230: 76-78

23. Marks F, Bertsch S, Fürstenberger G et al. (1983) In: Psoriasis: Cell Proliferation. Wright NA, Camplejohn RS (eds), pp 173-188, Churchill Livingstone, Edinburgh etc.

24. Marks F, Fürstenberger G, Ganss M et al. (1983) Brit J Dermatol 109, Suppl 25: 18-21

25. Sisskin EE, Gray T, Barret JC (1982) Carcinogenesis 3: 403-408

26. Fürstenberger G, Marks F (1985) In: Arachidonic Acid Metabolism and Tumor Promotion. Fischer SM, Slaga TJ (eds), pp 50-72, Nijhoff, Boston

27. Castagna M, Takai Y, Kaibuchi K et al. (1982) J Biol Chem 257: 7847-7851

28. Ashendel CL (1985) Biochim Biophys Acta 822: 219-242

29. Slaga TJ, Fischer SM, Weeks CE et al.(1982) In: Cocarcinogenesis and Biological Effects of Tumor Promoters. Hecker E et al. (eds), pp 19-34, Raven Press, New York

30. Marks F, Fürstenberger G (1984) In: Cellular Interactions by Environmental Tumor Promoters. Fujiki H et al. (eds), pp 273-287, Japan Sc Soc Press Tokyo; VNU Science Press, Utrecht

31. Troll W, Wiesner R (1985) Ann Rev Pharmacol Toxicol 25: 509-528

32. Kensler TW, Bush DM, Kozumbo WJ (1983) Science 221: 75-77

33. Gschwendt M, Kittstein W, Marks F (1986) Carcinogenesis, in press

34. Kinzel V, Loehrke H, Goerttler K et al. (1984) Proc Natl Acad Sci USA 81: 5858-5862

35. Kinzel V, Fürstenberger G, Loehrke H et al.(1986) Carcinogenesis 7: 779-782

36. Mass MJ, Kaufman DG, Siegfried JM et al. (eds): Cancer of the Respiratory Tract, Raven Press, New York (1985)

37. Wynder EL, Hoffmann D, McCoy GD et al. (1978) In: Mechanisms of Tumor Promotion and Cocarcinogenesis, Slaga TJ et al. (eds), pp 59-77, Raven Press, New York

CHEMICAL CARCINOGENESIS : THE LIVER AS A MODEL

E. FARBER and D.S.R. SARMA[a]

Departments of Pathology and of Biochemistry, Medical Sciences
Building, University of Toronto, Toronto, Ontario M5S 1A8, Canada.

I. LIVER CELL CARCINOMA IN HUMANS

Liver cell cancer (LCC[b]) is one of the commonest cancers
world-wide, involving millions of people and ranking 2nd in the
world. Unlike most of the other cancers in the top 10 (1), it is
quite uncommon in the Western world including the U.S.A. and Canada.

Epidemiologically, there is a good (but not a perfect)
correlation between the incidence of HBV infections, especially
carrier states, and of liver cell cancer the world over (2,3).
However, there is also increasing evidence that in some locations
such as parts of China and Africa, at least one additional factor,
exposure to mycotoxins, may play an important role in the etiology
and/or pathogenesis of liver cancer (4). In the Western countries
and in some other parts of the world, a similar but less intimate
correlation between alcohol consumption, alcoholic cirrhosis and
liver cancer has been found. Thus, although infection with HBV is a
common associate of LCC, mycotoxins like aflatoxin and alcohol may
also be important factors (4).

The role or roles of each of the suggested etiological agents
in the pathogenesis of LCC are not clear. As with known chemicals,
such as vinyl chloride in humans and most chemical carcinogens and
some viruses in experimental animals, the development of LCC with
HBV infection is a very slow process, requiring 30 to 60 years after
the time of known exposure. The same is also true with alcohol and
probably also with mycotoxins. These observations, together with the
known association between cirrhosis and LCC, suggests that the

[a] The author's research included in this review was supported by
research grants from the National Cancer Institute of Canada, the
U.S. Public Health Service (CA-21157, CA 23958, CA 37077), awarded
by the National Cancer Institute, DHHS, and the Medical Research
Council of Canada (MT-5994).
[b] Abbreviations used are: LCC, liver cell ("hepatocellular")
carcinoma; HBV, hepatitis B virus; RH, resistant hepatocyte;
2-AAF, 2-acetylamino-fluorene; PH, partial hepatectomy.

pathogenesis of LCC in humans, as in experimental animals (5-7), is a slow multistep process.

Little is known concerning the nature of the steps in this long complex process. Although integration of portions of the HBV genome has been found in human cancers, similar integration has been found in the non-neoplastic portions of livers with cancer; also the segment of the HBV genome integrated into liver cancers and their sites of integration have been variable. Given these observations and the inordinately long time period for pathogenesis, it becomes questionable whether the HBV itself is truly oncogenic. By "oncogenic" is meant a virus (or other agent) that adds specific information to the genome of the target cell relating directly to one or more of the phenotypic expressions characteristic for malignant neoplasia. An equally plausible hypothesis is that it is some common tissue or cellular change induced by HBV, rather than the viral information per se, that plays the more important role in the pathogenic mechanism in humans.

Somewhat against this non-specific role are the interesting findings in the woodchuck, the duck and the ground squirell (4,8). In the woodchuck, a close association between infection with a DNA virus similar to HBV and LCC appearance is known. In the duck, LCC occurs in areas of high LCC incidence in humans and an HBV-like virus has been found in this species. However, a similar possibility of a correlation between a viral-induced tissue change and LCC rather than a specific oncogenic role of these viruses should be considered. Consistent with this alternative view are the well known clinical observations that LCC is rarely seen in an otherwise normal liver.

Given the great uncertainty concerning the pathogenesis of LCC in humans, and the many similarities between hepatocarcinogenesis and liver cancer in humans and in the rat, it seems reasonable to attempt to understand in much greater detail the pathogenesis of LCC in an experimental animal in order to generate testable hypotheses. For chronic disease in humans in general, any fundamental and integrated understanding of mechanisms at the molecular, biochemical, cellular and tissue levels of organization requires the availability of model systems that mimic closely the pathogenetic

TABLE 1

MODELS OF LIVER CANCER DEVELOPMENT IN THE RAT

A. <u>Single agent</u>

(i)   Long-term continuous exposure to a carcinogen
(ii)   Intermittent chronic exposure
(iii) The stop model

B. <u>Initiation-Promotion-Progression</u>

(iv)   Chronic enzyme induction model
(v)   Resistant hepatocyte model
(vi)   Choline-methionine-deficient model
(vii) Orotic acid model

C. <u>Dietary Deficiency</u>

(viii) Choline devoid low methionine diet without added carcinogens

----

sequence in humans. Such systems are becoming available in the rat
with many different chemicals as initiating factors.

We shall review the current status of liver cancer development
with chemicals in the rat and then return to the situation in
humans. Unlike the mouse, the reactions of the liver to hepatotoxins
and to hepatocarcinogens <u>in the rat</u> resemble quite closely those
seen in humans. Although some differences do seem to be present,
these appear to be of minor importance in the pathogenic sequence
for liver cancer. The morphological and biological behaviour of LCC
in the rat closely resemble those in humans such that they are often
indistinguishable.

II. THE STEPWISE DEVELOPMENT OF LIVER CELL CARCINOMA IN THE RAT

A. MODELS

There are at least 8 models for the study of liver cancer
development with chemicals (Table 1) (9). (i) The original model,
first developed by Sasaki and Yoshida in 1933-1935 (10), and studied
in great detail by Kinosita (11) and others since, involved
observations of liver alterations at many time points during the
long-term continuous exposure to a carcinogen in the diet. Azo dyes
(o-aminoazotoluene and p-dimethylaminoazobenzene) were most
frequently used initially. The lack of synchrony in the development
of new cell populations and therefore the inability to dissect
step-by-step the possible relevant changes from the many irrelevant

ones makes this model virtually non-analyzable for sequence. At best, information about what <u>might</u> happen, but not what <u>does</u> happen, could be generated; (ii) A modification of this model, intermittent chronic exposure to a carcinogen, has proven to be very useful in generating large hepatocyte nodules for biochemical and biological studies (12-14). This model suffers from the same deficiencies as does model (i); (iii) Bannasch and colleagues (15) have described what they call a "stop model" in which rats are exposed to an hepatic carcinogen, such as N-nitroso-morpholine, for several weeks and then returned to a basal diet without carcinogen; (iv) A new type of model, one using an initiator and a promoter, was introduced by Peraino and colleagues in 1971 (16) Phenobarbital has been the most common promoter used, although DDT, PCB's, cyproterone acetate, a-hexachlorocyclohexane, and other inducers of drug metabolizing enzymes in the liver are also effective (16-18). These <u>chronic enzyme induction models</u> suffer from a common deficiency, lack of synchrony of lesion development, making it difficult to analyze any possible sequence. Foci and nodules appear over many weeks or months, thus preventing the delineation of "<u>what precedes what</u>"; (v) A new concept for a model, <u>the resistant hepatocyte model</u>, was developed by Solt and Farber in 1976 (19). This was based on the hypothesis, since receiving abundant support, that many chemical carcinogens induce a rare <u>resistant</u> hepatocyte during initiation and that such resistant hepatocytes can be rapidly stimulated to develop into focal proliferations (foci) and nodules by brief non-initiating exposure to low levels of chemicals, such as 2-AAF (19,20), coupled with a mitogenic stimulus. The 2-AAF inhibits proliferation of the vast majority of hepatocytes, the uninitiated (sensitive) ones, but not the proliferation of the few resistant hepatocytes. In this model, the selection pressure to generate nodules is intense and the initiated resistant cells thus proliferate synchronously as a cohort. This synchrony lasts for several steps. The almost complete inhibition of cell proliferation ("mito-inhibition") of the vast majority of hepatocytes (the presumably <u>uninitiated</u> hepatocytes) is probably the reason why the 2 week-exposure to the dietary 2-AFF does not initiate carcinogenesis (21); (vi) Lombardi, Shinozuka and coworkers (22) and Newberne, Rogers and their colleagues (23) have described an additional model in which promotion is effected by the post-initiation exposure to diets deficient in choline and low in methionine or low in all lipotropic components. It appears that the development of nodules in this model is non-synchronous; (vii) Sarma, Rajalakshmi and Rao (24,25) have described a new model in which orotic acid, the natural precursor in pyrimidine synthesis, is used post-initiation as a promoter. This appears to be a model with good synchrony for foci and nodules; and (viii) Poirier and colleagues (26), Ghoshal and Farber (27) and Lombardi and associates (28) have found that rats fed diets deficient in choline and low in methionine without any known addition of a carcinogen develop quite a high incidence of liver cell cancer.

The following discussion of the known steps involved in the development of liver cell cancer is a composite derived from all of the models. However, because of its synchrony, and because of the brief time periods during which the animals were exposed to the agents, the resistant hepatocyte model (model v) has generated the largest number of steps and allowed the development of considerable mechanistic insight for some. The expression of options at certain steps indicates that the permanent "toxic" effects on many cell populations are probably minimal in this model.

B. INITIATION (Fig. 1)

Definition: On the basis of our experience in carcinogenesis, we propose the following definition (29): Initiation is a change in a target tissue or organ, induced by exposure to a carcinogen, that can be promoted or selected to develop focal proliferations, one or more of which can act as sites of origin for the ultimate development of malignant neoplasia.

This definition is singularly devoid of two properties often used in the definition - interactions with DNA and growth. Each of these two properties is presumptive or invalid. There are an increasing number of chemical carcinogens that do not seem to interact with DNA to form adducts either directly or indirectly. Also, acquisition of any "autonomy of growth" is a much later step in the carcinogenic process and is not seen to accompany the initiation step in any known organ.

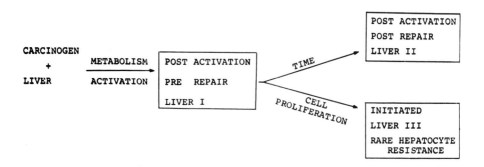

Fig. 1. Some key steps in initiation of carcinogenesis. (I-1 and I-2). (Modified from Chart 1, reference 30)

It should be emphasized that this definition seems appropriate only for those models of cancer development in which (a) initiation, promotion and progression can be observed and (b) the "product" of promotion is a focal proliferation such as a papilloma, polyp or nodule (9). Some other models of carcinogenesis do not seem to have the same pattern of stepwise development of cancer as do the commonly used ones such as in liver, skin, colon, urinary bladder and mammary gland (5,6,9).

Assays:

A major advantage of the rat liver, shared with the mouse skin, for the study of the stepwise development of cancer is the availability of assays for initiation. Scherer and colleagues in 1972 (31) were the first to show that the appearance of islands of hepatocytes with altered histochemical properties could be used as an assay for initiation and that the number of islands was related to the dose of the carcinogen used. This principle has been used to identify islands or foci of altered hepatocytes, "initiated hepatocytes", with many different carcinogens, in several models and with a variety of histochemical and other markers (32-36). The early histochemical indices, especially glucose-6-phosphatase and

"ATPase", were predominantly "negative" (31), i.e. <u>loss</u> of a property. Later, positive markers (gamma-glutamyltransferase (37), DT-diaphorase (38), epoxide hydrolase (39-41), glutathione-S-transferases (42) etc.) increased the versatility of this important approach (34,36).

In 1976, a second principle for the identification of initiated hepatocytes was introduced by Solt and Farber (19,43). They proposed that one type of initiated hepatocyte was an hepatocyte that acquires, during initiation, a resistance to the inhibitory effects of many carcinogens on cell proliferation ("mito-inhibition"). They developed an assay for such resistant cells and this assay has been used to test for potential carcinogenicity of many chemical carcinogens (19,21,44,45). The assay selects for carcinogen-induced resistant hepatocytes by rapid growth to form hepatocyte nodules (see below). This assay is the first in any system to use a <u>known</u> physiological change induced by a carcinogen during initiation (see 36).

A third principle for the assay for initiation utilizes the selection or expansion of islands or foci of altered hepatocytes by a promoting environment such as a long term exposure to (a) phenobarbital, DDT, PCB's or other liver enzyme inducers (16-18); (b) a diet deficient in choline and low in methionine (22,23), or (c) orotic acid (24,25). In these assays, the nature of the property or properties used to select or stimulate the initiated hepatocytes and the basis for the selective effects on these hepatocytes are unknown (29).

<u>Initiation has a minimum of 2 steps</u> - the genesis of a biochemical or molecular lesion or lesions (Fig. 1,I-1) and the fixation of one or more biochemical changes by a round of cell proliferation (Fig. 1, I-2). This stepwise process is sharply defined in the adult liver, because of the quiescent nature of this organ with respect to cell proliferation. In organs or tissues in which cell proliferation is an ongoing property, (a minority of tissues such as colon, skin, bone marrow), the stepwise nature of initiation is more difficult to establish. However, the evidence for its occurrence is impressive, nevertheless.

1. I-1. Biochemical Lesion(s) (DNA) (Fig. 1)

The majority of chemical carcinogens, either before ("direct acting" carcinogen) or after metabolic activation, interact with many cell constituents including DNA, RNA and proteins and various cell organelles. Most known carcinogens are metabolically converted to reactive derivatives by microsomal mixed function oxygenase systems associated with the cytochromes P-450 which are located predominantly in the microsomes but also in nuclei. However, it should be emphasized that this is by no means the only system for activation. Reduction with diaphorase (e.g. nitrofurans, nitroquinoline N-oxide), reaction with glutathione (e.g. dibromoethane, dichloroethane), hydrolysis with specific enzymes, e.g. intestinal bacterial B-glucosidase (e.g. cycasin) and oxidation via the prostaglandin synthesis system (e.g. polycyclic aromatic hydrocarbons) or via reactive oxygen species are four such examples of additional mechanisms.

The exact nature of the biochemical lesion or lesions related to initiation in any cell is unknown. However, there is considerable circumstancial evidence that alterations in DNA, including DNA adducts with many carcinogens, are probably closely linked to the initiation process (see 46, 47 for reviews). Although a mutation is a popular view of this biochemical change, other possibilities including translocations and inactivation of regulatory genes have not been excluded by any means. Also, there is a growing list of chemicals that are carcinogenic for the liver and do not seem to interact chemically, either directly or indirectly, with DNA in the liver. If liver cancer development with these agents is similar to that seen with the many carcinogens that show chemical interactions with DNA, perhaps some more subtle form of DNA alteration may be involved in initiation.

In the liver, the relevant biochemical change has a relatively short lifespan. Since cell proliferation is essential for initiation, since the induction of cell proliferation is easily controlled if the chemical or agent does not induce necrosis and since there are now available assays for initiation in the liver, as noted above, it becomes possible to "time" the lifespan of the biochemical lesion or lesions relevant to initiation (48,49). Repair of the key lesions is virtually complete by 96 hours, i.e. cell proliferation is no longer effective in initiation if delayed for 96 hours after the single injection of the initiating carcinogen (48-50).

2. I-2. Fixation by Cell Proliferation (Fig. 1)

In the liver, there is an absolute dependence upon one round of cell proliferation for initiation. In the adult animal, this can be induced by chemical mitogens (51), partial hepatectomy (17,19,21,31,51,52) or induction of liver cell necrosis and the subsequent liver cell proliferation (53). This need for cell proliferation is fulfilled "automatically" in the neonate or very young, since the liver contains many dividing hepatocytes at this early time (34,35). Many chemical carcinogens do not initiate liver cancer development because they do not induce liver cell death (necrosis) followed by liver cell proliferation. This is the basis for the need for partial hepatectomy or chemical mitogens in order to initiate (17,32,33,54) or to induce liver cancer (55) with brief exposure to a chemical carcinogen. An interesting example of this relates to 1,2-dimethylhydrazine which ordinarily induces mainly colon carcinoma with some angiosarcoma of the liver and few if any hepatocellular neoplasms. However, when administered after partial hepatectomy, even in a single dose, hepatocellular neoplasms now become frequent.

A complication in initiation with chemicals is introduced by the common inhibitory effects of original forms of carcinogens or of their metabolic products on cell proliferation (56). This effect tends to antagonize any cell proliferative effects and could complicate the interpretation of initiation or carcinogenicity with some chemicals.

It must be emphasized that the formation of adducts of carcinogens with DNA is not sufficient to initiate carcinogenesis. Thus, the majority of chemical carcinogens generate DNA adducts in the liver but do not initiate carcinogenesis in the absence of a round of cell proliferation. Only those carcinogens that are mitogenic or necrogenic for the liver initiate hepatocarcinogenesis in the absence of partial hepatectomy or other forms of liver cell mitogenesis. For unknown reasons, most chemical carcinogens do not induce liver cell death and thus do not initiate by themselves.

C. PROMOTION (Fig. 2)

Definition. We continue to define promotion operationally, as is appropriate until the mechanism or more properly mechanisms are understood. Promotion is the process whereby an initiated tissue or organ develops focal proliferations (such as nodules, papillomas, polyps etc.), one or more of which act as precursors for subsequent steps in the carcinogenic process (29).

During the process of promotion in liver as well as in many other organs including the skin, the urinary bladder and the colon, one observes the expansion by growth of phenotypically altered cells. These by definition, are called initiated cells and they generate the hepatocyte nodules in the liver, the papillomas in the skin and in the urinary tract and the polyps in the colon.

In the liver, one first sees microscopic islands or foci of hepatocytes (P1) some or all of which may grow to form visible nodules of altered hepatocytes (P2). Two kinetic patterns of promotion (selection) appear to occur: (a) In the RH model (model (v)); virtually every island or focus, if not every one, grows rapidly during selection to form nodules, such that an early end point is the appearance of visible nodules (0.5 to 2 mm), designated by us by the neutral non-interpretative term hepatocyte nodules. These are often called "hyperplastic nodules", "neoplastic nodules" or "adenomas"; (b) In models (iv), (vi) and (vii) (Table 1), one observes the appearance of microscopic foci or islands for relatively long periods of time during the fairly prolonged promotion phase with only a few developing into hepatocyte nodules after many weeks of promotion. Thus, microscopic islands or foci may appear transitorily during rapid nodule formation (RH model) or may dominate the liver for weeks or even some months, depending upon the nature and intensity of the promoter and promoting environment.

1. P1 - Microscopic Foci or Islands (Fig. 2)

The nature, properties and biological potential of foci of altered hepatocytes are subjects of active study (57-60). They are often called "preneoplastic", even though very few develop into hepatocyte nodules in most models (with the exception of the RH model) and even fewer can be related to any ultimate cancer. Under

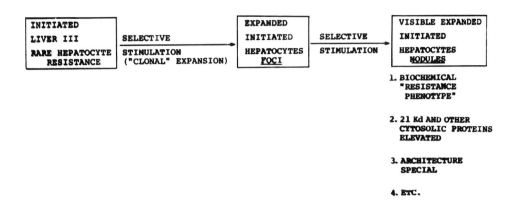

Fig. 2. Promotion of liver carcinogenesis in the RH model as at least 2 steps, P-1 and P-2 (Modified from Chart 2, reference 30).

some circumstances, they appear to be stable over many weeks, at least in so far as numbers are concerned (59,61). Whether this is the result of a balance between rates of appearance and disappearance or a reflection of true stability of each lesion has not been established (57-59,61,62). However, under other circumstances, especially in model (iv) with the use of phenobarbital, foci may show considerable instability (62,63).

This stability in numbers is in apparent contrast to the dynamic nature of individual hepatocytes within the foci. These show relatively high levels of labeling with thymidine without any comparable increase in the size of the foci (18,58,62). Also they show single cell death ("apoptosis") (62,64). Thus even though the foci or islands may appear to be stable, they may show a relatively large increase in cell proliferation and cell turnover in some models, when compared to the surrounding liver.

Microscopic islands or foci show reproducible histochemical and/or biochemical changes. Changes in glucose-6-phosphate dehydrogenase, and some other components of the pentose shunt as well as changes in glycolytic enzymes (65,66), in cytochromes P-450 and related enzymes (66-68,82) in glutathione (69) and in epoxide hydrolase (40,41) have been reported. Unfortunately, so far, the changes in glycolytic and shunt enzymes, unlike the phenotype associated with resistance (19,43,68), offer no obvious mechanisms for the clonal expansion of carcinogen-induced hepatocytes by cell proliferation. How these changes might confer relative resistance on these cells or some other functional or behavioural advantage has not been suggested (65,66).

Whether microscopic foci or islands can evolve into hepatocellular carcinoma without first expanding to hepatocyte nodules is an interesting question with no answer at the present time. Although investigators have on occasion expressed the opinion that microscopic foci may lead to cancer without first growing to non-cancerous nodules (57), the evidence remains to be presented. The finding of histologic or cytologic focal changes in hepatocytes inside foci without any evidence of biological neoplasia or malignancy is not convincing evidence of cancer arising in foci or islands. Late persistent nodules regularly show more advanced changes, nodules in nodules, without any biological behaviour of cancer. The latter is seen only much later. So far, no model has been described in which hepatocellular cancers occur without a prior appearance of hepatocyte nodules. Also the precursor role of hepatocyte nodules for cancer has been established in some instances (see Section II-E).

2. P2 - Hepatocyte Nodules (Fig. 2)

(a) Biological properties and options:

By nodules is meant visible focal proliferations of hepatocytes that are different from and compress the surrounding liver. They are larger than 0.5 to 1 mm in diameter and may measure up to 1 cm or more. They show a whole array of differences from the normal, control or surrounding liver (13,30,65,66,70,71), including differences in arrangement and architecture of their hepatocytes, blood supply, cytologic and histologic appearance, and biochemical properties. Unlike the findings in foci with some apparently casual histochemical markers that cannot be related at this time to any mechanism for initiation or promotion (34,59,65,66), the metabolic patterns in nodules are remarkably uniform from model to model and largely from nodule to nodule (70,71). This commonality refers both to the majority of nodules that remodel by redifferentiation and to the small minority that persist and become precursors for subsequent steps to cancer (see II C 2.b).

The most striking property of early hepatocyte nodules is the capability of expressing one of two options - remodelling by redifferentiation by the majority (95 to 98%) and persistence by a small minority (2-5%). The remodelling nodules show a major reorganization and rearrangement of their component hepatocytes and blood vessels to form normal-looking liver (72-74). Although phenotypic maturation or phenotypic reversion had been described previously (57,75,76), progressive replacement of nodule hepatocytes by ingrowth with different hepatocytes from the surrounding liver was not ruled out. It was only recently proven that the nodule hepatocytes themselves undergo a process of redifferentiation to adult-like hepatocytes during remodelling (74). This was a very critical finding in that it demonstrated that a majority of carcinogen-induced initiated or altered hepatocytes, if not all, possess and express a genetic program for such a complex redifferentiation process. This observation clearly points to the physiological nature of many of the earlier steps in the carcinogenic process (6,9).

A small subset of the nodules do not undergo the more or less rapid redifferentiation process but rather remain as persistent nodules. Some of these do appear to undergo slow remodelling, since there occurs a slow progressive decrease in the number of persistent nodules over many weeks (73,74,77). The persistent nodules retain the characteristic architecture, organization, blood supply and biochemical pattern of the precursor nodules before remodelling (72,73). Conceivably, the only difference between the few persistent nodules and the majority of remodelling ones is one of rate or kinetics, i.e. quantitative rather than qualitative. This decrease in the rate of redifferentiation may allow time for a next step to occur and this may be sufficient to commit this small population to the pathway of evolution toward cancer.

The persistent nodules acquire a new property - "spontaneous" or seemingly "autonomous" cell proliferation of their hepatocytes

(72,73,77) and become the origin for a slow evolution to hepatocellular carcinoma (see below).

Thus, once the foci enlarge by selection to form nodules, new options seem to appear - redifferentiation leading to remodelling and persistence with cell proliferation and evolution to cancer (9,30).

In the studies using the RH model and some other models, the inbred Fisher (F-344) strain of rat has been used. This strain is particularly useful in experiments with 2-AAF, because of its sensitivity and responsiveness to this agent.

In another strain of rat, the Wistar, the sensitivity to 2-AAF is considerably less and therefore the selection pressure created by 2-AAF plus PH or CCl_4 is less. The nodules generated are smaller than in the Fischer animals and fewer. Under these conditions, a two-step selection for nodules is more effective, with the use of 2-AAF plus PH, followed by dietary phenobarbital (78-80).

(b) Biochemical properties:

As has been recently emphasized (70,71,81), hepatocyte nodules have a very distinctive metabolic pattern in common, even when induced in six different models of liver carcinogenesis. The same metabolic pattern is present in the nodules both before remodelling begins and in the persistent ones.

The nodules show large decreases (75 to 90%) in total microsomal cytochromes P-450 and cytochrome b_5 and in several mixed function oxygenase activities (see references 30,70,71,67,82 for all the detailed references). These decreases in phase I enzymes are associated with marked decreases in metabolism and activation of carcinogens (83,84) and other xenobiotics. Accompanying the large decrease in metabolism are relatively large increases (2 to 15 fold) in glutathione (reduced, oxidized and bound), in several cytosolic glutathione-S-transferases and DT-diaphorase, in microsomal epoxide hydrolase and UDP-glucuronyltransferase I and in membrane gamma-glutamyltransferase. All of these components play a role in the detoxification of several types of xenobiotics and their metabolic derivatives including the generation of mercapturic acids. In addition, the nodules from different models show a special polypeptide with a molecular weight of 26 Kd in the cytosol. This has recently been identified as being the same as the placental glutathione-S-transferase of Sato and colleagues (85-88).

The biochemical pattern is unusually relevant to the resistance of nodule hepatocytes to xenobiotics (6,9,30,33,54,70,71,81). The properties are such as to make it very likely that a common gene regulator or regulating gene is intimately involved in mechanism (see below under II).

D. PROGRESSION (Fig. 3)

Definition: We define progression as the process whereby one or more focal proliferations, such as papillomas, polyps and nodules, undergo a slow cellular evolution to malignant neoplasm. Included in this term are the series of changes which a malignant neoplasm may undergo as it becomes more malignant, and more prone to show invasion and then to metastasize.

One of the most positive features of the RH model is its ability to distinguish the few persistent nodules from the large number of remodelling nodules and thus to allow a study of the nodule to cancer sequence. Early studies of the persistent nodules have already delineated two new steps in the sequence, PC-1 and PC-2.

1. PC-1. Cell Proliferation Plus Cell Death (Fig. 3)

In the RH model, the persistent nodules at 2 months continue to show an unusual degree of synchrony, certainly no less than in the surrounding or control liver, at least in their response to partial hepatectomy (77). This continuation of synchrony makes it possible to study a presumptive step-by-step sequence during the nodule to cancer phase of progression.

Unlike the early hepatocyte nodules generated during promotion or selection (89), the small subset of persistent hepatocyte nodules show "spontaneous" cell proliferation from their beginning (72-74,77). At 2 months post-initiation, (PC-1) the percentage of hepatocytes in the persistent nodules undergoing cell proliferation is about 4% and this increases to 8% by 6 months (PC-2). This is in contrast to the hepatocytes in the liver surrounding the nodules which show a growth fraction of about 0.4%.

At 2 months, not only is there about a 10 fold increase in cell proliferation over the surrounding liver but there is another new phenomenon - cell loss or cell death. Cell loss or cell death during the promotion phase of nodule formation (P-2) was virtually absent, with a growth fraction of over 80% (89). The growth of the nodules matched very well with the rate of cell proliferation and the duration of the cell cycle (89). In the early persistent nodules (PC-1), there now appears cell loss or cell death as a quantitatively significant property of nodules (77). The 4% growth fraction is almost balanced by a 3% cell loss, thus accounting for a slow rate of enlargement of the nodules (73,74,77). This appears to be the first clear-cut appearance of cell death in the sequence in the RH model and is present throughout the whole nodule-to-cancer sequence as well as in the cancers themselves (64,77).

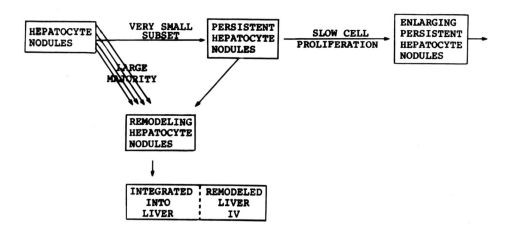

Fig. 3. Progression of liver carcinogenesis in the RH model. The early precancerous steps are indicated (PC-1, PC-2 etc.) (Modified from Chart 4, reference 30).

Despite the appearance of a "spontaneous" or "autonomous" cell proliferation and cell death, the hepatocytes in the hepatocyte nodules at 2 months show at least some normal control patterns. The cell cycle shows a diurnal rhythm similar to the normal (77). Also, the nodule hepatocytes respond to the mitogenic stimulus of partial hepatectomy both quantitatively and qualitatively as do normal control or the surrounding liver hepatocytes (77). The response to partial hepatectomy is vigorous and brisk, and the hepatocytes return to the base line level (4%) by 14 days. The cell cycle phases of the hepatocytes at 2 months, unlike those during the developing nodules during promotion (89), are "normal" in that they are identical to those in control untreated animals. At an earlier time, during P-1 and P-2, the nodule hepatocytes showed a considerable prolongation of the S phase (89) but this is no longer present in the 2 month persistent nodule.

At 2 months, the proliferating hepatocytes appear to be a more or less discrete subset of the total nodule hepatocyte population. Instead of showing a random scatter of hepatocytes, each undergoing an occasional episode of cell proliferation, the available evidence suggests that the same subset of hepatocytes in these nodules undergo more than one cell cycle (77). If future evidence continues to suggest the existence of a proliferating subset, it should become possible to separate such a subset of hepatocytes from the majority of the nodule hepatocytes by flow cytometry. The fact that 60 to 80% of nodule hepatocytes respond to partial hepatectomy by cell proliferation suggests that the majority of these cells have retained the same basic controls of their proliferative potential as have the hepatocytes of control young adult liver.

2. PC-2. Cell Proliferation, Cell Death and Altered Shut-off of the Cell Cycle (Fig. 3)

In the RH model at 6 months, the hepatocytes in the nodules have retained their ability to respond briskly and vigorously to partial hepatectomy (77). Starting from a baseline cell proliferation (growth fraction) of 8%, 60 to 80% of the nodule hepatocytes respond as do the surrounding and age/sex matched control liver hepatocytes to a mitogenic stimulus. However, some nodule hepatocytes have acquired an additional property - lack of shut-off of the cell cycle. Unlike control untreated or surrounding liver or 2 month nodule hepatocytes, a measurable number of 6 month nodule hepatocytes do not return to the baseline level of cell proliferation, but continue to show repeated cell proliferation, for at least 3 weeks, in excess of the basal level, in response to partial hepatectomy (77). Although these findings might be a reflection of a heterogeneous response to a mitogen on the part of the nodule hepatocytes, the available evidence favors the acquisition of a new property by some nodule hepatocytes - a failure to stop cycling once the cell cycle is begun. Again, flow cytometry could prove very useful in obtaining this new subset of nodule hepatocytes.

The persistent nodules at 6 months also show another new property - generation of nodules and hepatocellular carcinoma on transplantation to the spleen (90). This is in contrast to the behaviour of the early nodules. The early nodules will mostly remodel and grow slowly in the spleen like normal liver hepatocytes with gradual replacement of the splenic pulp by liver but without nodules or cancer (91).

3. Subsequent Steps

Although two new steps relating to the control of cell proliferation have been identified at 2 and at 6 months post-initiation, the nature of any subsequent steps remain only speculative and conjectural. Even up to 6 months, the nodule hepatocytes, although showing progressively altered cell cycle control, remain highly predictable and seemingly still under a reasonably rigid control. However, at 2 and 6 months, it is already evident that subsets of nodule hepatocytes are showing new properties that could be interpreted as approaching closer to a more autonomous and more uncontrolled state. Thus, the RH model is showing what has been suspected for a long time - cellular evolution with small numbers of cells participating or at risk (92-94). Since the nodule to cancer segment of liver cancer development appears to be quite synchronous at least until 6 months, it is anticipated that synchrony might continue and this would allow a sequential analysis from 6 months to the time of cancer formation.

Despite its obvious importance, the nodule-to-cancer sequence has been little studied. One of the most evident problems in this area is the lack of synchrony of nodule development and of cellular evolution in most models. As with any multistep process, no sequence analysis is possible unless one can be certain that the presumptive steps are arranged "in order" and are synchronized. This is particlularly important when several or many different lesions occur at each step (95).

As yet, there is virtually no insight into the phenomenon of nodule evolution to cancer, let alone any solid evidence for mechanims. Work in progress in our department has indicated that whereas estradiol and progesterone can either inhibit or stimulate respectively the growth of the early nodules, neither treatment has any effect on cancer development (96). A similar situation has been found with orotic acid (1% in diet) and with the calmodulin inhibitor trifluoropyrazine (0.01%). Interestingly, choline chloride (1% in the diet) appears to delay considerably the nodule to cancer progression.

E. HEPATOCELLULAR CARCINOMA

Minimum of Three Steps - HC -1, HC-2 and HC-3 (Fig. 4). In most models of hepatocellular carcinoma development with chemicals in adult rats, including the RH model, one usually sees unequivocal malignant neoplasia by 9 to 12 months post-initiation. However, no detailed study of the later steps to cancer has been possible to date. Our experience with the RH model suggests that it may now become feasible, providing the synchrony of lesion development seen at 2, 4 and 6 months is maintained for an additional 2 to 4 months.

It is known that the hepatocyte nodules are precursors for hepatocellular carcinoma in at least 5 studies with different models (see 30 for references). This observation provides clear convincing evidence that cancer can arise inside hepatocyte nodules. Whether this is an obligatory requirement for liver cell cancer is, of course, unknown and may well remain so for a long time. However, these observations indicate the utility of studying the nodule to cancer sequence as one established sequence.

It is generally seen that the expressions of advanced invasion and metastasis are not always present, by any means, with every unequivocal cancer. In fact, it appears that these are relatively late manifestations of a malignant neoplasm.

However, until the fundamental basis for each property is better understood and until sensitive assays are available for the fundamental alterations, it is impossible to discuss intelligently how the properties relate to a step-wise sequence. Is the order fixed or variable? Is there an interdependence among the three properties in that altered growth must be acquired <u>before</u> the ability to invade and the latter in turn must be acquired <u>before</u> the ability to metastasize? Until a model is developed for a step-wise analysis, these questions will continue to remain speculative and abstract.

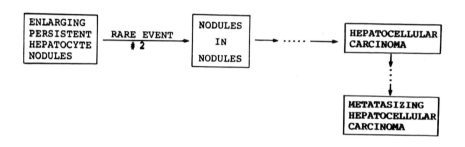

Fig. 4. Progression of liver carcinogenesis in the RH model. The later steps, including at least 3 relating directly to cancer, are indicated. (Modified from Chart 5, reference 30).

III. MECHANISMS AT DIFFERENT STEPS

A. INITIATION

There is considerable circumstantial but inconclusive evidence that DNA is <u>a</u> major target macromolecule if not <u>the</u> target. Yet, the many dozens or hundreds of molecular changes induced by interactions of a highly reactive ultimate carcinogen with virtually all portions of the cell including the nucleus, mitochondria, endoplasmic reticulum, membranes etc. and DNA, RNA's and proteins make the scientific evidence for the exclusive role of any single target in carcinogenesis unobtainable so far. Even if it is assumed that DNA is the major or only target, the number of chemical, functional and steric alterations in the DNA of target tissues (46,47) again offers a virtually insoluble problem if a relationship between any single change or even a single group of chemical changes and initiation of carcinogenesis is sought. The number of parallel phenomena that accompany the critical one or ones is no doubt large (5,97).

Therefore, any conclusion concerning the role of mutation, gene rearrangement, gene amplification, gene suppression, gene activation, oncogene activity etc. must remain at best highly speculative and premature.

Biologically, initiation in vivo is associated with the appearance, in a rare cell, of a change that can be made "permanent" or relatively so by a round of cell replication (98). These properties per se are consistent with a mutation-like change in DNA that can be fixed by one round of DNA replication. However, other types of DNA - associated phenomena, such as gene rearrangements, translocations or activations might also fit the biological "facts" as presently known. Whatever the nature of the relevant molecular lesion, it is not related directly to any "autonomous" or "spontaneous" growth.

In the liver, one or more of these presumed changes in DNA must generate a new biochemical pattern, one which is associated with resistance to xenobiotics, to the potential for a new state of differentiation and to a genetic program for redifferentiation. Clearly, this can only reside in some regulatory gene or genes of a major type. This regulator gene could be structurally altered by a mutation or functionally altered by a change in some related region of the DNA. By allowing for a biochemical program for resistance to the cytotoxicity of xenobiotics including carcinogens, this may be sufficient to explain the first major phase of carcinogenesis, the genesis of focal proliferations or hepatocyte nodules.

Thus, by an intensive search for the relevant genes for one or more phenotypic components of hepatocyte nodules, it becomes theoretically possible to begin to focus on the key gene or genes, the alteration of which relate to initiation. The 26 Kd polypeptide in nodule cytosol (85) which appears to be closely related to the glutathione-S-transferase P of Sato and colleagues (42,86-88) could be one such penetrating probe. From the current perspective, it appears much more realistic and profitable to work "backwards" (5) from the known to the unknown if we are to understand the essential nature of the key interactions of a chemical carcinogen with DNA that relate to the first phases of cancer development. The "forward" "head-on" approach, by looking for changes in DNA without a guide, could be an excellent example of the "needle in the haystack".

B. PROMOTION

The liver offers one established mechanism for promotion, "differential inhibition" (33). By providing a stimulus for cell proliferation (partial hepatectomy or cell death by CCL_4) and by inhibiting cell proliferation of the vast majority of uninitiated susceptible hepatocytes by the brief exposure to 2-AAF, the few rare resistant hepatocytes, the "initiated ones", are able to respond to the mitogenic stimulus and rapidly generate focal proliferations or nodules. Thus, in this system, promotion is essentially by inhibition, not by selective stimulation. Since, in humans, cancer often arises in an atrophic, not a hyperplastic organ or tissue (e.g. stomach, liver, pancreas), it is likely that this overall mechanism may well be a common one. This is certainly most likely in animals and in humans where cancer arises in response to repeated long term exposure to one or more carcinogens, i.e. the carcinogen is both initiator and promoter. This pattern appears to be much commoner in nature than is the initiation-promotion pattern that is being used more and more experimentally.

Other patterns of promotion have been proposed. For example, "differential stimulation" or "differential recovery" are two feasible possibilities (33).

It should be emphasized that the current research approaches for the study of promoters, like that of initiators, is the "forward one". By cataloguing what biochemical, molecular, genetic, immunologic or biophysical changes are induced by a particular agent, it is hoped to understand the mechanism of promotion. To date, this approach has generated virtually no insight into the mechanisms of promotion. The prospects that it may do so soon do not seem promising. However, this approach has reinforced in a clear manner the existence of synergisms among promoters and has dissected promotion in mouse skin into at least two biological steps neither of which have been delineated mechanically so far (99).

The likelihood of understanding a mechanism before a phenomenon is delineated seems unrealistic. For example, since differential inhibition is one mechanism for promotion in liver carcinogenesis, it would be irrational to focus on the presence of a selective proliferative response by the initiated hepatocytes and ignore the failure to respond by the majority. A more rational approach, which is productive, is to study the biochemical and genetic basis for the resistance by the initiated hepatocytes.

From the RH model, it is also apparent that populations derived from the same cells, presumably by clonal expansion, show different properties at different steps during expansion. Initiated resistant hepatocytes are stable for months as small invisible or visible cells or foci (98). However, on expansion to nodules, the resistant initiated hepatocytes demonstrate a new biological option - remodelling by redifferentiation (74). Thus, clones of the same cells, expanded to different degrees, show two different patterns of behaviour.

In this context, it is interesting to consider the comparison between foci and nodules with respect to cell proliferation and cell turnover. In the RH model, the foci appear as a brief transitory population of hepatocytes during the rapid expansion from initiated cells to nodules during a period of some 4 weeks (2 to 6 weeks post-initiation). During this phase of hepatocarcinogenesis, cell proliferation dominates the cell dynamics (89). Almost no cell loss or turnover is seen until the appearance of persistent nodules at about 8 weeks post-initiation. This dominance of cell proliferation and the virtual absence of cell loss or cell death ("apoptosis") is in striking contrast to what has been found in foci of altered hepatocytes with model (iv). Schulte-Hermann and colleagues (18,62,66) have found that foci appearing during the slow promotion by phenobarbital after initiation show much more labelling of their hepatocytes with thymidine than do hepatocytes in the surrounding liver. However, the rate of growth or expansion of these foci is minimal during the time period studied, indicating that the cell proliferation is largely balanced by a more or less equal rate of cell loss. The latter could be by a process of individual cell death ("apoptosis").

Thus, at least two patterns of cell proliferation and cell loss are seen in foci in two different models, either (a) continual cell proliferation without cell loss leading to progressive expansion of foci to generate nodules, or (b) balanced cell proliferation - cell loss with little or no net expansion of foci and with only very slow development of nodules. However, if the crucial property for evolution to cancer is the number of cell proliferations any single hepatocyte undergoes, rather than the pattern of growth, then conceivably expansion to nodules or not could be unimportant. Continual "unbalanced" cell proliferation without cell loss generating nodules or "balanced" cell proliferation and cell loss may be equivalent with respect to further steps in the development of cancer, so long as some cells participate in many or several rounds of cell proliferation and so long as each cell undergoing cell proliferation does not die at some phase in the cell cycle. Viewed from this perspective, a comparison between the cell dynamics of hepatocytes in foci and in nodules could be rewarding.

It is well known in embryology or developmental biology that clonal expansion plays an important role in differentiation (100). In muscle and other types of cells, the concept of quantal cell cycle is very attractive. Cells seem to require a certain number of cell divisions before a new pattern of gene expression can become manifest. This could well be the pattern in the carcinogenic process where different degrees of clonal expansion of a similar cell population generate new focal proliferations of different biological behaviour. If this is applicable to the process of cancer development (100), it is not surprising that smaller foci or islands of initiated cells may have quite different biological options available than do larger nodules. This principle should be explored further both in vivo and in vitro.

C. PROGRESSION

The RH model has brought into focus two aspects of the possible mechanisms of progression to cancer: (a) cell death either as a trigger or as a consequence of cell proliferation, and (b) the production of growth factors and stimulation of oncogene expression.

(a) The "sudden" appearance of cell death at the earliest observable time in the persistent nodule, i.e. in the nodule-to-cancer sequence, introduces an important component in carcinogenesis in vivo. Can cancer development occur without cell death? Does the cell death _trigger_ the "spontaneous" or "autonomous" cell proliferation in step PC-1 or is cell death a consequence of the cell proliferation? The new availability of a model to study this might lead to some answers.

(b) Another important consideration linked to (a) is whether step PC-1 is associated with the new production of growth factors, perhaps on an autocrine basis (101). Since some oncogenes are related to some growth factors (101,102), it is possible that one or more oncogenes may become expressed or may show increased expression at step PC-1. Again, the RH model makes it now possible to pose this question.

Regardless of the basis for the "spontaneous" cell proliferation in steps PC-1, PC-2 and later, the continual proliferation of a small population in the persistent nodules without constant shedding of the progeny, (such as occurs on a mucous or cutaneous surface or from bone marrow) may now make these steps open to a process of cell evolution (92) by mutation and selection (93) or clonal evolution (94) and these may well become the major overall mechanisms for the progressive pressure toward more and more malignant behaviour.

An important aspect of this phase of carcinogenesis is the study of increasing growth, invasive properties and metastasis as separate sets of mechanisms. It is well known that these three sets are acquired separately and seriatim. Without a knowledge of these three apparently separable phenotypic expressions, any hope of studying the basis for the malignant behaviour of cancer and for the great diversity and heterogeneity of malignant neoplasms seems remote. So far, virtually all the studies on malignant neoplastic populations, be they monoclonal or polyclonal, have generated little new insight into the essential nature of malignancy, with one notable exception - the possible genesis of growth factors (so-called transforming growth factors, etc) and the interesting possibility of autocrine control of cell proliferation by malignant neoplastic cells (101). The vast majority of phenotypic changes seen in cancer might well be epiphenomena, "noise", on a fundamental base of growth, invasion and metastasis. Studies of cell populations in which these are not delineated and controlled as variables are not

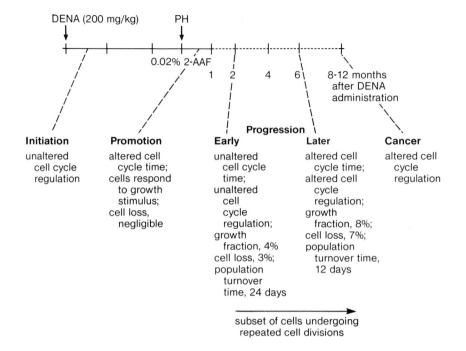

Fig. 5. Diagrammatic representation of our current understanding of the steps involved in the development of liver cancer with chemicals. Two new steps, early and later progression, have been added recently (77)

likely to be fruitful of new insights.

Current studies have added two new steps to our understanding of the step-by-step development of liver cancer with chemicals (Fig. 5). In addition to at least two steps in initiation (I-1, I-2) and two in promotion (P-1, P-2), there are now two steps in the early phases of progression (PC-1, PC-2) in the pre-cancerous persistent hepatocyte nodules. These two new steps now offer a new model to begin to dissect some of the major phenotypic manifestations of cancer cells, increasingly "autonomous" growth, without the accompanying complicating and complex associations of invasiveness and ability to metastasize. It appears that the RH model remains synchronous well into the pre-cancerous phase and therefore is potentially amenable to scientific analysis in increasing depth. The occurrence of the steps long after the discontinuation of the exposure to any exogenous agent, be it initiating, promoting or otherwise modulating, may make it possible to understand the basic changes and response patterns in relevant cells in carcinogenesis in the absence of an ongoing overlay with the acute responses of cells to carcinogens and promoters. Another important feature is the ability to identify grossly the small number of crucial nodules that persist and that are at least one type of cancer precursor.

IV. COMPARISONS WITH OTHER ORGANS AND TISSUES

The pattern of multistep carcinogenesis in the rat liver is remarkably similar in principle to multistep development of cancer in the mouse skin (99), in the urinary bladder (103), in the colon in humans and in mice (104,105), in the pancreas (106-109), in the breast and mammary gland (110) and in the respiratory tract (111). The interactions with DNA and other cell constituents, the importance of cell proliferation, and the clonal expansion during the promotion phase appear to be very common. The reversibility of many focal proliferations (papillomas, nodules and polyps) appears to be a common phenomenon in some systems (5,6). Also, the multistep (at least 2 steps) nature of the promotion phase in the skin is well documented (99). The stepwise nature of progression has been poorly studied and begs for increased emphasis if we are ever to understand the steps between focal proliferations and malignant neoplasia.

The genesis of melanoma in the human (112) also has many resemblances to the basic patterns in the rat liver. In fact, some of the steps in the human melanocyte and rat hepatocyte systems seem almost superimposable. These similarities are encouraging in that they support the thesis that the detailed elucidation of _any_ system, be it human or animal, will almost certainly act as a blueprint and a model , in principle for many other systems, both clinical and experimental.

V. SOME CENTRAL QUESTIONS IN MULTISTEP ANALYSIS OF CANCER DEVELOPMENT

Given the relatively undeveloped understanding of the multistep nature of cancer development in all systems, it becomes important to formulate some of the key questions that must be studied for clarification of the most fundamental aspect of cancer research, the stepwise development of cancer.

A. OVERALL PATTERNS

The studies in experimental animals are focused almost exclusively on one pattern of cancer development, the multistep pattern with focal proliferations (9). There are at least three patterns of cancer development (9), only one of which has papillomas, polyps etc. as key precursors. Are there truly systems of cancer development without such focal proliferations as cancer precursors?

B. INITIATION

To date, initiation has been demonstrated in many tissues or organs as well as in in vitro. However, a central issue concerns the relation of the initiated events to cancer. What are the essential phenotypic and genotypic characteristics of initiated cells in each major system? Does an initiating exposure to a carcinogen "convey any message" that pertains to the ultimate cancer or does it only induce the first step in the few initiated cells - i.e. the potential to become the site for a focal proliferation? The simplest hypothesis is the latter - an initiator inducing a change that allows that cell to become clonally expanded by a further exposure to the same or a different carcinogen or to a promoter. Intuitively, most cancer researchers assume that an initiating carcinogen not only initiates but induces some effect that relates more directly to cancer.

C. PROMOTION

In most models of carcinogenesis, focal or clonal expansion of the few "initiated" target cells is the only immediate visible concomitant of promotion. If the expansion is sufficient in degree, is this all that is associated with promotion or must there be some additional alteration in the expanding cell population that relates to cancer? Additional so-called "hits" are commonly discussed in this context, without any conclusive experimental evidence (32,113). A two-hit concept is quite popular. The possible nature of the so-called multi-hits have not been discussed, other than as additional mutations. The "multi-hit model" follows naturally from the current paradigm of chemical carcinogenesis. Mutations, with the genesis of "abnormal" or "pathologic" new cells, coupled with selection form the basis of the current paradigm (95). It would be expected on this basis that multiple "hits" are required to generate the repeated mutations.

It should be pointed out that obvious mechanisms for "multiple hits" are not readily apparent in models (iv) (vi) and (vii) for liver carcinogenesis, unless the promoters or promoting environments are participating in unsuspected effects on DNA or on some other important component of the genomic organization. Free radicals and their possible effects on DNA generated by promoters are being discussed increasingly.

However, there is increasing evidence that the current paradigm of chemical carcinogenesis is not compatible with many of the observations being made in liver carcinogenesis. An alternative hypothesis, that of a physiological adaptative nature (6,9,62) is becoming attractive to explain many of the phenomena in hepatocarcinogenesis specifically and chemical carcinogenesis in general. There is increasing data to show that, despite the many chemical differences between the many agents used in the different models of liver carcinogenesis, the tissue changes and response patterns of the liver, such as foci and nodules, are remarkably similar in their many phenotypic properties. Also, a major response during liver carcinogenesis, the hepatocyte nodule, is beneficial to the host in a hazardous environment by virtue of being composed of cells resistant to cytotoxic effects of many xenobiotics. In addition, this same common response is associated with a complex new pattern of gene expression, redifferentiation. This phenomenon is clearly due to the expression of a new pattern of genes. Thus a key step in the sequence of events during liver cancer development exercises a major option based upon a complex genetic program. Clearly, much of the early events in carcinogenesis are genetically programmed and are part of a normal physiological pattern of adaptation to some xenobiotics which we call carcinogenesis (6,9,62).

D. PROGRESSION

What is the underlying mechanism for the subset of persistent nodule hepatocytes or similar subsets in other systems to begin to undergo cell proliferation? The fundamental issue is: is this secondary to cell death as a new acquired property at the PC-1 step or are the "new" cells now generating growth factors, perhaps because of the activation of some selected oncogenes? The step PC-1 and PC-2 are the places to ask these questions, since the system is uncomplicated by uncontrolled growth, invasion and metastasis and by the many epiphenomena that in concert contribute to the bewildering array of phenotypic expressions in any fully developed cancer.

VI. POSSIBLE RELATIONSHIPS BETWEEN THE PATHOGENESIS OF LIVER CANCER IN THE RAT AND THE HUMAN

Given the relatively large fraction of the normal life-span that it takes to develop hepatocellular carcinoma in the rat and in the human, and the many similarities between the ultimate malignant neoplasms in each species, it is reasonable, as a first approximation, to consider that the carcinogenic processes may be similar in the two species.

If this is a reasonable position, it is attractive to consider that the identification and elucidation of the mechanisms underlying each step in the rat may offer testable hypothesis for the steps in the human. Such an eventuality reinforces the potential importance of studying step by step how liver cell cancer develops in the rat so that new markers, new ways to interrupt the process and new modulating influences for the human disease may be uncovered. Also, given the many similarities, in principle, between the stepwise development of cancer in several organs and tissues, it is likely that any clarification of one or more steps in liver cancer evolution may well have applications to the neoplastic process in other organs or tissues.

Particularly relevant may be the suggestion that the pathogenesis of hepatocellular carcinoma in humans in association with HBV may involve the induction of resistant hepatocytes (R cells) and the selection of such hepatocytes for growth by virtue of an effect of the virus on the majority of hepatocytes that are susceptible or sensitive (S cells) (114). This suggestion, so close in principle to that previously suggested for hepatocarcinogenesis with chemicals in the rat (6,19), has been discussed by others since

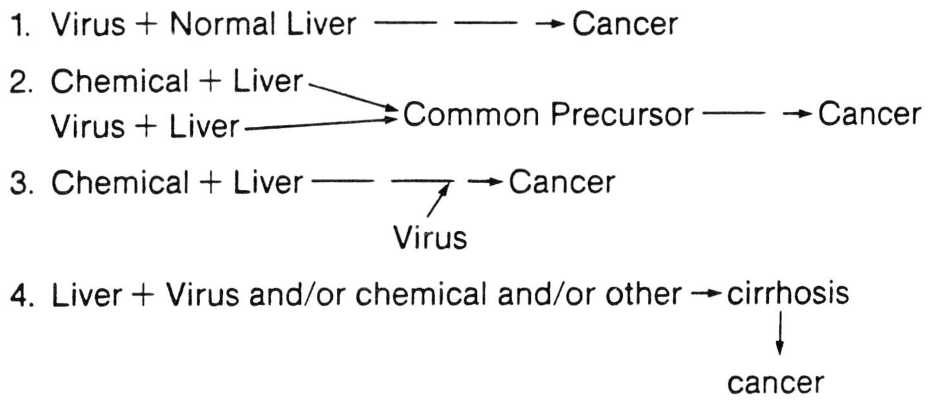

1. Virus + Normal Liver ⎯⎯ ⎯⎯ ➤ Cancer

2. Chemical + Liver
   Virus + Liver ⎯⎯⎯⎯➤ Common Precursor ⎯⎯ ➤ Cancer

3. Chemical + Liver ⎯⎯ ⎯⎯➤ Cancer
                    Virus

4. Liver + Virus and/or chemical and/or other ➤ cirrhosis
                                                  ↓
                                               cancer

Fig. 6. Schematic representation of possible relationship between hepatitis B virus, chemical carcinogens and liver cancer.

then in relation to the pathogenesis of human cancer (4,115).

With respect to the possible interplay between different etiological factors in human cancer development, several various combinations can be considered (Fig. 6). As insight is generated in regard to identifiable steps in the genesis of liver cell cancer in the rat, conditions for the testing of such considerations may well become available.

VII. PERSPECTIVES AND CONCLUSIONS

Clearly, the stepwise analysis of a carcinogenic process opens up many possibilities for study and generates new critical and crucial questions relating to our understanding of the way in which cancer develops mechanically.

The remarkable similarities between many models in different organs and tissues and with different carcinogens and in humans and mice, rats and other animals, coupled with the paralyzing diversity and heterogeneity of any end stage cancer, point clearly to the importance of studies in cancer development as basic to our ultimate understanding of cancer. This obvious conclusion seems not to have been taken to heart by the vast majority of cancer researchers, given the relative paucity of studies in the stepwise analysis of cancer development. The experience with one system, the liver, indicates that new analyzable features of neoplasia will continue to be generated by expanded studies on the steps through which cells evolve as they slowly move toward cancer.

REFERENCES

1. Waterhouse J, Muir C, Powell J (1982) Cancer incidence in five continents. Vol. IV, IARC Publications, N° 42, World Health Organization, Lyon

2. Mackay J, Okuda K (eds) (1984). UICC workshop on hepatocellular carcinoma, UICC Technical Report Series, N° 74

3. Beasley RP, Hwang LY, Lin CC, et al. (1981) Lancet 2: 1129-1133

4. Harris CC, Sun T (1984) Carcinogenesis 5: 697-701

5. Foulds L (1969 and 1975) Neoplastic development, Vols 1 and 2, Academic Press, New York

6. Farber E, Cameron R. (1980) Adv Cancer Res 35: 125-226

7. Emmelot P (Coordinator) (1980) Biochim Biophys Acta 605: 149 -304

8. Popper H, Gerber MA, Thung SN (1982) Hepatology 2: 1S-9S

9. Farber E (1984) Biochim Biophys Acta 738: 171-180

10. Sasaki T, Yoshida T (1935) Virchow's Arch Pathol Anat Physiol Klin Med 295: 175-200

11. Kinosita R (1937) Trans Jpn Pathol Soc 27: 665-729

12. Reuber MD (1965) J Natl Cancer Inst 34: 697-723

13. Epstein S, Ito N, Merkow L, et al. (1967) Cancer Res 27:1702-1711

14. Teebor GW, Becker FF (1971) Cancer Res 31: 1-3

15. Bannasch P, Moore MA, Klimek F, et al. (1982) Toxicol Pathol 10: 19-34

16. Peraino C, Fry RJM, Staffeldt E (1971) Cancer Res 31: 1506-1512

17. Pitot HC, Sirica AE (1980) Biochim Biophys K Acta 605: 191-215

18. Schulte-Hermann R, Ohde G, Schuppler J et al. (1981) Cancer Res 41: 2556-2562

19. Solt DB, Farber E (1976) Nature (Lond) 263: 702-703

20. Ito N, Tatematsu, M, Nakaniski K et al (1980) Gann 71: 832-942

21. Tsuda H, Lee G, Farber E (1980) Cancer Res. 40: 1157-1164

22. Sells MA, Katyal SL, Sell S, et al. (1979) Br J Cancer 40: 274-283

23. Newberne PM, Rogers AE, Nauss KM (1983) In: Nutritional Factors

in Oncogenesis and Maintenance of Malignancy. Buterworth PE and Hutchinson ML (eds), Academic Press, New York, 247-271

24. Rao PM, Nagamine K, Ho RK et al. Carcinogenesis 4: 1541-1545

25. Laurier C, Tatematsu M, Rao PM et al. (1984)   Cancer Res 44: 2186-2191

26. Mikol YB, Hoover KL, Creasia D et al. (1983)   Carcinogenesis 4: 1619-1629

27. Ghoshal AK, Farber E (1984) Carcinogenesis 5: 1367-1370

28. Yokoyama S, Sells MA, Reddy TV et al. (1985)   Cancer Res 45: 2834-28

29. Farber E (1982) in: Cancer: A Comprehensive Treatise, Becker FF (ed) Vol 1, 2nd Ed, Plenum Publ Corp, New York, pp 485-506

30. Farber E (1984) Cancer Res 44: 5463-5474

31. Scherer E, Hoffman M, Emmelot P, et al. (1972) J. Natl Cancer Inst 49: 93-106

32. Emmelot P, Scherer E (1980) Biochem Biophys Acta 605: 247-304

33. Farber E (1980) Biochim Biophys Acta 605: 149-166

34. Peraino C, Staffeldt EF, Carnes BA et al. (1984) Cancer Res 44: 3340-3347

35. Peraino C, Richards WL, Stevens FJ (1983) In: Mechanism of Tumor Promotion, Vol I. Tumor Promotion in Internal Organs, Slaga TJ (ed), CRC Press Inc, Boca Raton, Florida

36. Tatematsu M, Kaku T, Medline A et al. (1983) In: Application of Biological Markers to Carcinogen Testing, Millman HA and Sells S (eds), Plenum Publ Corp, New York, pp 25-42

37. Kalengayi MMR, Ronchi G, Desmet VJ (1975) J Natl Cancer Inst 55: 579-588

38. Schor NA, Ogawa K, Lee G et al. (1978) Cancer Lett 5: 167-171

39. Novikoff AB, Novikoff PM, Stockert RJ et al. (1979) Proc Natl Acad Sci USA 76: 5207-5211

40. Enomoto K, Ying TS, Griffin MJ, et al. (1981) Cancer Res 41: 3281-3287

41. Kuhlmann WD, Kirschan R, Kuntz W, et al. (1981) Biochem Biophys Res Commun 98: 417-423

42. Tatematsu M, Mera Y, Ito N et al. (1985) Carcinogenesis 6: 1621-1626

43. Solt DB, Medline A, Farber E. (1977) Am J Pathol 88: 595-618

44. Solt DB, Cayama E, Tsuda H et al. (1983) Cancer Res 43:188-191

45. Leonard TB, Dent JG, Graichen ME et al. (1982) Carcinogenesis 3: 851-856

46. Grover PL (ed) (1979) Chemical Carcinogens and DNA, CRC Press Inc, Boca Raton, Vols I and II

47. Rajalakshmi S, Rao PM and Sarma DSR (1982) In: Cancer: A Comprehensive Treatise, Becker FF (ed), Plenum Publ Corp New York, Ed. 2, Vol 1, pp 335-409

48. Scherer E, Steward AP, Emmelot P (1977) Chem biol Interact 19: 1-11

49. Ying TS, Enomoto K, Sarma DSR et al. (1982)   Cancer Res 42: 876-880

50. Padmore R, farber E (1985) Proc Am Assoc Cancer Res 26: 117

51. Cayama E, Tsuda H, Sarma DSR et al. (1978) Nature (Lond) 275: 60-62

52. Columbano A, Rajalakshmi S, Sarma DSR (1981) Cancer Res 41: 2079-2083

53. Ying TS, Sarma DSR, Farber E (1981) Cancer Res 41: 2096-2102

54. Farber E (1984) Cancer Res 44: 4217-4223

55. Craddock VM (1976) In: Liver Cell Cancer, Cameron HM, Linsell DA and Warwick GP (eds), Elsevier Press Inc, Amsterdam, pp 152-201

56. Farber E (1976) In: Liver Cell Cancer, Cameron HM, Linsell DA and Warwick GP (eds), Elsevier Press Inc, Amsterdam, pp 243-277

57. Williams GM (1980) Biochim Biophys Acta 605: 167-189

58. Schulte-Hermann R, Schuppler J, Timmermann-Trosiener J et al. (1983) Environ Health Persp 50: 185-194

59. Goldsworthy T, Campbell HA, Pitot HC (1984) Carcinogenesis 5: 67-71

60. Pugh TD, Goldfarb S (1978) Cancer Res 38: 4450-4457

61. Scherer E, Emmelot P (1975) Europ J Cancer 11: 698

62. Bursch W, Lauer B, Timmerman-Trosiener J et al. (1984) Carcinogenesis 5: 453-458

63. Glauert HP, Schwarz M, Pitot HC (1986) Carcinogenesis 7: 117-121

64. Columbano A, Ledda-Columbano GM, Rao PM et al. (1984) Am J Pathol 116: 441-446

65. Bannasch P, Hacker HJ, Klimek F et al. (1984) Adv Enzym Regul 22: 97-121

66. Schulte Hermann R, Timmerman-Trosiener I , Schuppler J (1984) Models, Mechanisms and Ethiology of Tumor Promotion, Brzsnyi W, Day NE, Yamasaki H (eds), Int Agency Res Cancer Sci Publ, Lyon, pp 67-75

67. Buchmann A, Kuhlman W, Schwarz M et al. (1985) Carcinogenesis 6, 513-521

68. Hanigan MH, Pitot HC (1985) Carcinogenesis 6: 165-172

69. Deml E, Oesterle D (1980) Cancer Res 40: 490-491

70. Farber E (1984) Can J Biochem Cell Biol 62: 486-494

71. Roomi MW, Ho RK, Sarma DSR et al. (1985) Cancer Res 45: 564-571

72. Ogawa K, Medline A, Farber E (1979) Br J Cancer 40: 782-790

73. Enomoto K, Farber E (1982) Cancer Res 42: 2330-2335

74. Tatematsu M, Nagamine Y, Farber E (1983) Cancer Res 43: 5049-5058

75. Kitagawa T (1971) Gann 62: 207-216

76. Kitagawa T, Sugano H (1973) Cancer Res 33: 2993-3001

77. Rotstein JB, Sarma DSR, Farber E (1986) Cancer Res, 46: 2377-2385

78. de Gerlache J, Lans M, Taper H et al. (1982) In: Mutagens in our Environment, Vaino H and Sorsa M (eds), Alan R Liss Inc, New York, pp 35-46

79. de Gerlache J, Lans M, Preat V et al. (1984) Toxicol Pathol 12: 374-382

80. Preat V, de Gerlache J, Lans M et al. (1985) Carcinogen Mutagen 5: in press

81. Eriksson LC, Ahluwalia M, Spiewak J et al. (1983) Environ Health Perspect 49: 171-174

82. Hanigan MH, Pitot HC (1985) J Natl Cancer Inst 75: 1107-1112

83. Rinauds JAS, Farber E (1986) Carcinogenesis 7: 523-528

84. Farber E, Parker S, Gruenstein M (1976) Cancer Res 36: 3879-3887

85. Eriksson LC, Sharma RN, Roomi MW et al. (1983) Biochem Biophys Res Commun 117: 740-745

86. Sato K, Kitahara A, Satoh K et al. (1984) Gann 75: 199-202

87. Kitahara A, Satoh K, Sato K (1983) Biochem Biophys Res Commun 112: 20-28

88. Roomi MW, Satoh K, Sato k et al. (1985) Proc Am Assoc Cancer Res 26: 302

89. Rotstein J, Macdonald PDM, Rabes HM et al. (1984) Cancer Res 44: 2913-2917

90. Lee G, Tatematsu M, Makowka L (1983) Proc Am Assoc Cancer Res 24: 106

91. Lee G, Medline A, Finkelstein S et al. (1983) Transplantation 36: 218-221

92. Farber E (1973) Cancer Res 33: 2537-2550

93. Cairns J (1975) Nature (Lond) 255: 197-200

94. Nowell PC (1976) Science (Wash.), 1984: 23-28

95. Farber E (1973) In: Current Research in Oncology 1972, Anfinsen CB, Potter M and Schecter AN (eds), Academic Press, New York, pp 95-123

96. Ho RK, Mishkin S, Farber E (1982) Proc Am Assoc Cancer Res 23: 52

97. Farber E (1976) Cancer Res 36: 2703-2705

98. Solt DB, Cayama E, Sarma DSR et al. (1980) Cancer Res 40: 1112-1118

99. Slaga TJ (ed) (1984) Mechanisms of Tumor Promotion, Vol II. Tumor Promotion and Skin Carcinogenesis, CRC Press, Boca Raton

100. Holtzer H, Dienstman S, Holtzer S et al. (1974) In: Differentiation and Control of Malignacy of Tumor Cells, Nakahara W, Ono T, Sugimura T, Sugano H (eds), University Park Press, Baltimore, pp 389-400

101. Sporn MB, Roberts AB (1985) Nature (Lond.) 313: 745

102. Heldin CE, Westermark B (1984) Cell 37: 9-20

103. Cohen SM, Murasaki G, Ellwein LB et al. (1983) In: Mechanism of Tumor Promotion, Vol. I. Tumor Promotion in Internal Organs, Slaga TJ (ed), CRC Press, Boca Ranton, pp 131-149

104. Morson BC (ed) (1978) The Pathogenesis of Colorectal Cancer, WB Saunders Co, Philadelphia

105. Maskens AP (1983) In: Precancerous Lesions of the Gastro -intestinal Tract, Sherlock P, Morson BC, Barbara L and Veronesi V (eds), Raven Press, New York, pp 223-240

106. Denda A, Inui S, Sunagawa W et al. (1978) Gann 69: 633-639

107. Scarpelli DG, Rao MS (1981) Cancer (Phila.) 47: 1552-1561

108. Pour PM, Donnely T, Stepon K et al. (1983) Am J Pathol 110: 75-82

109. Roebuck, BD, Longnecker DS, Yager JD (1983) In: Mechanisms of Tumor Promotion, Vol. I: Tumor Promotion in Internal Organs, Slaga TJ (ed), CRC Press, Boca Raton, pp 151-171

110. Russo J, Tait L, Russo IH (1983) Am J Pathol 113: 50-66

111. Steele VE, Nettesheim P (1983) In: Mechanism of Tumor Promotion, Vol I Tumor Promotion in Internal Organs, Slaga TJ (ed) CRC Press, Boca Raton, pp 91-105

112. Clark WH Jr, Eder DE, Guerry D et al. (1984) Human Pathol 15: 1147-1165

113. Potter VR (1984) Cancer Res 44: 2733-2736

114. London WT, Blumberg BS (1981) In: Cancer Achievements, Challenges and Prospects for the 1980s, Burcheval JH and Oettgen, HF (eds), Grune and Stratton, New York, pp 161-183

115. Popper H, Gerber MA, Thung SN (1982) Hepatology 2: 15-95

© 1987 Elsevier Science Publishers B.V. (Biomedical Division)
Concepts and theories in carcinogenesis. A.P. Maskens et al. eds.

221

MULTISTEP CARCINOGENESIS IN THE COLORECTAL MUCOSA

A.P. MASKENS

Université Catholique de Louvain, Centre de Coloproctologie, rue Boduognat 15, 1040 Brussels, Belgium

I. INTRODUCTION

During the period of time, usually long, which separates the action of a carcinogenic insult on a normal tissue from the emergence of a cancer, many events can be observed. Stepwise modifications have been noted, with the final production of fully transformed cells remaining a rare event compared with the number of cells at risk. Most pertinent questions therefore are: (1) how many essential steps can we identify during carcinogenesis, and (2) what are their biological properties? This paper will review data obtained in the rat colon carcinogenesis model, an experimental system characterized by some unique features which make it a particulary valuable tool in the study of carcinogenesis in general (1-3). The meaning of these observations will then be discussed against other models as well as human data. It will be shown that the concepts of <u>initiation</u>, <u>completion</u> (which is being introduced here), and <u>modulation</u> constitute strong bases upon which to build our understanding of carcinogenesis.

II. SOME DEFINITIONS

What is meant by "essential steps"?

We will, in this paper, restrict the use of "step" to situations where a) the modification is unequivocal, i.e. involving an all or nothing type qualitative change; b) the modification has a relatively low probability of occurring (4). Such a definition indeed distinguishes key changes (or rate limiting changes) from other ones in chain processes.

On the other hand, events observed during carcinogenesis can fall into 3 main categories : essential, determining, or incidental (Table 1). Essential events are those which are necessary for the process to succeed. Carcinogenesis cannot occur in their absence. On the other hand, one can think of other

TABLE 1

TYPES OF EVENTS OBSERVED DURING CARCINOGENESIS

----

1. ESSENTIAL EVENTS

2. DETERMINING EVENTS

3. INCIDENTAL EVENTS

----

events which are not essential, but the presence of which can
greatly modify the rate of occurrence of the essential steps.
Finally, some facts observed during carcinogenesis can be just
incidental, i.e. entirely unrelated to the process while
coinciding with it in time. These distinctions can be illustrated
in another highly hazardous process, namely lottery winning. In
such a process, one essential step is obviously the buying of
tickets. The quality of the person selling the tickets, although
not at all _essential_ to the process, can nevertheless represent a
determining factor (fig. 1).

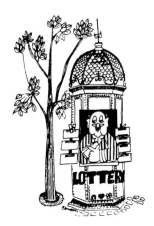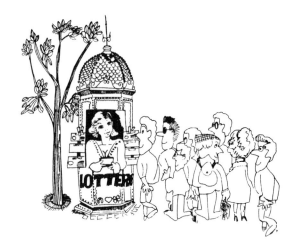

Fig. 1. In the process of winning on the lottery, the first
essential step is buying a ticket. The quality of the person
selling the ticket, while not essential, can nevertheless be a
determining factor and greatly modulate the possibility of
occurrence of the first essential step.

Obviously, if we are to understand the mechanisms of carcinogenesis, we have to try to establish the number and nature of its essential steps. However, equally important in terms of preventive action can be the search for determining factors or changes - even if not essential.

III. THE MATHEMATICAL CONSEQUENCES OF THE "MULTISTEP" CONCEPT

One advantage of restricting the analysis of carcinogenesis at the essential step level as defined above, is that, within a stable experimental system, much can be learned about these steps from the observation of their visible consequences, i.e. the timing and magnitude of cancer occurrence. Experimental cancer models can indeed be viewed as closed cell systems in which there are several compartments defined by the degree of neoplastic transformation. At one extreme are the normal cells, which in ideal models should be amenable to quantitative estimates. At the other extreme is the fully transformed cancer cell, the number of which corresponds to the number of observed tumors (assuming a clonal origin of tumors (5)). The number of intermediate stages is unknown, but will be directly connected with the relation observed between time and tumor incidence, as clearly shown by Armitage and Doll (6) and by Peto (4), amongst others.

Let "N" be the number of normal cells at risk for cancer transformation, N1, N2 ..., the number of cells in the 1st, 2nd..., stages of malignant change, Nc the number of cells having undergone the final change towards cancer phenotype, "n" the number of stages, R1, R2..., Rn the respective rates at which cells will undergo the next change, "t" the time from first carcinogen treatment, and let us assume that the order in which the changes must occur is fixed:

$$N \xrightarrow{R1} N1 \xrightarrow{R2} N2 \xrightarrow{R3} \dots \xrightarrow{Rn} Nc$$

then it can be shown that:

$$Nc = (1/n!) \, N \, R1 \, R2 \, \dots \, Rn \, t^n \qquad (1)$$

Thus, if R1, R2, ..., Rn are constant throughout the experiment, the relation $Nc = kt^n$ must be verified.

What we actually observe in clinical or experimental conditions is not Nc but the number of visible tumors, so that the relation becomes:

$$P = K (t-w)^n \qquad (2)$$

where 'P' is tumor prevalence at time 't', and 'w' is the time needed for a cancer cell to become a visible nodule. If only a fraction of fully transformed cells eventually give rise to tumors, due, for instance, to elimination of some of them by immune or other mechanisms, the value of 'k' will accordingly be affected, without however modifying the applicability of the relation defined in equation (2).

In the specific situation where exposure to the initial carcinogenic stimulus (responsible for the first change from 'N' to 'N1') is not constant but limited in time, then N1 becomes constant and a function of the dose of carcinogen, and the relation between prevalence, time, and number of stages becomes:

$$P = k' (t-w)^{n-1} \qquad (3)$$

The derivatives of formulas (1), (2) and (3) give the corresponding tumor incidence per time unit.

Thus, in situations of two-step carcinogenesis initiated by a short-term exposure to a carcinogen, the number of observed cancers will increase linearly with time, with the incidence rate remaining constant, proportional to the dose of carcinogen (see illustration in fig. 2)

IV. AN EXPERIMENTAL MODEL

1. The animal

The model consists of one animal, the BD IX rat, and one chemical carcinogen, symmetrical 1,2 dimethylhydrazine.

It was on the BD IX rat that the first dimethylhydrazine (DMH) carcinogenesis experiments were performed by Druckrey in

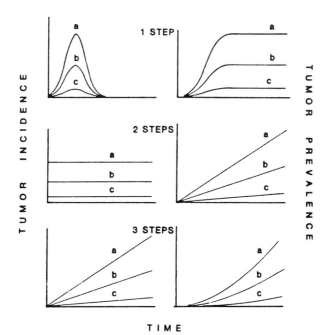

Fig. 2. Examples of the shape of tumor prevalence (right) and incidence (left) curves according to time, in a theoretical system where the test animals were given one injection of a carcinogen in a dosage varying from 1 (c) to 4 (b) to 8 (a). Upper figure shows the curves obtained for a one-step model, middle figure shows the curves in a two-step model, and lower figure in a three-step model.

1967 (7). Druckrey soon reported a high tumor yield and a high specificity for the colon when administering DMH to this breed (8). Tumors were reported to arise in sufficient numbers before killing the animal, thus allowing adequate quantitative analyses to be performed. In addition to being highly susceptible, the BD IX strain is characterized by an excellent genetic homogeneity. Further experiments with this compound revealed that the tumors produced were also quite homogeneous, with a vast majority being adenocarcinomas. These features make the DMH/BD IX model a unique system, as they have allowed, for perhaps one of the first times in carcinogenesis research, accurate quantitative studies in carcinoma production to be performed.

The basic histological architecture of the intestinal wall of BD IX rats is comparable to that reported for other rodent species. The mucosa is essentially composed of a regular succession of cylindrical glands perpendicular to the intestinal lumen, the "crypts of Lieberkuhn". These glands are lined by a simple columnar epithelium. In adult male BD IX rats, the number of crypts present in the colorectal mucosa amounts to about 5.9 x 10^5. The total number of epithelial cells is close to 375 millions (3).

2. The carcinogen

Dimethylhydrazine belongs to a well studied class of carcinogens. It has been shown to acquire powerful alkylating properties after metabolic activation (9-13), and to exert mutagenic effects. Alkylation affects electronegative centers from cell constituents including DNA, RNA, proteins. Most affected in rats are cells from the liver and from the intestinal epithelium (9). In their nucleic acids, formation of 7-methylguanine, O^6-methylguanine, and methylated adenine substitutes have been described (9,11,12,14,15). Other severe DNA alterations, as evidenced using ultracentrifugation techniques, are also widely present (16).

While DMH was not detected as a mutagen in previous studies using the Salmonella/microsome test (17), it was clearly mutagenic in the host mediated assay (18). More recently, DMH was shown to be mutagenic in vitro when incubated in the presence of several bile acids (19,20), or epithelial cells (21).

3. The encounter

Obviously, the events that will immediately follow the contact between the active metabolite of DMH, and the colon epithelium, are of major importance in the carcinogenic process. After earlier reports had indicated that they were characterized by histological evidence of nucleotoxicity (22-26), we have attempted to document the quantitative aspects of these acute effects by simply scoring the karyorrhectic figures (karyorrhectic index, KI) at several intervals after one injection of the carcinogen (27). In the intestines, a severe karyorrhectic reaction was observed, with a maximum at 6 h. The highest KI values were observed in the mucosal glands of the duodenum, ileum, and transverse colon with 16.7 to 28.6% of the nuclei being destroyed. The mean KI for the entire colon and rectum was 12.2%. By 24 h., most fragmented muclei had been eliminated.

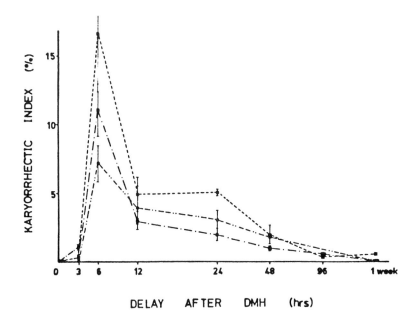

Fig. 3. Variation of the karyorrhectic index at various intervals after a single injection of DMH in 3 segments of the large intestine: □ , transverse colon; ■, caecum; ●, rectum. Vertical bars indicate standard errors (6 rats for each point).

The variation of the KI values in three segments of the large intestine is illustrated in Fig. 3. In villi of the small intestine, where no mitotic activity was observed in the controls, the KI remained very low (max. 0.43%), especially when compared with the crypt values. In the stomach, characterized by a moderate proliferative activity, karyorrhectic nuclei were rare findings (maximum 0.06%). In the kidney and liver, where mitoses are much less frequent, the karyorrhectic indices, although extremely low (maximum of 0.12% and 0.10% respectively), were slightly higher than in the stomach.

Thus, the KI probably reflects the occurrence of both DNA alkylation and cell proliferation. Indeed, although a high degree of DNA alkylation is induced by DMH in the liver as well as in the intestines (see discussion above), almost no karyorrhectic figures were found in the liver or in the non-proliferative compartment of the intestines. This would indicate that, in organs with a high degree of DNA alkylation, karyorrhexis is probably a direct consequence of proliferative activity.

Secondly, this nucleotoxic reaction, although well correlated with carcinogenicity (as will be shown in the following paragraphs), probably represents for the main part a highly unspecific effect, having no consequences on further tumor development. Indeed, one single s.c. injection of 20mg DMH-HCl/kg in an adult rat represents about 2.7×10^{19} alkylating molecules: it will result in about 45 million karyorrhectic figures and many more DNA alterations in the colorectal epithelium (12.2% of 375 million cells); and yet, only a few tumors will eventually develop. It is therefore probably impossible to observe and characterize those relatively few cells which have undergone a specific change that will ultimately lead to cancer growth. Their behavior can however be postulated from observations on the subsequent behavior of the tumors themselves.

4. The latency period

When BD IX rats are given weekly s.c. injections of DMH, intestinal nodules will develop in all instances, after however an average latency period inversely related to the total amount of the carcinogen administered. This latency before the appearance of naked-eye visible tumors is about 40 weeks after one single injection, and 18 weeks after 16 or more doses (2). Part of this period is occupied by a phase of microscopic growth of carcinomatous foci, which however remain rare findings among normal-looking or hyperplastic mucosa (1).

5. Tumor production

The tumors arise predominantly in the large intestine, with a majority along the flexura major, between the ascending and descending segments (1,28). This, interestingly, is also the site of highest KI immediately following an injection of DMH. Tumor sizes vary from a few mm^3 to several cm^3 (up to 35); multiple tumors are frequently observed (up to 20 per large intestine).

In the framework of various experiments (28,29), we have analyzed a total of 864 naked-eye visible neoplasms of the large bowel. Of these, 843 were suitable for histological analysis. The findings are summarized in Table 2.

TABLE 2

HISTOLOGICAL ANALYSIS OF MACROSCOPIC TUMORS OBSERVED IN THE LARGE INTESTINE OF DMH-TREATED BD IX RATS

Histology	Number		Proportion (%)	
Glandular neoplasms	800		94.9	
invasive		747		88.6
non-invasive		53		6.3
Signet ring cell carcinomas	30		3.6	
Undifferentiated carcinoma	1		0.1	
Non-neoplastic polyps	12		1.4	
Total	843		100.0	

Two major conclusions can be drawn here. The first is that the rat DMH model yields a rather uniform type of lesion, i.e. adenocarcinomas. They represent 88.6% of the 843 tumors of the large intestine analyzed in the present work. This finding, together with the large number of carcinomas produced in each animal, indicates how interesting this model can be in carcinogenesis studies. The second relates to one of the major questions presently being asked in the field of histogenesis of colorectal cancer: do carcinomas obligatorily arise in pre-existing benign adenomas? Our histological observations represent strong evidence against this mandatory filiation. As many as 92.5% of all glandular tumors were invasive carcinomas. Even the smallest tumors already showed invasive properties (90% of tumors <3mm). Microscopic invasive carcinomas were regularly found in flat mucosa (Fig. 4). Finally, benign polyps actually developed later than did carcinomas (28).

6. Kinetic analysis of tumor production

What are the quantitative observations during carcinogenesis in this model? In a careful experiment, in which rats were submitted to 4 different levels of DMH exposure (1, 4, 8, or 16 weekly injections of DMH-HCl, 20 mg/Kg s.c.), several points could be established (2) (Fig. 5).

a) While none of the controls developed colon carcinomas, DMH exposure resulted in tumor production in all 4 experimental groups, even those receiving one single injection of the carcinogen.

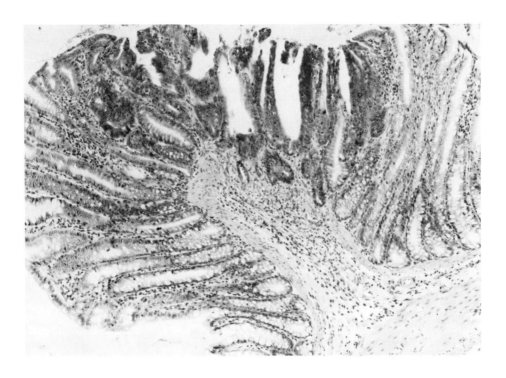

Fig. 4. Histological preparation of a microscopic adenocarcinoma at the tip of a mucosal fold in the colon of a DMH-treated BD IX rat. The carcinoma comprises only a few carcinomatous crypts. Invasion of the muscularis mucosae is present.

b) In all 4 groups, the number of carcinomas continued to increase in a constant way, even after a delay of more than one year. Thus, new tumors constantly arose in the mucosa, long after cessation of the biochemical interference between the carcinogen and the mucosa, and long after the time needed for tumors to grow from one cell to a visible nodule.

c) Tumor incidence in the 4 groups was dose-related. In animals given a short exposure to DMH (1 to 8 weeks), the number of adenocarcinomas per animal increased linearly with time, at a rate proportional to the total dose of DMH. Tumor incidence was about 1.4×10^8 per cell at risk per dose of DMH per year. In animals given a prolonged exposure to DMH (16 weeks), the number of colorectal carcinomas per rat increased as a function of the

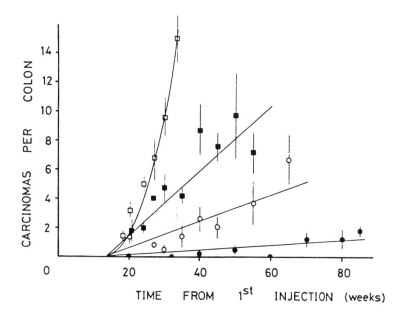

Fig. 5. Mean number (± S.E.) of macroscopically visible adenocarcinomas observed in the large intestine of rats sacrificed per groups of 3 to 6 at various intervals after 1 (●: group I), 4 (○: group II), 8 (■: group III), or 16 (□: group IV) weekly injections of DMH. The lines represent the best-fitting regression curves of tumor prevalence versus $(t-w)^1$ for the three first groups, and versus $(t-w)^2$ for the 4th group, where 't' is the time from 1st injection, and 'w' the average time needed for tumors to grow from a volume of 1 cell to a visible nodule (93 days) (From ref. 2)..

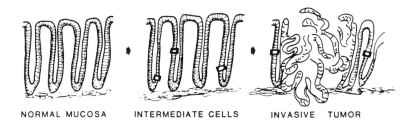

NORMAL MUCOSA   INTERMEDIATE CELLS   INVASIVE TUMOR

Fig. 6. The two essential steps in experimental colon carcinogenesis. DMH induces a first specific change in a fraction of the epithelial cells ("intermediate cells"). These cells have no phenotypic expression in terms of proliferative advantage, but are at risk for a second transformation capable of initiating tumor growth.

2nd power of time. Tumor incidence rose to more than one per large intestine per week.

d) Such incidence data do in fact correspond to a process in which only two essential steps are present (cfr. fig. 2 and refs. 2,3). The first such step in these experiments is clearly constituted by the specific carcinogenic insult caused by DMH in a fraction of the epithelial cells. The final step will obviously be the one which initiates a process of continuous clonal growth in a few of the DMH-affected enterocytes, resulting in the emergence of a visible tumor (Fig.6).

V. INITIATION AND COMPLETION : TWO ESSENTIAL EVENTS IN CARCINOGENESIS

These two essential events observed during colon carcinogenesis are of a rather general nature. Although several additional intermediate steps have been postulated in many other situations, the process always begins with the interference between an "initiator" and normal cells. It has always to be completed by at least one additional event which makes it possible for one of the "initiated" cells to express its potential for uncontrolled, invasive growth. The first step in carcinogenesis is called "initiation". We suggest the last specific step, as defined here, be called "completion". What are their properties in the experimental colon model?

It is a general observation in chemical carcinogenesis that in some of the target cells, the initiator induces dose-dependent specific changes which are irreversible, and transmissible upon cell renewal. These changes however are not sufficient to allow the expression of the cancer properties. The same situation applies in DMH-induced colon carcinogenesis.

On the other hand, the properties of the "completion" step in carcinogenesis are generally poorly documented. In the rat colon model, however, they can be easily illustrated :

- it does not require the presence of the carcinogen,

- it can only operate on initiated cells (no cancers in controls),

- it is a rare event (one tumor per dose of DMH per colon per year) randomly affecting some of the initiated cells,

- its rate is rather constant, for a given dose of the carcinogen,
- the resulting cell change is transmitted upon cell renewal.

Such a two-step mechanism, with one step being caused by an external agent and one resulting from an intrinsic property of the system, is reminiscent of the process of winning on the lottery. One first has to buy tickets (initiation). This is a highly determined, dose (money)-dependent step. But bought tickets have no different values from the others. Then comes the draw, which is a random process. Unsold tickets, if drawn, will not be affected. Only those tickets which have been bought ("initiated") will become winners ("completion") if drawn.

VI. POSSIBLE BIOLOGICAL BASES FOR THE LOTTERY SEQUENCE

The observed properties of initiation and completion in the DMH-colon model do in fact considerably narrow the speculative possibilities about the nature of each of the two steps. Since the first change is stable and transmissible in the renewing mucosa, without however being expressed, and since DMH has alkylating and mutagenic properties well correlated with its carcinogenic effect (3,9,14,18), the most logical assumption is that initiation here is represented by a somatic mutation. As for the second, carcinogen-independent step, it is known that mitotic errors occur in all renewing tissues at a given, tissue-specific, average rate. They represent rare events randomly affecting proliferating cells. Some such errors can lead to the expression of recessive mutations (e.g. somatic recombination of homozygous genes), (see Harnden, this volume). They will have no consequence in the normal cells, while causing the expression of the recessive mutation in initiated cells. Thus, the couple carcinogen induced mutation/mitotic error is one possible candidate to fit the observed lottery type characteristics of initiation/completion in experimental colon carcinogenesis.

Two step carcinogenesis based on the expression of a recessive mutation has also been postulated in a variety of hereditary cancers, in which the recessive mutation is being inherited (30). This implies that presence of one normal allele is sufficient to protect against the occurrence of a given cancer

- hence its proposed name of "antioncogene" (31).

VII. MODULATION

The present approach to the two-stage essence of carcinogenesis differs from the classical "initiation-promotion" experiments. The major significance of the latter type of observation is that carcinogenesis occurs as a multi-step process, in which the first step is possibly mutational and the other, or one (or several) of the others, can be promoted by a variety of agents which are not carcinogenic per se. This however is often presented as if promotion in itself constituted the essence of the second (or ulterior) step(s) (see ref. 32 for a review on tumor promotion). In our opinion, "promotability" might just be one of the characteristics of some of the steps involved in carcinogenesis, and therefore any analysis aimed at decoding the essential steps in cancer transformation ought to be carried out in the absence of added promoting factors, as we did in the present study.

In fact, having defined the two necessary and sufficient steps involved in experimental colon carcinogenesis, several ways in which promotion could act can be immediately envisaged. Any factor multiplying the number of intermediate cells will increase the risk of cancer. Activators of carcinogen metabolism, presence of an increased proliferative status at the time of carcinogen treatment, as well as hyperplasia and benign tumor formation, will be some of these factors. Any agent increasing the mitotic activity will on the other hand also increase the probability that a mitotic error affects one of the intermediate cells. It has been shown that colorectal tumorigenesis can indeed be enhanced by such promoters of epithelial proliferation as bile acids (33-36), non-specific injury (32), or transmissible murine colonic hyperplasia (38).

In the same way as they can be promoted, the rate of the essential steps in carcinogenesis can be negatively affected by various factors, and research in this field is of high priority in terms of cancer prevention. For instance, the anti-initiating activity of N-acetylcysteine in experimental colon cancer has been recently demonstrated (39).

Thus the concept of a process in which each of the two essential steps (INITIATION /COMPLETION) can be either promoted or inhibited (i.e. "MODULATED" - see the paper of Roberfroid in this volume) is in good accordance with the observed experimental data, and a valuable tool for the design and understanding of possible preventive strategies.

VIII. HUMAN COLON CANCER

It would be extremely difficult to determine exactly how many essential steps are involved in human colon carcinogenesis. Indeed, human beings are submitted to a variety of carcinogenic as well as modulating factors during their entire lifetime.

We would only like here to draw the attention upon two points of major importance.

Based on epidemiologic observations that prevalence of human colorectal cancer varies with the 5.0^{th} to the 6.3^{th} power of age (6,40-42), it has been concluded by some authors that this indeed represents the number of steps that separate a normal enterocyte from a carcinomatous cell (6,40,42). This however does not take into account the fact that the above-described mathematical relationships between tumor incidence and number of steps hold only if the transformation rates from one stage to the next one remain constant over the observation period, i.e. in this instance over the entire lifespan of individuals. This is certainly not the case, as changes in exposure to carcinogens (4), in metabolism or susceptibility to the carcinogen (43,44), in hormonal or physiological status of the host, proliferative status of the affected tissues (45,46), DNA repair mechanisms, immune mechanisms and probably other factors, are all likely to occur. In fact, on pure mathematical grounds, a two-step mechanism in which both steps are submitted to modulatory factors which vary with age will show age/incidence relationships of the type observed in epidemiological studies (47).

Human observations on the other hand confirm the importance of cell proliferation as well as the capacity of clonal expansion, as strong promoters of carcinogenesis. While cancer risk is minimal in normal crypts, conditions characterized by increased proliferation (e.g. dysplasia) represent a much higher risk. When clonal expansion is present (adenomas, villous tumors), the risk is even higher.

In other words, colon adenomas, while not mandatory steps in the carcinogenesis process (28,48), can however by nature greatly promote its essential steps. They therefore fit into the category of "determining factors".

A consequence in terms of preventive research is that the value of proliferative parameters in the colonic mucosa as potential markers of modulatory activity deserves to be further investigated, and that the search for agents capable of reducing abnormal proliferative conditions should be actively pursued (49).

IX. OTHER MODELS

If one compares experimental colon carcinogenesis with the skin and liver models (32,50-58) it soon appears that the first step is quite comparable in all three instances. In each case indeed,

1. the process of malignant transformation is initiated by the application of a chemical which, after metabolic activation, is capable of reacting with nuclear DNA;

2. cell proliferation is present or has to be induced at the time of carcinogen application;

3. one single application of the carcinogen is sufficient to induce tumors;

4. a "memory effect" is present, i.e. the changes induced by the carcinogen are retained in the tissue for prolonged periods, even if apparently unexpressed.

The main differences between the colon and the other two systems are to be found in the steps of carcinogenesis which follow initiation. In skin and liver indeed, numerous benign neoplasms are usually induced before appearance of invasive cancers, a finding not observed in the rat colon. This dissimilarity can be interpreted in two different ways. One possibility is that, due to tissue peculiarities, the intermediary benign growths are mandatory and specific steps towards cancer in skin and liver, but not in colon. Another interpretation is that these benign neoplasms, while not specific nor mandatory, do in fact greatly enhance the probability that one induced cell will undergo the final cancer change. Although complete discussion of this point is beyond the scope of the present work, it should be stressed here that one of the major characteristics of the benign neoplasms observed prior to cancer formation in the skin and liver models, is that their proliferative activity is increased as compared with the corresponding normal tissue. In the liver model, it has been well established that the proliferative activity of the presumptive preneoplastic lesions is a prerequisite for their further malignant transformation (50,51,59). As the colon mucosa is a tissue with a high degree of spontaneous proliferative activity, a possible explanation again is that cell proliferation in itself increases the probability of the last steps of carcinogenesis, be it natural or in the frame of a benign neoplasm.

X. CONCLUSION

In conclusion, the two essential steps observed in colon carcinogenesis , "initiation" and "completion", both amenable to modulation, constitute useful conceptual bases for our understanding of carcinogenesis in general. Amongst modulating factors, increased cell proliferation is perhaps one of the most important.

REFERENCES

1. Maskens AP (1976) Cancer Res 36:1585-1592

2. Maskens AP (1981) Cancer Res 41:1240-1245

3. Maskens AP (1982) Kinetic Analysis of Experimental Colon Carcinogenesis, Thesis, University of Louvain, School of Medicine, Brussels, 126 pages.

4. Peto R (1977) In: Origins of Human Cancer, Hiatt HH, Watson JD, Winsten JA (eds), New York, Cold Spring Harbor Publications, pp 1403-1428

5. Fialkow PJ (1979) Ann Rev Med 30:135-143

6. Armitage P, Doll R (1954) Br J Cancer 8:1-12

7. Druckrey H, Preussmann R, Matzkies F, et al. (1967) Natur-wissenschaften 54:285-286

238

8. Druckrey H (1970) In: Carcinoma of the colon and antecedent epithelium, Burdette WJ (ed), Springfield: Charles C Thomas, pp 267-279

9. Hawks A, Magee PN (1974) Br J Cancer 30:440-447

10. Hawks A, Swann PF, Magee PN (1972) Biochem Pharmacol 21:432-433

11. Likhachev AJ, Margison GP, Montesano R (1977) Chem-Biol Interact 18:235-240

12. Rogers KJ, Pegg AE (1977) Cancer Res 37:4082-4088

13. Shank RC, Magee PN (1967) Biochem J 105:521-527

14. Cooper HK, Buecheler J, Kleihues P (1978) Cancer Res 38:3063-3065

15. Swenberg JA, Cooper HK, Buecheler J, et al. (1979) Cancer Res 39:465-467

16. Kanagalingam K, Balis AE (1975) Cancer 36:2364-2372

17. Mc Cann J, Choi E, Yamasaki E, et al. (1975) Proc Natl Acad Sci US 72:5135-5139

18. Moriya M, Kato K, Watanabe K, et al. (1978) JNCI 61:457-460

19. Wilpart M, Mainguet P, Maskens A, et al. (1983) Carcinogenesis 4:45-48

20. Wilpart M, Mainguet P, Maskens A, et al. (1983) Carcinogenesis 4:1239-1241

21. Oravec CT, Jones CA, Huberman E (1986) Cancer Res 46:5068-5071

22. Deschner EE (1978) Z Krebsforsch 91:205-216

23. Hawks A, Hicks R, Holsman J, et al. (1974) Br J Cancer 30:429-439

24. Löhrs U, Wiebecke B, Eder M (1969) Z Ges Exp Med 151:297-307

25. Zedeck MS, Sternberg SS, Poynter RW, et al. (1970) Cancer Res 30:801-812

26. Zedeck Ms, Grab DJ, Sternberg SS (1977) Cancer Res 37:32-36

27. Maskens AP (1979) Cancer Lett 8:77-86

28. Maskens AP, Dujardin-Loits RM (1981) Cancer 47:81-89

29. Maskens AP (1978) In: Gastrointestinal Tract Cancer, Lipkin M, Good R (eds), New York, Plenum Press, pp 361-384

30. Knudson AG (1985) Cancer Res 45:1437-1443

31. Knudson AG (1983) Prog Nucleic Acid Res Mol Biol 29:17-25

32. Slaga TJ, Sivak A, Boutwell RK (Eds) (1978) Carcinogenesis, vol.2, Mechanisms of Tumor Promotion and Cocarcinogenesis, New York, Raven Press

33. Cohen BI, Raicht RF, Deschner EE, et al. (1980) JNCI 64:573-578

34. Deschner EE, Raicht RF (1979) Digestion 19:322-327

35. Reddy BS, Narisawa T, Weisburger JH, et al. (1976) JNCI 56:441-442

36.   Reddy BS, Watanabe K (1979)   Cancer Res 39:1521-1524

37.   Pozharisski KM (1975)   Cancer Res 35:3824-3830

38.   Barthold SW, Jonas AM (1977)   Cancer Res 37:4352-4360

39.   Wilpart M, Speder A, Roberfroid R (1986)   Cancer Lett 31:319-324

40.   Ashley DJB (1969)   J Med Gen 6:376-378

41.   Maskens AP, Vandenberghe A (1979)   Acta Endoscopica 9:155-160

42.   Utsunomiya J, Murata M, Tanimura M (1980)   Cancer 45:198-205

43.   Ebbesen P (1974)   Science 183:217-218

44.   Ebbesen P (1977) JNCI 58:1057-1060

45.   Lesher S, Sacher GA (1968)   Exp Geront 3:211-216

46.   Thrasher JD (1967)   Anat Rec 157:621-628

47.   Maskens AP (1982) In: Malt R, Williamson RCN (eds) Falk Symposium 31: Colonic Carcinogenesis, Lancaster: MTP Press, pp 211-219

48.   Maskens A (1982)   Acta Gastroent Belgica 45:158-164

49.   Buset M, Lipkin M, Winawer S, et al. (1986)   Cancer Res 46:5426-5430

50.   Barbason H, Betz EH (1981)   Brit J Cancer 44:561-566

51.   Barbason H, Smoliar V, Fridman-Manduzio A, et al. (1979)   Br J Cancer 40:260-267

52.   Berenblum I (1941)   Cancer Res 1:807-814

53.   Berenblum I, Shubick P (1949)   Br J Cancer 3:109-118

54.   Columbano A, Rajalakahmi S, Sarma DSR (1980)   Chem-Biol Interact 32:347-351

55.   Emmelot P, Scherer E (1980)   Bioch Biophys Acta 605:247-304

56.   Mottram JCA (1944)   J Pathol Bacteriol 6:439-484

57.   Peraino C, Fry RJM, Staffeldt E, et al. (1973)   Cancer Res 33:2701-2705

58.   Pitot HC (1977)   Am J Path 89:401-412

59.   Rabes H, Hartenstein R (1970)   Experientia 26:1356-1359

INTERNAL AND EXTERNAL ENVIRONMENT

© 1987 Elsevier Science Publishers B.V. (Biomedical Divison)
Concepts and theories in carcinogenesis. A.P. Maskens et al. eds.

REPRODUCTION, SEX STEROID HORMONES AND CANCER

J.D. POTTER

Senior Research Scientist, CSIRO Division of Human Nutrition, Kintore Avenue, Adelaide, South Australia 5000, Australia.

INTRODUCTION

There is evidence of a relationship between aspects of reproduction and steroid hormone metabolism and risk of cancer. This is true not only of breast and reproductive sites (particularly in women) but also of other less immediately obvious cancers. The evidence has resulted from a variety of study types - descriptive and analytic epidemiology, clinical studies, receptor and cell studies, and studies on animals.

This paper is built around an epidemiologic framework and will examine the risk of cancer in relation to four topics:

1) sex differences in cancer;

2) reproductive factors (including use of oral contraception);

3) receptors;

4) urinary and plasma sex steroids.

Rather than discuss each cancer site separately under these headings, I will attempt to identify both the hormonal influences held in common between sites and differences in order to elucidate possible common aetiology and, therefore, prospects for prevention.

SEX DIFFERENCES

Most neoplasms in humans have a male excess (1). Table 1 shows the male: female sex ratio for the common shared-site cancers. The male excess for four sites (lung, oesophagus, larynx and bladder) is consistent with the increased consumption of tobacco amongst men compared with women. Differences in alcohol consumption may also be relevant. Indeed, the commonest explanation for the general male excess is that males experience higher exposure to the relevant aetiologic agents. Lung cancer is typical with both smoking and occupational exposures being higher in males. Such differences in exposures are central to public health considerations but do not directly shed light on the biology of cancer. Cancers of interest in

TABLE 1

RATIO OF MALE:FEMALE AGE-STANDARDIZED INCIDENCE RATES OF VARIOUS CANCERS, SOUTH AUSTRALIA 1983.

CANCER	MALE/FEMALE RATIO
Oesophagus	2.5
Stomach	3.3
Colon	1.4
Rectum	1.8
Larynx	6.4
Lung	5.0
Malignant melanoma	0.8
Bladder	3.7
Brain	1.7*
Thyroid	0.4
All lymphomas	1.4
All leukaemias	2.1

* M:F ratio for meningioma approx. 0.7

this latter regard are typified by breast cancer where the relevant sex differences in risk appear to be related wholly to biology and more specifically to sex hormone differences - this cancer being uncommon not only in men but also in women with ovarian dysgenesis and other causes of sexual immaturity.

The other exceptions to the general pattern are thyroid cancer, malignant melanoma, cancer of the gallbladder and bile ducts, and meningioma, all of which occur more commonly in women (of these, only malignant melanoma has an obvious possible environmental exposure difference between men and women).

In general, the sex difference in the incidence of tumours other than breast cancer is likely to be explained by a mix of differences in exposure and differences in biology including differences in susceptibility.

Intriguingly, one common cancer with a sex ratio close to 1.0 - colon cancer - exhibits biologic differences between the sexes

(2,3); the sex ratio varies systematically with age - a female excess at premenopausal ages and a male excess thereafter (see Table 2). It has also been shown that there are differences in the relationship between dietary intake and age, sex, and colonic cancer subsite in ways consistent with differences in susceptibility between the sexes; whereas women have a higher rate of proximal colon cancer at all ages, men show a higher rate distally at older ages. The relative risk associated with higher consumption levels of fat, protein, and total calories is higher for proximal colon cancer in women but distal colon cancer for men; for younger ages in women but older ages in men (4).

TABLE 2

COLON CANCER: AGE-SPECIFIC INCIDENCE RATES BY SEX AND AGE-SPECIFIC SEX RATIOS, SOUTH AUSTRALIA 1977-81

SEX	AGE (yr)				
	25-34	34-44	45-54	55-64	65-74
MALE	16.5	89.0	300.0	682.0	1563.5
FEMALE	22.5	101.5	295.5	597.5	1234.0
MALE-TO-FEMALE RATIO	0.73	0.88	1.02	1.14	1.27

As yet no clear explanation for the significant male excess in stomach cancer has emerged but one animal experiment has demonstrated that sex steroids have a potent influence on carcinogenesis at this site (5).

Research to identify differences in exposure and biologic response will provide data useful for public health, for understanding aetiology, and for screening in high risk groups.

REPRODUCTION AND ORAL CONTRACEPTION

Major interest in the relationship between reproductive hormones and cancer has centred on the cancers obviously related to these factors - genital and breast cancers in women. More recently, attention has focussed on other sites in women, particularly colon, and some questions have been asked in relation to thyroid cancer, meningioma and malignant melanoma.

For breast, ovarian, endometrial, and colon cancer, there is a very consistent relationship between reproduction, exogenous hormone use and risk (see Table 3)

TABLE 3

REPRODUCTION, HORMONES AND CANCER RISK

	BREAST CANCER	OVARIAN CANCER	ENDOMETRIAL CANCER	COLON CANCER
Early menarche	+	0	+?	0?
Late menopause	+	+	+	0?
Nulliparity	+	+	+	+
Increasing parity	-	-	-	-
Late age at first live birth	+	+?	?	+
Oophorectomy	-	-*	?	?
O/C Use	0#	-	-**	-
Obesity	+	?	+	+
Postmenopausal oestrogens	0	0	+	?

```
*   Effect greater for unilateral oophorectomy than would be
    expected from the simple elimination of half the relevant tissue
#   Specific groups may have an elevated risk
**  Combined O/C; sequential O/C are associated with increased risk
+   Positive relationship with risk
-   Negative relationship
0   No relationship
?   Relationship not adequately described
Sources: refs 6-11
```

The relationship between reproductive status and other cancers is less clear (12-15) but appears at least to have prognostic significance (e.g. for malignant melanoma) (16). Meningioma, which shows a female excess, has been noted to occur more frequently in women with a previous breast cancer (and vice versa) (17) and, in one population study (15), but not another (18), brain tumours were shown to be inversely related to parity . Risks of some gastrointestinal tract cancers are positively related to increasing parity (15,18).

The significance of these reproductive findings for cancer prevention is not clear; it has encouraged some to consider seriously prospects for chemoprevention, at least in high risk groups. In relation to our understanding of carcinogenesis, the similarity between the pattern for colon cancer and that for female reproductive and breast cancers provokes questions regarding shared metabolic aetiology and challenges our current view of the causes of these apparently unrelated cancers. Previously the focus in relation to colon cancer has been on dietary factors and that for breast cancer has been on hormonal influences. There is now a sufficient body of evidence to argue for an integration of the environmental and the metabolic (4,19,20). There are further intriguing features, however in the relationship between reproductive history and both breast and colon cancer. There is evidence that some of the risk factors for breast cancer have a reversed relationship to risk at young vs old age. It has been shown that both single marital status and nulliparity - risk factors for breast cancer at older ages - are associated with reduced risks of the disease under age 40 years

TABLE 4

AGE-RELATED REVERSALS OF ASSOCIATIONS BETWEEN RISK FACTORS AND CANCERS

RISK FACTORS	ASSOCIATION WITH CANCER RISK AT YOUNG AGES	ASSOCIATION WITH CANCER RISK AT OLD AGES	REF
REPRODUCTION (BREAST CANCER)			
Married vs. Single	+	−	21
Parity	+	−	22,23
REPRODUCTION (COLON CANCER)			
Parity	+?	−	24
BODY WEIGHT (BREAST CANCER)			
Mean Weight	−	+	25
Quetelet's Index	−	+	26
Body Mass Index	−	+	27

(21-23). The reduced risk associated with higher parity in colon cancer may be present only in older women (24) (see Table 4). Obesity, a risk factor for post-menopausal breast cancer is associated with a lower rate of premenopausal disease (25-27) (see Table 4). (Wang, however, has argued that these apparent reversals may be due to a cohort effect) (28).

Although high parity and early age at first birth are associated with a reduced risk of breast cancer overall, among those women who do develop cancer, these factors are associated with a significantly earlier age at presentation (29-32). A similar observation has been made in relation to colon cancer (9) (see Table 5). Although breast and colon cancers at a young age are relatively infrequent and therefore perhaps of lower public health priority than the same cancers in the middle and later years, a complete explanation of the relationship between reproductive status and carcinogenesis must take these reversals of risk factor status (if they are not artefactual) (28) into account. One plausible explanation is that although the hormonal changes associated with pregnancy induce a "maturation" of breast tissue thus reducing risk of future malignant transformation, those same hormonal changes may act as a promotional stimulus to preexisting cancer cells. The argument is less clear for colon cancer as no "maturation" effect

TABLE 5

DIFFERENCES IN AGE AT PRESENTATION BETWEEN NULLIPAROUS AND PAROUS PATIENTS WITH BREAST AND COLON CANCER

STUDY (ref)	AGE AT PRESENTATION		P
	NULLIPAROUS	PAROUS	
BREAST CANCER			
(29, 30)	58.0	55.8	<0.04
(31)	63.1	57.9	<0.001
(32)	65.9	62.1	
COLON CANCER			
(24)	68.6	61.3	<0.01

has been noted. Obesity may exert different effects on the

premenopausal hormonal environment from that found after ovarian hormone production has ceased.

RECEPTOR STUDIES

Most receptor studies have been undertaken on cancerous tissue of breast and reproductive sites. They are related to the endocrine responsivity of tumours (33) although not consistently. Their relationship to prognosis is complex. Oestrogen receptor positivity is associated with longer survival (34) but the association with a longer interval to first recurrence is a matter of dispute (35).

Their aetiologic significance is less clear for two reasons. Firstly, the natural distribution and even function of receptors in normal tissue in the normal population has not yet been defined. Receptors are reported in a variety of normal animal (36, 37) and human (38-40) tissues but at least one human study has found no receptor in normal breast tissue (41). Secondly, until recently, little attention has been paid in aetiologic studies to the

TABLE 6

RELATIONSHIP BETWEEN OESTROGEN RECEPTOR (ER) POSITIVITY OF TUMOURS AND KNOWN RISK FACTORS BREAST CANCER

RISK FACTOR	RELATIONSHIP BETWEEN KNOWN RISK FACTORS AND ER+ STATUS	STUDIES REPORTED	STUDIES FINDING RELATIONSHIP	REF
Nulliparity	+	4	4	42-45
Late age at first birth	+	4	4	42-45
Late menopause	+	1	1	43
Family history of breast cancer	0	1	1	46
Obesity	+	3	3	43,44,47
Benign breast disease	+	1	1	42

relationship between the known hormonal and reproductive risk factors and breast cancers of differing receptor status. Where this has been investigated some surprising findings have been reported. For instance, nulliparity is associated with increased risk of oestrogen receptor (ER) positive tumours but not ER negative tumours (42-45). The breast cancer risk factors associated only, or more strongly, with ER positive than ER negative tumours are shown in Table 6.

ER negative tumours are both commoner at younger ages (42,43,48) and are associated with a poorer survival (34). Whether this latter explains the better survival associated with nulliparity (in turn associated with ER positivity) noted above or whether both are associated with yet another prognostic factor has not been investigated. What is clear is that the artificial distinction between the role of the epidemiologist in determining aetiologic factors and the role of the clinician in regard to prognostic factors can happily be abolished when each appreciates that the time of clinical presentation is an arbitrary one not bearing significantly upon the natural history of the disease and that factors acting before this time (aetiologic), can continue to be important after (prognostic). This has recently been demonstrated to be true, for instance, for dietary fat in relation to breast cancer (49).

The function of sex steroid receptors in other tumours - colon, lung, meningioma etc. and even reproductive tumours - is less well defined still but may prove important both for therapy and the understanding of aetiology.

URINARY AND PLASMA SEX HORMONES

The majority of human studies on sex steroid concentrations in relation to risk of cancers have been undertaken in relation to breast cancer risk. Such studies include population correlation studies and analytic studies of individuals with and without cancer.

Hormone levels have been used to compare populations or sub-populations with known major differences in rates of specific cancers. A number of studies have shown that cross-sectional measures of plasma (total or bound) and urinary (total or oestriol ratio) oestrogens in populations or subgroups at varying risks correlate positively with breast cancer risk. Thus, comparison of Japanese and British women shows more oestradiol bound to sex hormone binding globulin (SHBG) in the Japanese than the British and less bound to albumin (50). International comparisons of urinary oestriol ratio (51,52) and oestriol excretion (52) relate to risk of breast cancer but differences are not explained by dietary constituents (52).

A number of cross-sectional studies of vegetarians - a low risk group for breast cancer - have shown that they are exposed to lower levels of plasma (54) and urinary (55,56) oestrogens possibly as a result of higher faecal output (56). Not all studies have found differences between vegetarians and non-vegetarians (57). Vegetarians have higher plasma SHBG than non-vegetarians (56).

Trichopoulos found no relationship between urinary oestrogens and height, weight or obesity index in a study of 200 women (58).

Nulliparous women, who are at higher risk of breast cancer have lower urinary oestriol ratios (59,60) higher plasma oestrogens, and lower SHBG levels (61) than parous women.

A family history of breast cancer is associated with increased serum (62,63) and urinary (63,64) oestrogens but not consistently (65).

There are a number of recent studies showing a relationship between oestrogen levels and risk of breast cancer itself (see for example refs. 66-69) but the results are not entirely consistent. This reflects at least in part the failure to ensure that timing (within the menstrual cycle) of specimen collection was consistent. Other methodologic problems are obvious also.

Androgens may be protective against ovarian cancer (70) but some work has suggested that, while higher progestin levels are associated with lower risk of breast cancer, the reverse is true of androgen levels (71).

At present, the above data are fairly consistent in that higher total plasma oestrogens or free oestrogens are associated with specific risk factors for breast cancer although there are different hypotheses to explain this pattern. A generally higher exposure to oestrogenic stimulation - whether via specific oestrogen fractions or free (as opposed to bound) oestrogen - is consistent with explanations offered for the association between risk of cancer and aspects of reproductive history.

CONCLUSION

The current hypothesis to explain the relationship between reproductive and hormonal factors and cancer suggests that oestrogens facilitate the proliferation of tissue, either before malignant transformation or subsequently, and that the first (and possibly each subsequent) pregnancy induces a permanent change in oestrogen profile which allows breast tissue maturation and reduces subsequent proliferative activity (72). Whether other tissues are similar is not established. Further modifications of the theory have been proposed to account for the reversals of risk between young and old and to explain the associations with colon cancer. As yet, the role of receptors in relation to reproductive risk factors and possible aetiology is unclear; the role of receptors in cancers not thought to be related to sex steroids has been little investigated either in relation to treatment or causation; and the exploration of the relationship between aetiologic and prognostic factors awaits the meeting of minds between clinicians and epidemiologists. Perhaps the most significant aspect of the relationship between hormonal factors and cancer at a variety of sites is that it provides evidence for a growing realization that cancer in humans is less the result of specific alien exposures than it is of disturbances in the balance of internal metabolic and regulatory function.

REFERENCES

1. Waterhouse J, Muir C, Shanmugaratnam K, et al (1982) Cancer incidence in Five Continents, Vol IV IARC, Lyon

2. McMichael AJ, Potter JD (1980) JNCI 65: 1201-1207

3. McMichael AJ, Potter JD (1983) Am J Epidemiol 118: 620-627

4. McMichael AJ, Potter JD (1985) NCI Monogr 69: 223-228

5. Furukawa H, Iwanaga T, Koyama H, et al (1982) Cancer Res 42: 5181-5182

6. Armstrong B (1982) In: Host Factors in Human Carcinogenesis. Bartsch H, Armstrong B (eds), IARC, Lyon, pp 193-221

7. Kelsey JL, Hildreth NG (1983) Breast and Gynecologic Cancer Epidemiology, CRC Press, Boca Raton, pp 5-115

8. Hildreth NG, Kelsey JL, Li Volsi VA et al (1981) Am J Epidemiol 114: 398-405

9. Potter JD, McMichael AJ (1983) JNCI 71: 703-709

10. Howe GR, Craib KJB, Miller AB (1985) JNCI 74: 1155-1159

11. Nomura A, Heilbrun LK, Stemmermann GN (1985) JNCI 74: 319-323

12. McTiernan AM, Weiss NS, Daling JR (1984) Am J Epidemiol 120: 423-435

13. Green A, Bain C (1985) Med J Aust 142: 446-448

14. Holly EA, Weiss NS, Liff JM (1983) JNCI 70: 827-831

15. Plesko I, Preston-Martin S, Day NE et al. (1985) Int J Cancer 36: 529-533

16. Elwood JM, Coldman AJ (1978) Lancet 2: 1000-1001

17. Schoenberg BS, Christine BW, Whisnant JP (1975) Neurology 25: 705-712

18. Miller AB, Barclay THC, Choi NW et al. (1980) J Chron Dis 33: 595-605

19. Mc Michael AJ, Potter JD (1985) JNCI 75: 185-191

20. Mc Michael AJ, Potter JD (1986) Dietary Influences Upon Colon Cancer, Proceedings of 16th International Symposium of the Princess Takamatsu Cancer Research Fund (in press)

21. Janerich DT, Hoff MB (1982) Am J Epidemiol 116: 737-742

22. Ron E, Lubin F, Wax Y (1984) Am J Epidemiol 119: 139-140

23. Pathak DR, Speizer FE, Willett WC et al (1986) Int J Cancer 37: 21-25

24. Potter JD, McMichael AJ. Age-related variation in risk of colon cancer in women associated with reproductive events (In preparation)

25. Choi NW, Howe GR, Miller AB et al (1978) Amer J Epidemiol 107: 510-521

26. Paffenbarger RS, Kampert JB, Chang H-G (1980) Am J Epidemiol 112: 258-268

27. Helmrich SP, Shapiro S, Rosenberg L et al. (1983) Am J Epidemiol 117: 35-45

28. Wang DY, Rubens RD, Allen DS et al. (1985) Int J Cancer 36: 427-432

29. Juret P, Couette JE, Brune D et al (1974) Europ J Cancer 10:591-594

30. Juret P, Couette J-E, Brune D et al (1975) Bull Cancer 62: 165-174

31. Woods KL, Smith SR, Morrison JM (1980) Brit Med J 2: 419-421

32. Alderson M (1981) Brit Med J 283: 9-10

33. Lippman ME, Allegra JC (1978) New Engl J Med 299: 930-933

34. Howell A, Barnes DM, Harland RNL et al (1984) Lancet 1: 588-591

35. Editorial. (1984) Lancet 1: 887-888

36. Markaverich BM, Roberts RR, Alejandro MA et al (1984) Cancer Res 44: 1575-1579

37. Haslam SZ, Gale KJ, Dachtler SL (1984) Endocrinol 114: 1163-1172

38. Gay G, Jozan S, Marques B et al (1983-84) J Recept Res 3: 685-701

39. Cao Z-Y, Eppenberger U, Roos W, et al (1983) Arch Gynecol 233: 109-119

40. Kauppila A, Vierikko P, Isotalo H et al (1984) Acta Obstet Gynecol Scand Suppl 123: 45-49

41. Gomez P, Rivadeneyra J, Rabago M et al (1980) Arch Invest Med (Mex) 11: 303-313

42. Hildreth NG, Kelsey JL, Eisenfeld AJ et al (1983) JNCI 70: 1027-1031

43. Pascual MR, Lazo R, Fernandez L et al (1982) Neoplasma 29: 453-461

44. Nomura Y, Tashiro H, Hamada Y et al (1984) Breast Cancer Res Treat 4: 37-43

45. Lage A, Rodriguez M, Pascual MR et al (1983) Neoplasma 30: 475-483

46. Skinner JR, Wanebo HJ, Betsill Wl et al (1982) Ann Surg 196: 636-641

47. Donegan WL, Johnstone MF, Biedrzycki L (1983) Am J Clin Oncol 6: 19-24

48. Romic-Stojkovic R, Gamulin S (1980) Cancer Res 40: 4821-4825

49. Gregorio DI, Emrich LJ, Graham S et al (1985) JNCI 75: 37-41

50. Moore JW, Clark GMG, Takatani O et al (1983) JNCI 71: 749-754

51. MacMahon B, Anderson AP, Brown J et al (1980) Eur J Cancer 16: 1627-1632

52. Gray GE, Pike MC, Hirayama T et al (1982) Prev Med 11: 108-113

53. Trichopoulos D, Yen S, Brown J, Cole P et al (1984) Cancer 53: 187-192

54. Schultz TD, Leklem JE (1983) Nutr Cancer 4: 247-259

55. Goldin BR, Adlercreutz H, Gorbach SL et al (1982) New Engl J Med 307: 1542-1547

56. Armstrong BK, Brown JB, Clarke HT et al (1981) JNCI 67: 761-767

57. Gray GE, Williams P, Gerkins V et al (1982) Prev Med 11: 103-107

58. Trichopoulos D, Polychronopoulou A, Brown J et al (1983) Oncology 40: 227-231

59. Cole P, Brown JB, Mac Mahon B (1976) Lancet 2: 596-599

60. Trichopoulos D, Cole P, Brown JB et al (1980) JNCI 65: 43-46

61. Bernstein L, Pike MC, Ross RK et al (1985) JNCI 74: 741-745

62. Henderson BE, Gerkins V, Rosario I et al (1975) New Engl J Med 293: 790-795

63. Pike MC, Casagrande JT, Brown JB et al (1977) JNCI 59: 1351-1355

64. Trichopoulos D, Brown JB, Garas J et al (1981) JNCI 67: 603-606

65. Boffard K, Clark CMG, Irvine JBD et al (1981) Eur J Clin Oncol 17: 1071-1077

66. England PC, Skinner LG, Cottrell KM et al (1974) Br J Cancer 30: 571-576

67. Morreal CE, Dao TL, Nemoto T et al (1979) JNCI 63: 1171-1174

68. Moore JW, Clark GM, Bulbrook RD et al (1982) Int J Cancer 29: 17-21

69. MacMahon B, Cole P, Brown JB et al (1983) JNCI 70: 247-250

70. Cuzik J, Bulstrode JC, Thomas BS et al (1983) Int J Cancer 32: 723-726

71. Secreto G, Toniolo P, Berrino F et al (1984) Cancer Res 44: 5902-5905

72. Russo J, Tay LK, Russo IH (1982) Breast Canc Res Treat 2: 5-73

© 1987 Elsevier Science Publishers B.V. (Biomedical Divison)
Concepts and theories in carcinogenesis. A.P. Maskens et al. eds.

IMMUNOLOGICAL SURVEILLANCE OF TUMORS AND THE MAJOR HISTOCOMPATIBILITY COMPLEX

P.C.DOHERTY

Department of Experimental Pathology , John Curtin School of Medical Research, Canberra, ACT 2601, Australia.

IMMUNOLOGICAL SURVEILLANCE

The Burnet/Thomas (8) concept of immunological surveillance has been of undoubted value in stimulating both thinking and experiments. However a great deal of new information concerning the specificity and function of thymus derived lymphocytes (T cells) has emerged over the past 10 or 15 years, which has in turn led to a basic re-evaluation of T cell surveillance (16). Much of this is concerned with the requirement for effector T cells to focus onto self major histocompatibility complex (MHC) glycoproteins, the phenomenon known as MHC restriction (66). It is now apparent that tumor cells can escape immunological surveillance by mechanisms which involve the modulation of MHC glycoprotein expression (18). In contrast, some highly antigenic tumor cells express modified MHC molecules (38). Further confusion is added by the fact that a propensity for tumor metastasis may sometimes be correlated with presence of more MHC molecules on cell surface (29).

MHC RESTRICTION AND T CELL RECOGNITION

Immune T cells are specific for neoantigen presented in the context of one or another self MHC glycoprotein (self + x). In broad terms, the cytotoxic T lymphocytes (CTL) recognize cell-surface changes associated with the class I MHC molecules (H-2K, D, L in the mouse, HLA-A, B in man), the so-called strong transplantation antigens, while helper/delayed-type hypersensitivity (DTH) lymphocytes are targeted onto class II MHC determinants (I-A, I-E/C in mouse, HLA-D, DR in man), commonly known as the immune response (Ir) gene products (Ia molecules). In fact, the term Ir gene is equally applicable to the class I genes, as different class I and class II MHC glycoproteins are associated with varying levels of T cell responsiveness to particular non-self antigens. The term

MHC must also be regarded as historical as, if it were to be rediscovered now, we would probably describe it as a "self-surveillance complex". Monitoring the integrity of self is likely to be of more contemporary significance to mammals than is rejection of allografts, though the latter may be important for primitive life forms such as corals and sponges (23,24) and may thus be of phylogenetic interest for man.

Recent studies with T cell clones have established quite clearly that the generalization that CTL are class I MHC-restricted while helper/DTH cells are targeted onto class II molecules is far from absolute. There are now a number of examples of virus-immune, class II MHC-restricted CTL clones (28,40). Class I MHC-restricted T cells may also produce lymphokines and cytokines such as gamma interferon, interleukin 2 (Il-2) and Il-3 (31,41) . The one paradigm that does seem to hold fairly true is the correlation between the T lymphocyte Lyt (in the mouse) or OKT (in man) phenotype and MHC-restriction pattern for self-monitoring T cells (59). It is possible that the L3T4, OKT4 molecules expressed on the T cell are involved in binding to constant regions of the class II MHC glycoproteins of the target, while the same may be true of the Lyt2, OKT8 glycoproteins and the class I determinants (48). This may only be of importance if the affinity of the T cell for the target antigen is relatively low (37). The MHC molecules themselves cannot now be regarded as differential 'signalling' channels for the delivery of "kill" or "help" messages.

In fact, recent studies have made it obvious that the MHC molecules are irrelevant if effector CTL can be appropriately targeted onto cell surface. Hybrid immunoglobulin molecules made using antibodies to the T cell receptor (or the associated T3 molecule) and to almost any cell-surface glycoprotein on the target can be used to bring the two cells in sufficiently close apposition for the target to be killed (46,59). Cells expressing a monoclonal antibody specific for the clonotypic CTL receptor are lysed even if the target presenting the antibody is MHC-negative (32).

This seems to leave us with two possible reasons for the fact of MHC-restriction. One proposal is that the T cell receptor repertoire is basically specific for variants of class I or class II

MHC glycoproteins, as suggested originally by Jerne (26) and argued in our formulation of the "single T cell receptor-altered self" model (17,66). The alternative is that interaction with the MHC molecule is associated with the delivery of a 'signal' for triggering T cell precursors even though, as described above, recognition of MHC can be circumvented at the effector phase.

TUMOR CELLS MAY EXPRESS MODIFIED MHC GLYCOPROTEINS

There have been a number of reports over the past 10 years that tumor cells may express modified class I MHC molecules (reviewed in 16). Much of this information has been difficult to evaluate because of the lack of precision of serological probes, and the possibility of cell contamination. However, recent studies from the laboratories of Schreiber, Rovner and colleagues have established beyond any reasonable doubt that the tumor-specific transplantation antigens (TSTA) on a UV-induced fibrosarcoma (1591) are indeed modified MHC molecules (38,47). Apparently the 1591 fibrosarcoma expresses at least two aberrant class I MHC glycoproteins. Monoclonal antibodies raised against this tumor cross-react with MHC determinants that would normally be considered allogeneic: one of the TSTA's is apparently very similar to a naturally-occurring MHC molecule, $H-2L^d$.

Tumors bearing these variant molecules are readily rejected by syngeneic C3H ($H-2K^kD^k$) mice. However, antigen-negative variants selected in the fluorescence activated cell sorter with one of the monoclonal antibodies do not express either of the novel TSTA molecules, indicating that the expression of the two aberrant MHC glycoproteins is closely linked at the genetic level. Such variants grow progressively in mice and are no longer recognized by tumor-specific CTL in vitro.

At this stage it is not clear whether the novel MHC molecules expressed in the 1591 tumor are a direct consequence of the mutagenic effect of UV-irradiation, or if 'silent' class I MHC genes have been activated. Application of molecular biology techniques has revealed the existence of numerous, 'orphan' class I MHC genes that have not yet been assigned any biological function (34). The products of at least some of these genes are antigenic when transfected into L cells (53).

The UV-induced tumors have been known for some time to be highly antigenic (33). Changes in even a few key amino acids of an MHC molecule as occurs, for instance, in H-2-mutant mice that have been selected on the basis of reciprocal skin graft rejection, promotes very strong CTL responses. Obviously, this mechanism provides the basis for an effective form of immunological surveillance.

ESCAPING T CELL SURVEILLANCE BY MODULATING MHC GLYPROTEIN EXPRESSION

The best characterized examples of tumours escaping immunological surveillance by modulating the expression of one or another of the MHC molecules that they normally express are provided by two virus transformation systems, SV40 and adenovirus (Ad). In these situations the MHC molecules in question serve as Ir genes for the TSTA recognized by CTL.

The identity of x in the self + x equation for the SV40 transformation system is the virus-coded large T antigen (43,45,61). Mice of the H-2^d haplotype, which make little (if any) CTL response to SV40 TSTA, develop tumors following inoculation with the virus while those of the H-2^k haplotype, which respond strongly, do not (1). The Ir gene for SV40 in the H-2^k haplotype is H-$2D^k$ not H-$2K^k$: Gooding (19) was able to select a tumor cell line which expressed H-$2K^k$ but not H-$2D^k$ and grew progressively in H-2^k mice. There is thus a clear correlation between class I-MHC Ir gene expression, CTL function and growth or elimination of the tumor.

The Ad 2 early virus protein, E19, complexes to class I MHC glycoprotein (2). However, these complexes cannot be demonstrated on cell surface by serological means. The net effect of the interaction between E19 and MHC is to prevent further insertion of class I MHC glycoproteins in the cell membrane, with the complexes accumulating in the perinuclear region. As a consequence, class I MHC glycoproteins are gradually lost from the cell plasma membrane.

Rat cells transformed with Ad5 or Ad12 grow progressively in athymic nu/nu mice. However the Ad5-induced tumors are rejected in immunologically intact syngeneic (MHC-identical) rats, while the Ad12 clones grow progressively. The difference is that the Ad12, but not the Ad5, lines modulate the expression of class I MHC glycoprotein (7,54). This is evidently a general property of Ad12, as exactly the same situation is found for the mouse (18). In this case, the level of class I H-2 mRNA in the Ad12 tumors is from 5 to 20% of that found in the Ad5 cells. However, as shown previously for some brain cells that express low levels of class I MHC glycoproteins (13), the amount of H-2 in the Ad12 mouse tumors can be greatly enhanced by exposure to gamma interferon (18). This raises interesting questions concerning the role of inflammatory process, as many CTL produce gamma interferon (41).

Tumor cells that have escaped from immunological surveillance by modulating a class I MHC Ir gene product can be rendered immunogenic by transfection with the gene in question. An AKR (H-2^k) leukemia line that grows progressively in AKR mice and is resistant to T-cell-mediated lysis does not express the H-2^k molecule. Tumor cells that have been transfected with the H-2K^k gene express the H-2K^k glycoprotein and are rejected by syngeneic H-2^k mice (25). Similarly, Ir gene defects associated with class II MHC glycoproteins can be corrected by transfecting the missing gene into appropriate stimulator cells (35).

It should also be recognized that tumor cells may escape from immunological surveillance by modulating the expression of non-MHC molecules. In, for instance, Epstein-Barr virus-positive lymphoma cells, tumor clones may emerge which express a normal complement of MHC glycoproteins, but are no longer recognized by CTL (50).

INCREASED LEVELS OF MHC EXPRESSION ON SOME TUMORS

There are some situations where higher levels of MHC glycoprotein expression are associated with enhanced metastatic capacity (30). Variants of a murine lymphoma, which is apparently not recognized by immune T cells in syngeneic mice, proved much less metastatic when selected for reduced levels of surface MHC glycoprotein (29). This was associated with enhanced susceptibility to natural killer (NK)-mediated lysis. It is thus possible that the rules for the more 'primitive', NK-surveillance mechanisms are the converse of those for CTL recognition, thus presenting an alternative mode for host resistance.

Tumors induced by endogenous viruses in, for instance, AKR mice, may show high levels of MHC glycoprotein expression in association with relatively large amounts of viral gp70 on cell surface (44). Exposure to high levels of MHC + virus during T cell development in thymus would, presumably, drive potential effector clones to either deletion or suppression. The 'antigenicity' requirements for establishing tolerance early in T cell ontogeny, and immunity for mature T cell populations, may be similar (15).

MHC EXPRESSION ON HUMAN TUMORS

Much of the interest in MHC expression on human tumors has been concerned with the class II molecules (6,16). The reason for this is that it is easy to look for abnormal induction as the class II glycoproteins are normally found on only a few categories of cells, such as B lymphocytes, monocyte/macrophages and some T cells (in man). Greaves et al. (20) have seriously questioned the overall biological significance of finding such class II MHC glycoprotein expression in tumors. However, it is possible that the presence of class II molecules may serve to promote the development of inflammatory process. The question that then arise is whether such inflammation is beneficial or deleterious to the host, especially as it will involve T cells that secrete growth factors such as Il-2 and Il-3.

Screening human tumors for variations in the level of class I MHC glycoprotein expression may be of value in situations where, for instance, a viral aetiology is suspected. Otherwise, in the absence of any information concerning the identity of MHC Ir genes, such an approach may prove essentially unproductive in situations where (like the UV-induced tumors (33)) there is the possibility of a number of different TSTA's. It is instructive in this regard that strong correlations between MHC phenotype and development of particular forms of cancer have not generally emerged, though Hodgkin's disease, Kaposi's sarcoma and, perhaps, melanoma may be exceptions (see Immunological Reviews Vol. 70, 1983, and 16). At this stage, it would seem worthwhile to continue the search for association between HLA phenotype and susceptibility, using as wide a variety of probes as possible, in the hope that this may allow the identification of putative Ir genes. More precise analysis by restriction fragment length polymorphism mapping is likely to prove of great value in this regard.

WHAT ARE TSTA'S ?

While it now seems clear that abnormally expressed (or modified) class I MHC glycoproteins may be TSTA's in some experimentally-induced tumors, and that recognition of class I MHC glycoproteins is certainly required for CTL function (reviewed in 16), the molecular nature of the TSTA in the great majority of situations is still something of a mystery.

Gene transfection studies with the SV40 model have shown that different regions of the large T molecule are required to form immunogenic cell-surface changes in the context of different class I MHC glycoproteins (43). This is readily interpreted on the basis of an antigen association model, as postulated in our original formulation of the 'altered self' concept (17,66), though it could equally reflect some other form of post-translational effect on the MHC glycoprotein. The adenovirus 2 early glycoprotein, E19, has been shown to associate directly with both rat and human class I MHC glycoproteins (27). The half-life of E19 is much shorter than that of the class I molecules, which may reflect continued re-cycling of the complex from the cell-surface and degradation of E19 in lysosomes.

It is instructive that, in the influenza CTL system, a significant number of virus-immune T cell clones recognize cells transfected with the viral nucleoprotein (NP) gene (63). The NP does not have the characteristics of an integral membrane protein and only very small amounts of the molecule can be found serologically on the surface of the transfected L cell (62). This emphasizes the potential for divergence in the identity of tumor associated surface antigens (TASA) detected by antibody molecules, and the TSTA's seen by the T cell receptors. Cells infected with influenza express very large quantities of viral haemagglutinin and neuraminidase on their surface but these molecules seem to be much less immunogenic for CTL than is the NP. What is it, then, that makes a molecule of interest to the CTL compartment? All current evidence indicates that T cell recognition is mediated via a single, clonotypic receptor, consisting of an alpha and beta chain organized in much the same way as an Ig molecule (12). These two chains define the specificity of the binding site, and thus the components of both the MHC and non-MHC molecules that are recognized (65). It seems inescapable that T cell recognition depends on there being an appropriate interaction between, for instance, viral and MHC molecules on cell surface (16,66). The non-self molecules that determine T cell specificity would, therefore, appear to be those that can in some way bind to MHC glycoprotein, and allow the formation of a stable ternary complex with the T cell receptor (3,4). One suggestion is that the non-MHC proteins that stimulate T cells are those capable of organizing as amphipathic structures, i.e. with separated hydrophilic and hydrophobic surfaces (11). These would then interact with MHC glycoprotein to constitute a stable entity on cell surface.

Most of the present evidence indicates that the complex between self (MHC) and non-self (e.g. virus) on the target cell forms in the absence of specific T cell effectors (4,5). However, recent studies, using fluorescence transfer protocols to assess the proximity of molecules on cell surface, are considered to support the idea that the T cell receptor plays a part in stabilizing the antigenic complex (64). Which ever ultimately turns out to be true, the realization that the MHC and non-self molecules must interact explains why, for instance, different regions of the influenza virus NP are associated with CTL recognition in the context of different MHC glycoproteins (62). The capacity to form this ternary complex between the T lymphocyte receptor, nominal antigen and MHC glycoprotein would seem to be basic to both Ir gene effects and T cell surveillance.

MHC RESTRICTION AND PROSPECTS FOR T CELL THERAPY

The fact that T cells are targeted onto neoantigen that is in some way associated with self MHC molecules seemed to create considerable problems for any therapeutic model involving cell-mediated immunity. It did not, of course, preclude the idea that a better understanding of immune regulation might allow us to manipulate the host so that tumor-specific T cells that had for some reason been down-regulated might be activated (42,54). The success achieved in some tumor systems with re-infusing an individual's own lymphocytes that have been incubated _in vitro_ in the presence of excess IL-2 may reflect, at least in part, the operation of such effectors in addition to the less specific lymphokine activated killer cells (51). Also, some form of therapy might cause the tumor cells to become more antigenic: gamma interferon offers possibilities as it may greatly enhance the level of expression of both class I and II MHC glycoproteins on tumor cells (18,56).

However, we now know that the physiological requirement for MHC-restricted T cell recognition to achieve target cell killing can be subverted by various mechanisms. A promising avenue would seem to be the use of heteroantibody duplexes made by covalently joining monoclonal antibodies to the T3 molecule (which is closely associated with the human T cell receptor) and to antigen on the surface of the tumor, in order to target any T lymphocyte as an effector of T cell mediated lysis (36,46). Analysis to date with monoclonal antibodies has provided little evidence that tumors, other than those induced by viruses, express unique antigenic determinants that do not also occur elsewhere in the organism, or at some stage during ontogeny (22,52). Even so, the relative level of expression of such an antigen on the tumor may be sufficient for preferential targeting of monoclonal antibody following _in vitro_ inoculation (21).

However, achieving appropriate interactions between effector T cells, antibody heteroduplexes and tumors in other than cell culture systems may not prove to be easy. Simple injection of large amounts of the heteroantibody duplex would, presumably, result in binding to all T cells: will these lymphocytes then recirculate normally, or might they be destroyed in liver or lung? The same difficulty arises if activated lymphocytes are first incubated with the antibody _in vitro_ and then injected. Obviously, it will be necessary to use immunoglobulins that do not fix human complement, and will not target effector macrophages onto the T cells as a consequence of Fc binding (21).

A different approach could be to use a heteroantibody duplex with one Ig binding site directed at the clonotypic receptor (not T3) of a killer T cell clone that is already growing _in vitro_ (59). The heteroantibody might be injected first and allowed to localize to the tumor, followed by the cloned T cells. Using T cells that are partially, if not fully, allogeneic could be an advantage in this case, as the host would be expected to eliminate these cells within a few days, thus avoiding the possibility that the T cell clones themselves might constitute the source of a new tumor. One difficulty is that (at least in the mouse) T cell clones that have been grown and maintained _in vitro_ do not generally home to the site of interest, unless this happens to be the lungs (9). That there is a way around this problem is suggested by the recent experiment of Matis _et al._ (39), who have succeeded in eliminating syngeneic murine leukemia cells from the mouse footpad by the intravenous inoculation of cloned, tumor-specific CTL that have first been activated _in vitro_ to express IL-2 receptors, followed by regular dosage with human, recombinant IL-2. Another potential limitation is that injected allogeneic, or partially allogeneic, lymphocytes may be eliminated very rapidly by mechanisms analogous to those operating in hybrid resistance (14,57). These phenomena are poorly understood in rodents (10,49) and even more mysterious in man.

We may thus need to develop a rather better understanding of the basic nature of T cell recirculation and localization, particularly with regard to activated lymphocyte populations and cell lines that have cultured _in vitro_, if such forms of therapy are to evolve. It may also be necessary to produce less cumbersome immunoglobulin, or immunoglobulin-like synthetic molecules, to avoid the involvement of untoward effector mechanisms that could eliminate the T cell. Even so, the successes to date with the non-specific lymphokine activated killers (51) indicate that more targeted effector T cell populations may be of value. The potential difficulties mentioned above would seem to be susceptible to analysis.

CONCLUSIONS

The central feature of the surveillance of tumor cell surface by T lymphocytes is the recognition of neoantigens presented in the context of self major histocompatibility complex (MHC) glycoproteins. This phenomenon is known as MHC restriction. Immune response gene effects, associated with the presence or absence of potential T cell effectors, are determined by the capacity to form a ternary complex between, on the one hand, the antigen-specific receptor on the T lymphocyte and, on the other, the tumor-specific determinant and the MHC glycoprotein on the tumor. Tumor clones can escape from immunological surveillance by modulating the expression of either the tumor-specific, or the MHC, molecules. Expression of the MHC glycoproteins may be restored by exposure to gamma interferon, which is secreted by many T cells. The requirement for MHC-restricted recognition to achieve T cell-mediated lysis can be circumvented by using heteroduplexes of monoclonal antibodies to bind effector T cells in sufficient proximity to the surface of the tumor cells. This procedure offers possibilities for the development of therapeutic protocols involving T cells, though the in vivo application of such an approach requires further analysis.

REFERENCES

1. Abramczuk J, Pan S, Knowles BB (1984) J Virol 49: 541-548.

2. Andersson M, Paabo S, Nilsson T, Peterson PA (1985) Cell 43: 215-222.

3. Ashwell JD, Fox BS, Schwartz RH (1986) J Immunol 136: 757-768.

4. Ashwell JD, Schwartz RH (1986) Nature 320: 176-179.

5. Babbitt BP, Allen PM, Matsuedo G, Haber E, Unanue ER (1985) Nature 317: 359-361.

6. Bernard DJ, Maurizis JC, Chassagne J, Cholet P, Payne R (1985) Cancer Res 45: 1152-1158.

7. Bernards R, Schrier PI, Houweling A, Bos JL, van der Eb AJ, Zijlstra M, Melief CJM (1983) Nature 305: 776-779.

8. Burnet FM (1970) In: Immunological Surveillance, Pergamon Press, Oxford.

9. Byrne, JA, Oldstone MBA (1986) J Immunol 136: 698-704.

10. Clarke , Harman (1980)

11. De Lisi C, Berzogsky JA (1985) Proc Natl Acad Sci USA 82: 7048-7052.

12. Dembic Z, Haas W, Weiss S, McCubrey J, Kiefer H, von Boehmer H, Steinmetz M (1986) Nature 320: 232-238.

13. Doherty PC (1985) Trends in Neurosciences 8: 41-42.

14. Doherty PC, Allan JE (1986) Immunology 57: 515-519.

15. Doherty PC, Bennink JR (1980) Scand J Immunol 12: 271-280.

16. Doherty PC, Knowles BB, Wettstein PJ (1984) Adv Cancer Res 42: 1-65.

17. Doherty PC, Zinkernagel RM (1975) Lancet i: 1406-1409.

18. Eager KB, Williams J, Breiding D, Pan S, Knowles B, Appella A, Ricciardi RP (1985) Proc Natl Acad Sci USA 82: 5525-5529.

19. Gooding LR (1982) J Immunol 129: 1306-1312.

20. Greaves MF, Janossy G (1978) Biochem Biophys Acta 516: 193-230.

21. Herlyn D, Powe J, Ross AH, Herlyn M, Koprowski H (1985) J Immunol 134: 1300-1304.

22. Herlyn M, Sears HF, Verrill H, Koprowski H (1984) J Immun Meth 75: 15-21.

23. Hildemann WH, Bigger CH, Johnston IS, Jokiel PL (1980) Transplantation 30: 362-367.

24. Hildemann WH, Jokiel PL, Bigger CH, Johnston IS (1980) Transplantation 30: 297-301.

25. Hui K, Grosveld F, Festenstein H (1984) Nature 311: 750-752.

26. Jerne NK (1970) Eur J Immunol 1: 1-9.

27. Kampe O, Larhammer D, Wiman K, Claesson L, Gustafsson K, Paabo S, Hyldig-Nielsen JJ, Rask L, Peterson PA (1983) In: Genetics of the Immune Response. Nobel Foundation Symposia, E & G Moller eds., Plenum Press, New York, pp 61-72.

28. Kaplan DR, Griffith R, Braciale VL, Braciale TJ (1984) Cell Immunol 88: 193-206.

29. Karre K, Ljunggren HG, Piontek G, Kiessling R (1986) Nature 319: 675-678.

30. Katzav S, De Baetselier P, Tarta Kovsky B, Feldman M, Segal S (1983) J Natl Cancer Res Inst 71: 317-321.

31. Kelso A, Glasebrook AL (1984) J Immunol 132: 2924-2931.

32. Kranz DM, Tonegawa S, Eisen HN (1984) Proc Natl Acad Sci USA 81: 7922-7926.

33. Kripke ML (1981) Adv Cancer Res 34: 69-106.

34. Lalanne J-L, Transy C, Guerin S, Darche S, Meulien P, Kourilsky P (1985) Cell 41: 469-478.

35. Le Meur M, Gerlinger P, Genoist C, Mathis D (1985) Nature 316: 38-41.

36. Liu MA, Kranz DM, Kurnick JT, Boyle LA, Levy R, Eisen HN (1985) Proc Natl Acad Sci USA 82: 8648-8652.

37. MacDonald HR, Glasebrook AL, Bron C, Kelso A, Cerottini J-C (1982) Immun Rev 68: 89-115.

38. Mc Millan M, Lewis KD, Rovner DM (1985) Proc Natl Acad Sci USA 82: 5485-5489.

39. Matis LA, Shu S, Groves ES, Zinn S, Chou T, Kruisbeck AM, Rosenstein M, Rosenberg SA (1986) J Immunol 136: 3496-3501.

40. Meuer SC, Hodgdon JC, Cooper DA, Hussey RE, Fitzgerald KA, Schlossman SF, Reinherz EL (1983) J Immunol 131: 186-190.

41. Morris AG, Lin YL, Askonas RA (1982) Nature 295: 150-152.

42. Naor D (1979) Adv Cancer Res 29: 45-125.

43. O'Connell KA, Gooding LR (1984) J Immunol 132: 953-958.

44. Oudshoorn-Snoek M, Demant P (1986) Int J Cancer 37: 303-310.

45. Pan S, Knowles BB (1983) Virology 125: 1-7.

46. Perez P, Hoffman RW, Shaw S, Bluestone JA, Segal DM (1985) Nature 316: 354-356.

47. Philips C, McMillan M, Flood PM, Murphy DB, Forman J, Lancki D, Womack JE, Goodenow RS, Schreiber H (1985) Proc Natl Acad Sci USA 82: 5140-5144.

48. Reinherz EL, Meuer SC, Schlossman SF (1983) Immunol Rev 74: 83-112.

49. Rolstad B, Ford WL (1983) Immunol Rev 73: 87-113.

50. Rooney CM, Rowe M, Wallace LE, Rickinson AB (1985) Nature 317: 629-631.

51. Rosenberg SA, Lotze MT, Muul LM, Leitman S, Chang AE, Ettinghausen SE, Matory YL, Skibber JM, Shiloni E, Vetto JT, Scipp CA, Simpson C, Reichert CM (1985) New Engl J Med 313: 1485-1492.

52. Ross AH, Cossu G, Herlyn M, Bell JR, Steplewski Z, Koprowski H (1983) Arch Biochem Biophys 225: 370-383.

53. Schepart BS, Woodward JG, Palmer MJ, Macchi MJ, Basta P, McLaughlin-Taylor E, Frelinger JA (1985) Proc Natl Acad Sci USA 82: 5505-5509.

54. Schirrmacher V (1985) Adv Cancer Res 43: 1-73.

55. Schrier PI, Bernards R, Vausen RTMJ, Houweling A, van der Eb AJ (1983) Nature 305: 771-775.

56. Shaw ARE, Chan JKW, Reid S, Sechafer J (1985) J Natl Cancer Inst 74: 1261-1268.

57. Shearer GM (1983) Immunol Rev 73: 115-126.

58. Spits H, Yssel H, Leeuwenberg J, De Vries JE (1985) Eur J Immunol 15: 88-91.

59. Staerz UD, Kanagawa O, Bevan MJ (1985) Nature 314: 628-631.

60. Swain SL (1983) Immunol Rev 74: 129-142.

61. Tevethia SS, Lewis AJ, Campbell AE, Tevethia MJ, Rigby PWJ (1984) Virology 133: 443-447.

62. Townsend AAM, Gotch FM, Davey J (1985) Cell 42: 457-467.

63. Townsend ARM, McMichael AJ, Carter NP, Huddleston JA, Brownlee GG (1984) Cell 39: 13-25.

64. Watts TH, Gaub HE, McConnell HM (1986) Nature 320: 179-181.

65. Yague J, White J, Coleclough C, Kappler J, Palmer E, Marrack P (1985) Cell 42: 81-87.

66. Zinkernagel RM, Doherty PC (1974) Nature 251: 547-548.

CARCINOGENESIS AND FACTORS MODIFYING AGING RATE

VN ANISIMOV

N.N. Petrov Research Institute of Oncology of the URSS Ministry of Health, Leningrad.

SUMMARY

Data concerning the effect of drugs on carcinogenesis, or their action in prolonging or decreasing the life span of animals, are discussed in the review. It has been shown that the influence delaying the aging rate and increasing maximum life span of animals inhibits spontaneous carcinogenesis. The increase in the mean life span, caused merely by the decrease in mortality at a young age, could result in a rise of tumor development. It is stressed that in working out measures of prolongation of human longevity, the possibility of the increase of cancer risk should be taken into account.

INTRODUCTION

Despite the fact that nobody denies the existence of the phenomenon of age-related increase in tumor incidence, at present there exists no common opinion on the nature of the relation between aging and development of cancer and on causes of this phenomenon. A decade ago Peto et al. (108) wrote that no relation exists between aging per se and cancer. Recently, it was affirmed that "there is no such thing as aging, and cancer is not related to it" (107). Cairns (41) supposed that aging and cancer are fundamentally different: cancer originated as a clone from a single transformed stem cell, while in aging the whole organism gets older. Aging is a continuous and irreversible process contrary to cancer, which has a beginning and is, in fact reversible.

Pitot (109) keeps a question mark in his paper entitled "Carcinogenesis and aging - two related phenomena?". Burnet (40) put forward a concept according to which the mechanism of immunological surveillance becomes less effective with age and less capable of removing "changed" cells prior to their proliferation with further tumor development. Dilman (51,52,54) proposed a hypothesis of "cancrophilia" as a syndrome, which is genetically programmed and develops in the process of natural aging, inevitably forming hormonal and metabolic shifts, facilitating age-related pathology formation, cancer included.

Dix et al. (57) and Ebbesen (61) do not doubt the existence of a deep interrelation between aging and carcinogenesis and give their arguments for the explanation of age-related increases in cancer incidence.

In one of his papers Martin (94) analysed 15 major ideas, which lie within the basis of various theories of aging. Justly noting changes in the genome as a primary substrate of aging, Martin suggests that all theories of aging could be divided into two classes. The first one includes theories emphasizing modifications in the structure of genes (stochastic theories). In compliance with these theories aging is a result of occasional non-repairable lesions of macromolecules (nucleic acids and proteins) induced by various exogenous and endogenous factors, such as free radicals, mutagens, etc. To the second class Martin (94) refers theories suggesting modifications in gene expression (theories of programmed aging, including regulatory, neurohumoral and immunological theories).

From the viewpoint of gerontologists supporting a hypothesis of this or that type, the increase of age-related tumour incidence could be considered a consequence of the summation of those occasional genomic lesions which lead to tumor transformation, or a result of "programmed" genome events which are realized in the process of natural aging.

From the viewpoint of oncologists, numerous hypotheses explaining the phenomenon of age-related cancer incidence arise from various viewpoints and these can eventually be divided into two groups. According to the first one, cancer incidence is conditioned by the accumulation of carcinogenic doses and/or increased exposure to their action. Supporters of the other hypothesis suggest that changes which appear in the organism in the process of natural aging, increase the probability of tumor occurrence and facilitate its growth and progression.

A large amount of data has now been obtained, both in

experiments on animals of various ages and species, and in epidemiological studies which could be interpreted in accordance with this or that hypothesis and used by supporters of each of the latter to confirm their viewpoint.

The first of these hypotheses is based on the well-known dependance of the effect, in experimental oncology, on the dose of carcinogen and time of exposure. This hypothesis suggests that all lesions induced by exogenous and endogenous factors, and leading to malignant transformations, are summed up, independent of the age of the host, at the moment of the damaging action. However, epidemiological data on some occupational groups of people exposed to carcinogenic action at different ages, as well as results of numerous experiments, where chemicals were administered to animals of different ages, are sometimes very contradictory: there was observed an increased carcinogenic effect in old age groups, absence of any age-related effect and significant age-related decrease of host sensitivity to action of carcinogens (13,14,17).

Differences in the results of such experiments are conditioned by many criteria, such as the type of carcinogen used (with direct or indirect action), their nature (chemical, radiation, hormonal, viral carcinogenic agent), methods of approach (kind of exposure, dosage, chronic or single administration, etc.), as well as host peculiarities (species, strain, sex, age group selected for comparison). Analysis is made elsewhere of material obtained on this aspect (13,14).

It was shown that age-related changes in the activity of enzymes activating and inactivating carcinogens, in the concentration of lipids and proteins exerting a transport of carcinogens in the cell or through its membrane, play an important role in the modifying effect of aging on carcinogenesis. The role of age-related alterations in the DNA repair has not yet been properly studied. However, available data suggest that they play a permissive role in the mechanism of age-related rise in cancer incidence.

A proliferative activity of a target tissue at the time of action of the carcinogens is evidently one of the most important factors in carcinogenesis. Age-related changes in the tissue proliferative activity and in the factors which control the proliferative activity, considerably modify carcinogenesis. Age-related shifts in the neuroendocrine system form conditions for metabolic immunodepression and are therefore an important factor of promotion and progression in carcinogenesis.

During the last few years the study of oncogenes have provided evidence that their activation might possibly be an important step in a multistage process of carcinogenesis (34,133,134). The oncogene activation could proceed through various pathways. The mechanism of these events induced by carcinogenic agents is not yet identified completely. Recently it was shown that one of the possible pathways of oncogene activation involved DNA hypomethylation, i.e. the decrease of 5-methylcytosine content in DNA (113,114).

It is worthy of note that DNA hypomethylation in animal tissues increased as age advanced (130). This process could lead to a spontaneous deamination of 5-methylcytosine to thymine, that is followed by 5-methylcytosine: guanine -- thymine: adenine transition (99). These transitions would accumulate over the life span of the animal. This mechanism may play a principal role in the age-related rise of spontaneous tumor incidence. If relevant controlling regions become completely unmethylated as result of such spontaneous deamination reactions, then the damaged cell might give rise to a spontaneous tumor. But even a partial methyl-depletion of multiple methylated controlling regions would increase the probability that action of carcinogens on DNA would result in a neoplastic effect (99). The authors suggested that if "old" DNA is undermethylated, fewer hypomethylating mutations would be required to put it over the regulatory threshold.

According to the first hypothesis on the cause of age-related increases in tumor incidence, the probability of spontaneous tumor development should be greater with increases in the life span of the organism and in the mean life span of populations, respectively. However, spontaneous tumor incidence does not correlate with the life span of a species and is approximately 30% for non-inbred rats that live for 3 years and for humans who live to the age of 70 years (19,125).

In accordance with data on the direct correlation between the duration of the life span of a species and the repair efficiency of DNA damaged by different carcinogens, and on the inverse correlation between the life span of a species and the ability of carcinogens to interrelate with DNA (65,71,121), direct quantitative comparison between data on spontaneous and induced carcinogenesis in different species cannot be made.

The question of the causes of the age-related increase in cancer incidence has another important theoretical and practical aspect. It should be stressed that preference for one of the mentioned viewpoints on causes of age-related increases of tumor incidence will determine the principal approach to the elaboration of preventive measures. Those who support the first hypothesis believe that these measures should imply prevention of contact with environmental carcinogens. The second hypothesis proclaims prophylactic measures aimed at prevention and inhibition of age-related changes, facilitating the appearance and growth of tumors.

In this connection, close attention should be paid to the suggestion of prophylactic employment of substances from the group of antioxidants and antimutagens decreasing the probability of lesions in macromolecules induced by carcinogens (132) on the one hand, and on the other hand, substances containing properties to normalize age-related hormone-metabolic and immunologic shifts in the organism (54). At the same time, there are data that some factors of the environment decrease the life span of animals, increasing the aging rate.

Comparative analysis of the efficiency of the influence of such agents on the incidence of spontaneous tumors and on the life span of animals could have helped to reveal mechanisms both common and different for aging and carcinogenesis and to understand the deeper nature of the interrelation of these two fundamental biological processes.

DEFINITION OF AGING RATE

Before turning to the factors that modify the rate of aging, this very term should be defined. The state of the art in gerontology evolved so that we now have a multitude of theories, elaborated with respect to different special questions, while fundamental terms still lack generally accepted definitions (124). At present, different definitions of the rate of aging exist, based on the consideration of processes that occur in an organism at different levels of its integration, or in a population.

For an individual organism, the concept of "biological age" is used together with such notions as "vitality", "vulnerability", etc. The rate of aging in this case will be determined by the rate of temporal changes in a set of parameters. The problem of the choice of these parameters is a matter of wide discussion (64,124). At different levels of integration in an organism, different parameters may be used:

(a) at the subcellular and cellular levels these may be the amount of lesions in DNA or the degree of collagen cross-links, the level of lipofuscine accumulation, enzyme activities, the number of receptors to a particular hormone or mediator, the number of possible cell divisions, etc;

(b) at the tissue and organism level, weight, cellularity, proliferative or some functional activity (muscle strength, sharpness of eye, secretion rate) may be considered;

(c) functional activity of motor, cardiovascular, nervous, endocrine, immune, hematopoietic and other systems and subsystems may be considered at the system integration level;

(d) on the level of the whole organism, the functions of the main integrative systems, which form the basis of the life cycle, for example the adaptational, reproductive and energy supplying systems, should be assessed.

Another approach to the estimation of the rate of aging is based on the analysis of the survival of the organism in a population. This problem is also far from being settled. At least 4 methods of estimating the rate of aging, with the help of survival data, are used at present (66):

(1) The rate of aging may be assumed to be the inverse of the mean longevity;

(2) If the dependence of cumulative mortality in the probit scale on the age is assumed to be linear, the rate of aging may

be estimated as the tangent of the angle between the graph and the abscissa;

(3) The rate of aging corresponds to the tangent of the angle between the graph representing the dependence of the logarithm of the probability of death on the age of the organism and the abscissa (Gompertz' function):

$$R = R_0 \, e^{\alpha t},$$

where R = mortality rate; R_0 R at the time $t = 0$, alpha = constant, which characterized the slope of the curve.

As for the aging rate of the population, when the living (maintenance) conditions of a population are identical and do not change with time, then it might be expressed by means of the death rate index as:

$$dR/dt = R_0 \, \alpha e^{\alpha t}.$$

It is evident that the aging rate of a population is determined by the constant alpha , which according to the Mildwan-Strehler theory of mortality is inversely proportional to LnR_0 (124).

(4) The rate of aging may be estimated as the age-related increase in specific mortality whatever mathematical model depicting this increase is chosen (66).

The analysis of the methods for estimating the rate of aging leads to the conclusion that all methods enumerated above are empirical and have no sound theoretical basis (66). One theoretical consideration nevertheless seems obvious. Any one of these methods must satisfy the following condition: the rate of aging in a non-aging population (without age-related increase in the rate of mortality) must be equal to zero. The number of organisms surviving to the age t in a non-aging population is described by the equation:

$$N_t = N_0 \exp (-kt),$$

where N_t is a number of animals surviving to age t; N_0 = number of members of a population at start; k = constant characterized rate of death.

The mean longevity in such a case is finite and equal to 1/k. The first of the enumerated methods for the estimation of the rate of aging as the inverse of the mean longevity appears to be unsatisfactory, since a value exceeding zero is obtained for the rate of aging in the case where there is no aging at all.

The second method is also incorrect because cumulative mortality will increase in any population including a non-aging one. The Gompertz equation is a satisfactory approximation to the kinetics of specific mortality in human populations in the age range of 20-80 years. It is suggested that the Gompertz equation (or its modification - the equation of Gompertz-Makeham) permits objective estimations to be made of the changes in the mortality in populations (75,118).

When the rate of aging is determined using the absolute age-related increase in the rate of mortality (the 4th method), the calculated parameter has the dimension not of rate, but of acceleration. It is worthy of note that its value had not markedly changed in the XXth century in human populations of different countries (67).

Thus, a brief representation of the problem of measuring the rate of aging demonstrates that this problem is far from the final solution. In the analysis of the factors modifying the rate of aging, we will assume that the value of alpha from Gompertz' equation may serve as an adequate measure of the aging of a population.

CARCINOGENS AS ACCELERATORS OF AGING

The capacity of carcinogenic and mutagenic agents to accelerate aging has been discussed for many years (2,6,13,53,54,60,89,118). The action of various mutagenic agents such as 5-bromodeoxyuridine (46), alkylating substances (45,59), carcinogenic polycyclic aromatic hydrocarbons and nitrosocompounds (6,10,84,101), ionizing radiations (2,89) decreases the life span of treated animals in direct proportion to dose and was considered as an acceleration of aging.

According to Ohno & Nagai (101) neonatal administration of DMBA decreased the life span of female mice from 608 down to 297 days. Premature cessation of estral function, greying of hairs, loss of weight etc. were observed with this. Dunjic (60) observed shortening of rat life span proportional to myleran dose and accompanied by such manifestations of old age as cataract, and testicle atrophy. In our experiments female rats submitted to 3-methylcholanthrene oral administration manifested early discontinuation of estral function, and a number of hormonal shifts which have allowed the suggestion of intensified aging, induced by the carcinogen (6).

In mice exposed to radiomimetics (nitrogen mustard or triethylenmelamine), a decrease of life span was observed which correlated with all types of disease associated with old age (44). Neonatal administration of 5-bromodeoxyuridine to rats significantly shortened the life span of animals. At the same time no tumors, which could have been responsible for this effect, developed (46).

Acceleration of aging by ionizing radiation could serve as an explanation of results obtained in studying "dose-effect" dependance on the action of ionizing radiation (2,118). On the other hand, the decrease of animal life span induced by irradiation or radiomimetic substances can not serve as an adequate model of normal aging (1,119).

Table 1 summarizes the data available in literature, and obtained in our experiments, on some hormonal-metabolic shifts in the organism and disturbances on tissue and cellular levels, observed in natural aging and in different types of carcinogenesis. Despite the incompleteness of the data, it is seen that there is a certain similarity between the shifts in aging and carcinogenesis. Carcinogens could be supposed to initiate a normal cell, interacting with its elements at the molecular level, on the one hand, and to produce diverse changes in the organism, facilitating promotion and progression of tumor growth on the other hand. This suggestion is expressed in Fig. 1, which gives a hypothetical scheme of carcinogenesis, where the effect of a carcinogenic agent on different levels of integration

TABLE 1

THE SIMILARITY OF CHANGES DEVELOPING IN ORGANISMS DURING AGING AND CARCINOGENESIS

Aging	Chemical Carcinogenesis	Ionizing Radiation	Exogenic Estrogens	Persistent estrus Syndrome
Hypothalamic catecholamine level and turnover decrease	Hypothalamic catecholamine level decrease	Hypothalamic catecholamine level decrease	Hypothalamic catecholamine level decrease	Hypothalamic catecholamine turnover changes
Decrease in hypothalamic estrogen binding	3-MCA changes binding of estradiol with receptors		Competition to estrogen receptors	Decrease in hypothalamic estrogen binding
Hypothalamic resistance to feedback effect of estrogen and glucocorticoids	Hypothalamic resistance to feedback effect of estrogens and glucocorticoids	Hypothalamic resistance to feedback effect of estrogens and glucocorticoids		Hypothalamic resistance to feedback effect of estrogens
Increase in serum estradiol level and nonclassic phenolsteroids excretion before switching off of reproductive function	Increase in nonclassic phenolsteroids synthesis and excretion	Increase in nonclassic phenolsteroids synthesis and excretion	Increase in serum estrogen level	Non-cyclic secretion of normal or enhanced amount of estrogens
Increase in persistent estrus incidence	In some cases the persistent estrus	Increase in persistent estrus incidence	Persistent estrus	Persistent estrus
Relative hypercorticism	Disfunction of adrenal cortex	Disfunction of adrenal cortex	Hypercorticism	Hypercorticism
Decrease in tolerance to carbohydrates	Decrease in tolerance to carbohydrates	Decrease in tolerance to carbohydrates	Decrease in tolerance to carbohydrates	Decrease in tolerance to carbohydrates
Hyperinsulinemia	Hyper- or normoinsulinemia	Decrease in insulin level		
Decrease in sensitivity to insulin	Decrease in sensitivity to insulin	Decrease in sensitivity to insulin		Decrease in sensitivity to insulin
Hypercholestrinemia	In some cases hypercholestrinemia	Hyperlipidemia	Decrease in cholesterol level	Normocholestrinemia

TABLE 1 (cont.)

Decrease in T-cell-mediated immunity	Decrease in T-cell-mediated immunity	Decrease in T-cell-mediated immunity	Decrease in T-cell-mediated immunity	Decrease in T-cell-mediated immunity
DNA repair lesions	Insufficiency of DNA repair	Insufficiency of DNA repair	Inhibition of induced DNA repair	
Increase in incidence of 'errors' in DNA	Mutagenic effect	Mutagenic effect	Diethylstilbestrol is covalently bound with DNA	
Increase in chromosome aberration incidence	Increase in chromosome aberration incidence	Increase in chromosome aberration incidence	Estrogens may induce the chromosome aberrations	
Changes in enzyme regulation	Changes in enzyme regulation	Changes in enzyme regulation	Enzyme inductio	
Changes in cell bioenergy	Change in cell bioenergy	Changes in cell bioenergy		
Decrease in proliferation activity of majority of tissues				
Clonal proliferation of some cells	Clonal proliferation of cells	Clonal proliferation of cells	Stimulation of proliferation of target tissues	Hyperplastic processes in some tissues
Age-related depression of oncoviruses and oncogenes	Activation of latent oncoviruses and oncogenes	Activation of latent oncoviruses and oncogenes	Activation of latent oncoviruses	
Increase in tumor incidence	Cancer induction	Cancer induction	Cancer induction	Increases in tumor incidence

TABLE 2

EFFECT OF AGING AND CARCINOGENIC AGENTS ON SOME PARAMETERS OF CARBOHYDRATE AND
LIPID METABOLISM IN RATS

Carcinogenic Agent	Serum concentrations					
	Tolerance to glucose	Insulin	Somatomedin activity	Cholesterol	Triglycerides	Ref
Aging	Decreases	Increases	Disturbances in regulation	Increases	Increases	21
NMU, i.v.	Decreases	Increases	"	No effect	No effect	20
NMU, transpla- centally	Decreases	No effect	"	Increases	No effect	
DMBA, i.v.	Decreases	Increases	N.E.(a)	No effect	No effect	19
DMH, s.c.	Decreases	Increases	N.E.	Increases	Increases	30
DES, transpla- centally	Decreases	Increases	Disturbances in regulation	No effect	Decreases	22
X-ray	Decreases	Increases	N.E.	N.E.	Increases	23

(a) N.E.: not estimated

TABLE 4

THE METHODS OF INDUCTION OF PERSISTENT ESTRUS IN FEMALE RATS

Target organ	Treatment
Pineal gland	Constant light regime
Hypothalamus	Electrolytic lesions of anterior and/or mediobasal hypothalamic area
	Neonatal administration of sex hormones
	Administration of diethylstilbestrol or testosterone during pregnancy
	Some chemical carcinogens
	Ionizing radiation
Liver	Ligature of portal vein
	Subtotal hepatectomy
	Carbon tetrachloride or some carcinogens
Ovary	Gonadotropic hormones
	Ionizing radiations
	Subtotal ovarectomy
	Ortotopic transplantation of an ovary into castrated animal
	Stitching an ovary with ligature
	Vessel-nervous bunch ligation
	Lubrication with iodine, phenol, etc.

into the organism is taken into account.

It was shown that chemical and radiation carcinogenic agents changed the level of activity of biogenic amines and neurosecretory elements in the hypothalamus (2,19,28,29,83). There are data on the capacity of some carcinogens to compete for specific steroid receptors in target tissues (73,81,137).

Great shifts in the function of pituitary, ovaries, adrenal and thyroid glands were found during early stages of chemical carcinogenesis in rats (129). The syndrome of persistent estrus followed disturbances in the reproductive system function developed in rats exposed to some carcinogens, for instance, polycyclic aromatic hydrocarbons and X-rays (6,79). It is worthy of note that persistent estrus inevitably completes the reproductive period in rats during the process of natural aging (32).

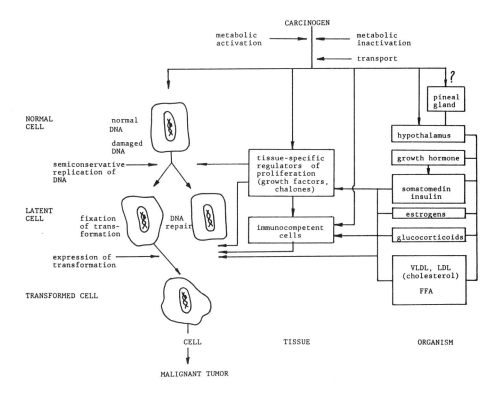

Fig.1. An integral scheme of carcinogenesis

Table 2 shows the results of studying the carcinogenic effect on some parameters of carbohydrate and lipid metabolism in rats. All experiments were performed during the period preceeding the finding of detectable tumors. All the models demonstrated the same similarity. Thus, lowered glucose tolerance was found, accompanied by more or less pronounced reactive hyperinsulinemia and disturbances in the regulation of serum somatomedin activity. Variations in serum cholesterol and triglyceride levels were not constant.

Lowered glucose tolerance in aflatoxin B1 - treated chickens was shown (111). These authors also showed that this carcinogen inhibits the activity of some glycolytic enzymes (hexokinase, phosphoglucoisomerase, pyruvate-kinase) and stimulates the activity of key enzymes of gluconeogenesis (pyruvate carboxylase and phosphoenol pyruvate carboxylase).

Regarding the data on the important role of cholesterol in cell proliferation (43), attention should be paid to the data on correlation between tissue sensitivity to a carcinogen (2-acetyl-aminofluorene) and src gene, determining disturbances in cholesterol level and increased DNA synthesis (112). It was also shown that such carcinogens as DMBA or benzo(a)pyrene stimulate development of atherosclerosis in chickens, inducing proliferation of atherosclerotic patches in the vessels (104).

In this connection, data on untimely development of atherosclerosis and increased incidence of deaths from acute vascular shifts in workers occupied in production of vinyl chloride and polyvinylchloride are very important (92). Increased secretion of growth hormone and obesity were observed in these workers. Vinyl chloride also blocked tissue activities of thyroid hormones.

During the past few years, extensive studies in the field of immunology of aging resulted in a large amount of evidence on the age-related changes in various chains of the system of immunity. Table 3 summarizes some of such data on immunosenescence and immune shifts occurring during carcinogenesis as well (35,49,77,80,102).

It should be noted that some data listed in the table are disputed by certain authors and require further elucidation. However, it is obvious that there are similarities in the direction

TABLE 3

THE DYNAMICS OF IMMUNOLOGICAL FUNCTIONS IN CANCER AND AGING

Parameter	Aging	Cancer
The number of stem cells in bone marrow	Decreases	Decreases
Migration of stem cells from bone marrow	No effect	Increases
The number of stem cells in spleen	Decreases	Increases
The number of B-cell precursors	No effect	Decreases
The number of T-cell precursors	Decreases	Decreases
Cooperation of T- and B-lymphocytes	Inhibited	Inhibited
Migration of B-cells from bone marrow	Inhibited	Inhibited
Migration of T-cells from thymus	Inhibited	Inhibited
Helper effect of T-cells	Decreases	Decreases
Killer effect of T-cells	Decreases	No effect
Suppressor effect of T-cells	Decreases	Increases
T-cell sensitivity to mitogens (PHA, conA)	Decreases	Decreases
Phagocytic activity of macrophages	Decreases	Decreases
Cytostatic function of macrophages	Decreases	Decreases
Interleukin 1 and 2 production	Decreases	Decreases

----

of shifts of many immunological parameters during aging and tumor development.

Comparative evaluation of disturbances in neuroendocrine regulation occurring in the organism during aging and due to carcinogens, as well as shifts in the immune system, gives an impression of earlier development and stronger pronouncement of age-related changes in radiation and carcinogenic effect.

CARCINOGENESIS WITH ACCELERATED AGING

The Hutchinson-Gilford syndrome, or progeria, is a rare genetic disease with a number of symptoms of precocious senility (to 15 - 17 years). At this age these patients develop marked thinning of skin with loss of subcutaneous fat, loss of hair, marked growth retardation, the signs of atherosclerosis with involvement of heart and brain. Death occurs at the median age of 12 years. There are no data on tumor incidence in such patients (76).

Werner's syndrome, as well as progeria, is characterized by signs of untimely aging, including atherosclerosis, diabetes mellitus, osteoporosis, and increased risk of cancer development (63). Cocayne's syndrome and ataxia telangiectasia are considered as segmental progeroid syndromes (94). Cocayne's syndrome is a progressive neurologic disease, characterized by retardation of physical and mental development, dwarfism, microcephaly, loss of adipose tissue, skeletal abnormalities and severe photosensitivity. Available data, recently summarized by Lehmann (87), suggest some alterations in the capacity of the cells of these patients to repair DNA, while in progeria and Werner's syndromes there are no data on DNA repair insufficiency.

It is worthy of note that no reports are available on an increased incidence of cancer associated with Cocayne's syndrome (87).

Ataxia telangiectasia commences with cerebellar ataxia and multiple telangiectases. Some immunological defects often occur in these patients. Death usually results from infections in the first two decades of life or from cancer in the third decade. Cancer incidence (mainly lymphomas and lymphocytic leukemias) is increased about 1200-fold over age-matched controls. The ataxia telangiectasia patients are characterized by hypersensitivity to ionizing radiation precluded by defective DNA repair (87).

Xeroderma pigmentosum patients have very high susceptibity to sunlight and 2000-fold excess in the incidence of skin cancer, melanomas of the skin, eyes, tip of the tongue at under 20 years of age. DNA in xeroderma pigmentosum patients is defective in the excision of damage produced in DNA, either by ultra-violet or by some carcinogens, but such patients have no sign of premature aging (87). It was recently shown that the xeroderma pigmentosum patients under 20 years of age had an estimated 12-fold increase in the occurrence of neoplasma in sites not exposed to ultra-violet irradiation (86).

In in vitro experiments it was shown that the classic promoter 12-O-tetradecanoylphorbol-13-acetate (TPA) had no significant transforming effect on skin fibroblasts of patients with defects of

DNA repair and/or genetic predisposition to cancer (xeroderma pigmentosum, Fanconi's anemia, trisomy 21, familial colon polyposis and retinoblastoma) in comparison to fibroblasts of normal donors (31). The authors suggested that skin fibroblasts of patients with genetic predisposition to cancer have not been in a status, preneoplastic or initiated, sensitive to oncogenic transformation. It is worthy of note that in this study the workers did not intend to test tissues which were predisposed to tumor development. On the other hand, a decrease was found of the rate of N-acetoxy-N-2-acetylaminofluorene-induced, unscheduled, DNA synthesis in the leukocytes of colorectal cancer patients (in remission) and in individuals genetically predisposed to cancer (106).

It was shown that in Down's syndrome patients there are signs of accelerated aging, first of all the immune system, and significantly increased incidence of malignancies in the lymphoid system (131).

The syndrome of Stein-Leventhal is usually formed in girls during puberty and is characterized by a bilateral sclerocystic enlargement of the ovaries, anovulation, sterility, hyrsutism and various disturbances of carbohydrate and lipid metabolism, particularly hyperlipidemia, lowered glucose tolerance, huyperinsulinemia, obesity, hypertensia. This disease is considered as an example of intensified aging (50). The incidence of breast and endometrial cancer is significantly increased in Stein-Leventhal syndrome patients.

Bokhman et al. (38) studied 80 patients with Stein-Leventhal syndrome and in 53 patients (66.2%) hyperplastic processes in the endometrium were found. Atypical hyperplasia of the endometrium was found in 8 patients (10%), and endometrial carcinoma in 12 patients (15%). These patients manifested obesity in 68.2% of the cases and lowered tolerance to glucose in 72.5% of the cases. The incidence of such disturbances should be considered high, because all the patients were young.

A convenient experimental model of the Stein-Leventhal syndrome in rats is presented by an autoimplantation of an ovary into the tail of ovariectomized female rats (6). In this case, the artificial mechanical obstacle to the rupture of follicules causes chronic disturbances in the hypotalamus-pituitary-ovaries system and the development of persistent estrus. The persistent estrus is formed in rats thus operated as early as 1-2 weeks following the operation and lasts for 1-2 years. A few months after the operation, the rats developed hormonal-metabolic disturbances which usually occurred in old female rats.

In addition, the rats with persistent estrus caused by the transplantation of an ovary into the tail, demonstrated pre-tumor and tumor development in the mammary gland, uterus and other organs. Total incidence of neoplasms in rats with persistent estrus was 61%, as compared to 33% in controls. The incidence of malignant tumors and tumor multiplicity in operated, persistent estrus, rats was also higher than in control ones. Mammary and uterus carcinomas were found only in rats with persistent estrus (6). In rats with persistent estrus induced by the above mentioned method, disturbances of carbohydrate and lipid metabolism were found. The pattern of these disturbances was similar to disturbances in Stein-Leventhal syndrome patients (19).

It should be stressed that in the experiment, the syndrome of persistent estrus normally completing the reproductive period of rodent life, might be induced in them by influences exerted on various chains of the neuroendocrine system by many other factors (Table 4). In practically all models it was shown that in the animals with persistent estrus the incidence of malignant and benign tumors is increased (12,79).

There are interesting data on the promoting effect of persistent estrus on carcinogenesis induced by various agents in rats. The induction of persistent estrus in rats by stitching of an ovary with silk ligature after one week following the injection of a sub-carcinogenic dose of DMBA, caused development of mammary neoplasms in a great number of experimental animals (128).

Subtotal ovariectomy after 2 weeks following the series of intravenous DMBA injections which induced persistent estrus in female rats, considerably shortened tumor latency and increased the incidence of mammary gland tumors in comparison with rats only with carcinogen (123). Constant lighting of DMBA-treated rats also induced persistent estrus in them and increased tumor yield in mammary glands (81).

In our experiments (3) rats were injected intraperitoneally with N-nitrosomethylurea on the 21st day of pregnancy. Tumors (mainly in the nervous system and kidneys) appeared in 37.5% of offspring. Then, pregnant rats were injected with the same dose of carcinogen, and their offspring at the age of 3 months were subjected to ovariectomy followed by autotransplantation of an ovary into the tail. As a result, persistent estrus was induced in these animals, and tumors were observed in 84% of the cases.

Obesity is another important factor promoting both the aging process and carcinogenesis. As age advances, the body weight and, which is extremely important, the percentage of fat in the body, is increased (36). It is well known that in obese individuals the death rate is higher than in that of individuals with normal weight (70). Atherosclerosis, diabetes mellitus and certain types of

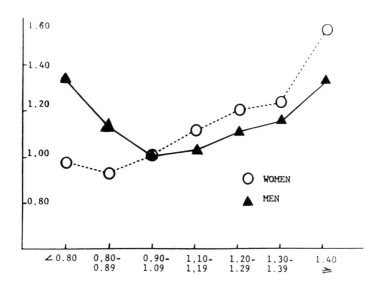

Fig. 2 : Cancer mortality ratios of men and women in the USA by weight index. Ordinate: mortality ratio for weight index in ranges 0.90-1.09; abscissa: weight index (actual weight divided by the average weight for people of similar weight and sex).

cancer are also more frequent in obese individuals (58,70). In the experimental studies it was also shown that in rats with excessive body weight, the risk of spontaneous tumor development is higher than in those with normal weight (117).

Fig.2 illustrates the death rate in 750,000 American men and women according to observations by Lew and Garfinkel (88). It can be seen that excessive body weight increases the risk of death from all types of cancer. The excess of body weight of 30-40% to the normal value increases the risk of death by 50% as compared to individuals with normal weight. If the weight of a subject exceeds the normal by more than 40%, then the risk of death in such humans is increased by 90% (88).

The high correlation between mortality and body weight was shown for endometrial and breast cancer in women. For some localizations of cancer this correlation was not clearly pronounced and sometimes was absent (58).

There is much evidence that a high fat diet promotes carcinogenesis induced by various agents in the skin, mammary gland, liver, intestines, pituitary and lungs (42,103,126). In old rats a high fat diet restores the susceptibility of mammary glands to the carcinogenic effect of NMU and DMBA (48,69).

It should be noted that an excess of carbohydrates in the diet, especially in the early postnatal period, might essentially influence carcinogenesis. In a recent study by Berstein and Alexandrov (37), pregnant rats were given a 10% glucose solution instead of drinking water beginning from the 7th day of their pregnancy. On the 21st day of pregnancy the rats were injected with NMU intraperitoneally at a dose of 20 mg/kg of body weight. For 1.5 months after the delivery, mother rats and their offspring were given a 5% glucose solution instead of drinking water. The authors observed a significant increase in tumor incidence in such progeny as compared to those that had not been given glucose. In male rats, a rise of tumor incidence was registered in the nervous system and kidneys, but in female rats - in mammary glands, pituitary and the hematopoietic system.

The data concerning the interrelation between hypertension and cancer (96) are also of great interest. The rise in arterial blood pressure is a disease closely connected with atherosclerosis and with aging. Pero et al. (105) reported on enhanced unscheduled DNA synthesis induced in lymphocytes by a carcinogen, the enhanced binding of a carcinogen with DNA, and the increased incidence of chromatide breaks in hypertensive patients. This, on the one hand, might contribute to the accumulation of DNA damage causing somatic mutations.

In the previous section, carcinogenic aging was discussed. In fact, sometimes carcinogenic substances promote intensified aging. However, if this is the case, apart from the induction of neoplasms in target tissues, carcinogenic agents must increase the incidence of tumors peculiar to a given strain of animals. In our experiments (10), female rats of the control group developed benign tumors of the mammary gland (fibroadenomas and fibromas, uterus (polyps), endocrine glands (adenomas) in the majority of spontaneous tumors. The total incidence of these spontaneous tumors was 26% and the mean latent period was equal to 738 $\pm$ 25.9 days. Female rats aged 3 months were injected with NMU 4 or 2 times. As a result, apart from mammary adenocarcinomas, kidney, colon and ovarian tumors, the benign tumors pertinent to control females not treated with the carcinogen, were developed by experimental animals in 38 and 25 % of cases, respectively. Their latent period was equal to 295 $\pm$ 24.5 days and 406 $\pm$ 18.0 days, respectively. In other words, NMU-treated female rats developed benign tumors in endocrine glands and hormone-dependent organs much earlier than control ones.

Similar results were obtained in our experiments involving a single injection of methyl(acetoxymethyl)nitrosamine into 3-month old female rats (15).

There is evidence for the enhancement of spontaneous carcinogenesis in F344 rats injected with low (less than 10 ppm) doses of NMU (90). Pregnant ICR/Jcl mice were treated with diethylstilbestrol on the 15th day of their pregnancy, and their offspring showed a significant increase in the incidence of tumors of the lungs and ovaries - i.e. neoplasms pertinent to oncological patterns of this strain of mice (98).

Thus, there is some evidence of the promoting effect of intensified aging on carcinogenesis.

EFFECT OF GEROPROTECTORS IN CARCINOGENESIS

One of the approaches to studying the mechanisms which underly the correlation between aging and tumor development may consist, in our opinion, of estimating the effect on tumor development of experimental influences and drugs, which increase the life span of experimental animals. These preparations are called geroprotectors. About 20 substances were suggested as geroprotectors on the basis of different theories of aging (100). Some of them inhibit tumor development, others affect only its latent period, the rest have no influence on tumor incidence or rate of growth or even cause an increase in these parameters (11).

Based on the analysis of the peculiarities of the geroprotector-induced slowing down of the aging process, Emanuel and Obukhova (62) suggested a classification of geroprotectors. According to this, all influences capable of increasing life span may be divided into three groups: 1) geroprotectors affecting equally the life span of all members of the population, resulting in a parallel shift of the survival curve to the right; 2) geroprotectors decreasing the mortality rate in long-lived individuals and thus increasing maximum life span; and 3) geroprotectors increasing the life span of short-lived individuals without affecting maximum life span.

The influence of geroprotectors on spontaneous carcinogenesis in general depends to a considerable extent on the type of geroprotector action they render (11; Fig. 3).

It may be seen in Table 5 that in mice, type I geroprotectors do not affect the incidence of tumors but only increase the latent period of their development. At the same time, type II geroprotectors decrease not only the rate of aging, but the incidence of tumors as well.

Two stages may be distinguished in the development of mammary adenocarcinomas in these mice. The first one is the stage of initiation when virus-induced cell genome modifications take place. The second one is the stage of promotion, the realization of which culminates in the expression of the malignant phenotype and which depends upon genetically-programmed age-related hormonal, metabolic and immunological changes. Probably it is at the promotion stage of MuMTV-induced mammary tumorigenesis when the antitumor effect of the selenium, the ability to suppress the replication of MuMTV was

TABLE 5

EFFECT OF GEROPROTECTORS ON DEVELOPMENT OF SPONTANEOUS MAMMARY
ADENOCARCINOMAS IN FEMALE MICE

Type of aging delay[a]	Geroprotector	Effect on Tumor latency	Tumor incidence	Ref
I	2-Mercaptoethylamine	Increases	No effect	69
	2-Ethyl-6-methyl-3-oxipyridine	Increases	No effect	62
II	Caloric restriction	Increases	Decreases	126
	Phenformin	Increases	Decreases	55
	Phenytoin	Increases	Decreases	55
	DOPA	No effect	Decreases	55
	Succinic acid	No effect	Decreases	18
	Pineal factor	Increases	Decreases	25
	Thymic factor	Increases	Decreases	25
	Levamisole	Increases	Decreases	39
III	Selenium	No effect	Decreases	95

[a] According to Emanuel and Obukhova (62)

suggested (95). It should be noted that other antioxidants such as
2-mercaptoethylamine or 2-ethyl-6-methyl-3-oxipyridine did not
affect the incidence of mammary tumors but only increased their
latent period.

In the rat, inherent spontaneous carcinogenesis seems to be
dependent on the realization of aging per se. The environmental
carcinogenic factors (background radiation, viruses, contamination
of food, water or air with chemical carcinogens or their precursors,
etc.) which are subjected to control, at least in principle, seem to
work at random. From this point of view, the apparent differences
in the characteristics of the effects of geroprotectors on the
development of spontaneous tumors (Table 6) seem to depend on the
mechanism of their geroprotector action.

According to this, all geroprotectors may be classified in two
main groups. The first group includes the preparations which

294

prevent stochastic injury of macromolecules. The theoretical basis
for using these preparations is provided for by variants of the
"catastrophe errors" theory, which regards aging as a result of the
accumulation of stochastic damage. The second group includes
preparations and influences which are thought to slow down the
program of aging and development of age-related pathology.

TABLE 6

EFFECT OF GEROPROTECTORS ON DEVELOPMENT OF SPONTANEOUS TUMORS IN
RATS

Type of aging delay(a)	Geroprotector	Effect on Tumor latency	Tumor incidence	Ref
I	Procaine (Gerovital)	No effect	No effect	33
II	Caloric restriction	Increases	Decreases	115,116
	phenformin	Increases	Decreases	12
	Buformin	Increases	Decreases	9
	Pineal factor	Increases	No effect	56
	Tryptophan-deficient diet	No data	Decreases	122
	Phenytoin	No effect	Decreases	9
III	EDTA	No data	Increases	59
	Tocopherol (Vit E):			
	benign tumors	Increases	Increases	110
	malignant tumors	Increases	Decreases	110
	Selenite: malignant tumors	No data	Increases	44,120
	Tritium oxide (low doses)	No data	Increases	97

(a) According to Emanuel and Obukhova (62)

Antioxidants are the most typical representatives of the first
group. Their geroprotector and antitumor effects depend upon the
age at which their administration is begun and inversely depend upon
the dose of the damaging agent. Antioxidants are sometimes thought
not to slow down aging *per se* but to inhibit the action of the
environmental factors which decrease the survival of control

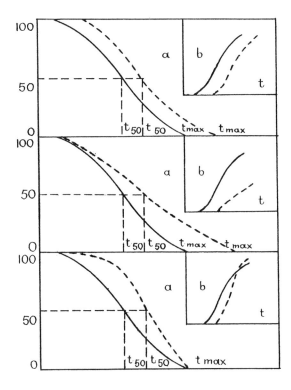

Fig. 3: Types of changes in survival (a) and tumor yield (b) curves
caused by geroprotectors. I - III: types of aging delay according
to Emanuel and Obukhova (62). Ordinate: a, surviving, %; b, tumor
yield, %; abscissa: time. Solid line - control, dashed line -
geroprotector.

(intact) animals by, say, preventing the action of dietary
components capable of producing free radicals (84). The tumor
inhibiting effect of antioxidants is more pronounced in the case of
carcinogenesis which is induced externally, by chemical carcinogens,
for example (13°).

The second group of geroprotectors is represented by
antidiabetic biguanides phenformin and buformin, pineal factor and
caloric restricted diet. These influences cause diverse effects on
the hormonal, metabolic and immunological parameters of an organism,
causing the normalization of their age-dependent shifts and thus
rendering their antitumor effect (10,13). It should be noted that
these influences were also capable of a pronounced inhibition of
chemical and radiation-induced carcinogenesis (Table 7).

TABLE 7

EFFECT OF SOME GEROPROTECTORS ON INDUCED CARCINOGENESIS IN RATS

Carcinogen	Drug	Total tumor incidence %	Main tumor localisation	Incidence of tumors of main site	Ref
DMBA, i.v.	Control	97.3	Mammary gland	81.1	27
	Buformin	54.4*		36.4*	
	Phenytoin	71.0*		55.3*	
	Pineal factor	80.0		25.7*	
	DOPA	50.0*		25.0*	
DMBA, i.v.	Control	96.9	Mammary gland	68.8	24
	Thymus factor	72.8*		18.2*	
NMU, i.v.	Control	100.0	Mammary gland	71.4	19
	Phenformin	75.0*		37.5*	
NMU,trans- placentally	Control	54.2	Nervous system	33.3	2
	Buformin	27.0		9.5*	
DMH, s.c.	Control	94.7	Colon	94.7	30
	Phenformin	90.8		90.8**	
Total body X-ray	Control	74.1	Malignant tumor at different sites	36.2	26
	Thymus factor	69.4		18.9*	
	Pineal factor	57.9		13.2*	
Total body X-ray	Control	78.0	Malignant tumors at different sites	42.0	23
	Phenformin	48.0*		30.0	

* Differences with control is significant, p > 0.05.
** Treatment with phenformin reduced the multiplicity of colon cancer and mean tumor size.

Of course, this classification is not absolute. It was shown, for instance, that some antioxidants were able to enhance immune reactions in old mice (72,91).

The comparison of the data on the type of the slowing-down of aging and the character of the antitumor effect of geroprotectors (Fig. 3) permits us to suggest that the tumor incidence of a certain age is the function of the rate of aging. Taking into consideration the exponential dependence of mortality on age and the data of Dix et al. (57) showing that the same dependency may exist between age and cancer incidence, we calculated a value of correlation between the parameters characterizing rate of aging and tumor development in animals (13,16).

A highly significant positive correlation was found between the aging rate of the rat populations and rates of age-related increase of tumor incidence in these populations (malignant tumors, in particular), while no positive correlation between mean life span and tumor incidence was found. Fig. 3 illustrates this conclusion. It may be seen that different types of slowing-down of aging may be associated with similar increases of mean life span. These results lead to the conclusion that the incidence of tumors and the rate of its age-related increase directly depend upon the rate of aging of a population. This dependence, together with the data that environmental factors which promote tumor growth (over-feeding, constant illumination, chemical carcinogens, ionizing radiation, etc.) may cause an acceleration of aging, suggests that the rate of aging in these cases may be a function of the dose of carcinogenic agent.

We believe that the data presented above permit us to consider possible causes of the increase in cancer incidence in the present century. The survival curves of human populations were noted to become more and more "rectangular" (47,75). This is caused first of all by the decrease in child and early mortality which is connected with tuberculosis and other infectious and non-infectious diseases. As a result, a significant increase in the mean life in human populations occurred, while the maximum of human life span has stayed the same for centuries (47).

Thus, the changes in the shapes of the survival curves of human populations respond to third type of aging delay according to the classification of Emanuel and Obukhova (62). The changes of this type were shown experimentally and epidemiologically to be associated with an increase in tumor incidence. In other words, for the increase in mean life span achieved by the decrease in mortality at an early age, mankind pays at a later age by an increased risk of cancer or some other disease of civilization like atherosclerosis or diabetes mellitus.

We believe that further progress in modern preventive medicine is impossible without radical changes in approaches to public health and to prolongation of the human life span. In the burst of industrialization, urbanization, and increasing environmental pollution, one may only hope for a partial alleviation of their unfavourable effects on human health. The achievement of more significant results in this field will require the solution of very complex scientific and technical problems as well as considerable economic expense.

It is probably true that, even at present, changes in life-style, i.e. dietary and sexual habits, smoking and alcohol consumption, etc., may be the most promising approach to achieving a decrease in cancer incidence and, hence, an increase in life-span (74,127). It seems to become more and more clear that the measures which normalize the age-related changes in hormonal status, metabolism and immunity, and thus slow down the realization of the genetic program of aging (not postponing aging but decelerating the rate of it) must be most effective in protection from aging and prevention of cancer development. The influences which protect from the initiating action of damaging agents (anti-oxidants, antimutagens) may be important additional means of prophylaxis of cancer and accelerated aging, especially under conditions of increased risk of being exposed to damaging environmental factors.

REFERENCES

1. Alexander P, Connell DI (1960) Radiat Res 12:38

2. Alexandrov SN (1982) In: Late Radiation Pathology of Mammals, Akademic-Verlag, Berlin

3. Alexandrov VA, Anisimov VN (1976) Vopr Onkol 11:98

4. Alexandrov VA, Anisimov VN, Belous NM, Vasiljeva IA, Mazon VB (1980) Carcinogenesis 1:975

6. Anisimov VN (1971) Vopr Onkol (1971) 8:67

7. Anisimov VN (1972) In: Blastomogenesis in persistent estrus rats. Diss Cand Med Sci, NN Petrov Research Institute of Oncology, Leningrad

8. Anisimov VN (1976) Vopr Onkol 8:98

9. Anisimov VN (1980) Vopr Onkol 6:42

10. Anisimov VN (1981) Exp Path 19:81

11. Anisimov VN (1981) Uspekhi Sovrem Biol 92:455

12. Anisimov VN (1982) Farmakol Toksikol 45:127

13. Anisimov VN (1983) Adv Cancer Res 40:365

14. Anisimov VN (1983) IARC Sci Publ 51:99

15. Anisimov VN (1983) In: Experimental study of peculiarities of carcinogenesis in different age periods. Diss Doc Med Sci, NN Petrov Research Institute of Oncology, Leningrad

16. Anisimov VN (1984) Dokl Acad Nauk SSSR 275:222

17. Anisimov VN (1985) IARC Sci Publ 58:123

18. Anisimov VN, Kondrashova MN (1979) Dokl Acad Nauk SSSR 248:1242

19. Anisimov VN, Lvovich EG (1976) Vopr Onkol 2:55

20. Anisimov VN, Belous NM, Vasiljeva IA, Dilman VM (1980) Eksp Onkol 3:40

21. Anisimov VN, Belous NM, Vasiljeva IA, Mazon VG (1980) Probl Endokr 5:70

22. Anisimov VN, Belous NM, Vasiljeva IA (1981) Akush Gynekol 5:53

23. Anisimov VN, Belous NM, Prokudina EA (1982) Eksp Onkol 6:26

24. Anisimov VN, Danetskaya EV, Morozov VG, Khavinson VKh (1980) Dokl Acad Nauk SSR 250:1485

25. Anisimov VN, Khavinson VKh, Morozov VG (1982) Mech Ageing Dev 19:245

26. Anisimov VN, Miretski GI, Morozov VG, Khavinson VKh (1982) Bull Exp Biol Med 94: 80

27. Anisimov VN, Ostroumova MN, Dilman VM (1980) Bull Exp Biol Med 88:723

28. Anisimov VN, Pozdeev VK, Dmitrievskaya AYu, Gracheva GM, Il'in AP, Dilman VM (1976) Bull Exp Biol Med 82:1473

29. Anisimov VN, Pozdeev VK, Dmitrievska AYu, Gracheva GM, Il'in AP, Dilman VM (1977) Vopr Onkol 7:34

30. Anisimov VN, Pozharisski KM, Dilman VM (1980) Vopr Onkol 8:54

31. Antecol MH, Mukherjee BB (1982) Cancer Res 42:3870

32. Aschheim P (1976) In: Hypothalamus, Pituitary and Aging, AV Everitt & Burgess JA, Eds, Thomas, Springfield, 376

33. Aslan A, Vrabiescu A, Domilescu C, Campeanu L, Costiniu M, Stanescu S (1965) Gerontol 20:1

34. Balmain A (1985) Br J Cancer 51:1

35. Bach JA, Vogel D (1984) Mech Ageing Dev 24:49

36. Berstein LM (1981) Human Physiol 7:360

37. Berstein LM, Alexandrov VA (1984) Cancer Lett 25:171

38. Bokhman JV, Anisimov VN, Volkova AT, Umenushkina LN, Polushina NA (1980) In: Oncological Aspects of Anovulation . Bokhman JV, Eds, Pskov:21

39. Bruley-Rosset M, Florentin I, Kiger N, Schulz JI, Mathé G (1980) Recent Results Cancer Res 75:139

40. Burnet FM (1970) Progr Exp Tumor Res 13:1

41. Cairns J (1982) Natl Cancer Inst Monograh 60:237

42. Carrol KK, Khor HT (1975) Progr Biochem Pharmacol 10:308

43. Chen HW (1984) Fed Proc 43:126

44. Cherkes LA, Aptekar SG, Volgarev MN (1962) Bull Exp Biol Med 53 (3):78

45. Conklin JW, Upton AC, Christenberry KW, McDonald TP (1963)

Radiat Res 19:156

46. Craddock VW (1981) Interactions 35:139

47. Cutler RG (1976) J Human Evolution 5:169

48. Dao TL, Chan PC (1983) J Natl Cancer Inst 71:201

49. Deichman GI (1983) IARC Sci Publ 51:113

50. Dilman VM (1968) In: Aging, Climateric and Cancer, Meditsina, Leningrad

51. Dilman VM (1971) Lancet 1:1211

52. Dilman VM (1978) Mech Ageing Dev 8:153

53. Dilman VM (1980) Vestnik Akad Med Nauk SSSR 7:86

54 .Dilman VM (1981) In: The Law of Deviation of Homeostasis and
Diseases of Aging, Wright, Boston

55. Dilman VM , Anisimov VN (1980) Gerontolgy 26:241

56. Dilman VM, Anisimov VN, Ostroumova MN, Khavinson VKh, Morozov
VG (1979) Exp Path 17:539

57. Dix D, Cohen P, Flannery J (1980) J Theor Biol 83:163

58. Doll R, Peto R (1981) J Natl Cancer Inst 66:1193

59. Dubina TL, Razumovich AN (1975) In: Introduction in Experimental Gerontology, Nauka i Tekhnika, Minsk

60. Dunjic A (1964) Nature 203:887

61. Ebbesen P (1984) Mech Ageing Dev 25:269

62. Emanuel NM, Obukhova LK (1978) Exp Geront 13:25

63. Epstein CJ, Martin GM, Schultz AL, Motulsky AG (1966)
Medicine (Baltimore) 45:177

64. Finch CE, Hayflick L, Eds (1977) In: Handbook of the Biology
of Aging, Van Nostrand Reinhold Co, New York

65. Francis AA, Lew WH, Regan JD (1981) Mech Ageing Dev 16:181

66. Gravilov LA (1984) In: Results in Sciences and Technique.
Ser. General Problems in Biology. Vol 4. Biological Problems
of Aging. NM Emanuel & TL Nadjarjan, Eds, All-Union Inst
Sci-Tech Inform, Moscow, 135

67. Gravilov LA, Gravilova NS, Nosov VN (1983) Gerontology
29:176

68. Gensler HLN, Berstein H (1981) Quart Rev Biol 56:279

69. Harman D (1972) Am J Clin Nutr 25:839

70. Harper AE (1982) Am J Clin Nutr 36:737

71. Hart RW, Setlow RB (1974) Proc Natl Acad Sci USA 71:2169

72. Heidrick ML, Hendricks LC, Cook DE (1984) Mech Ageing Dev
27:341

73. Hierowski M, Madon J (1968) Biochim Biophys Acta 170:425

74. Higginson J (1980) Arch Geschwulstforsch 50:498

75. Hirsch HW (1982) J Theor Biol 98:321

76. Hayflick L (1977) In: Handbook of the Biology of Aging, CE Finch & L Hayflick, Eds, Van Nostrand Reinhold Co, New York, 159

77. Horan MA, Fox RA (1984) Mech Ageing Dev 26:165

78. Ip C (1980) Cancer Res 40:2785

79. Ird EA (1966) In: Follicular Cysts and Dishormonal Tumors, Meditsina, Leningrad

80. Kay MMB, Makinodan T (1981) In: Handbook of Immunology of Aging, CRC Press, Boca Raton

81. Kensler TW, Busby W, Davidson NE, Wogan GN (1976) Cancer Res 36:4647

82. Khaetsky IK (1965) Vopr Eksp Onkol (Kiev) 1:87

83. Kienko LD (1968) In: Biology of Malignant Growth, Diagnostic and Treatment of Tumors. RE Kavetsky, Ed, Kiev, 55

84. Kodell RL, Farmer JH, Littlefield NA (1980) J Environ Path Toxicol 3:69

85. Kohn RR (1971) J Gerontol 26:378

86. Kraemer KH, Lee MM, Scotto J (1984) Carcinogenesis 5:511

87. Lehmann AR (1985) IARC Sci Publ 58:243

88. Lew EA, Garfinkel L (1979) J Chron Dis 32:563

89. Lindop PJ, Rorblat J (1962) Br J Radiol 35:25

90. Maekawa A, Ogiu T, Matsuoka C et al. (1984) Gann 75:117

91. Makinodan T, Albright JW (1979) Mech Ageing Dev 11:1

92. Makarov IA, Fedorova IV (1982) Abstr 4th All-Union Congress of Gerontologists and Geriatrics, Kiev, 239

93. Martin GM (1978) In: Genetic Effects on Ageing, Bergsma D & Harrison DE, Eds, Liss, New York, 5

94. Martin GM (1980) Mech Ageing Dev 7:5

95. Medina D, Shepherd F (1980) Cancer Lett 8:241

96. Miller DG (1980) Cancer 46:1307

97. Muksinova KN, Voronin VS, Kirillova EN et al. (1983) In: Biological Effects of Low-Level Radiation, YuI Moskalev, Ed, Moscow, 70

98. Nomura T, Kanzaki T (1977) Cancer Res 37:1099

99. Nyce J, Weinhouse S, Magee P (1983) Br J Cancer 8:463

100. Obukhova LK (1975) Uspekhi Khimii 44:1914

101. Ohno S, Nagai Y (1978) In: Genetics Effects of Ageing, D Bregsma & DE Harrison, Eds, Liss, New York, 501

102. Old LJ (1981) Cancer Res 41:361

103. Palmer S, Bakshi K (1983) J Natl Cancer Inst 70:1151

104. Penn A, Batastini G, Soloman J, Burns F, Albert R (1981) Cancer Res 41:588

105. Pero RW, Bryngelsson C, Mitelman F, Thulin T, Norden A (1976) Proc Natl Acad Sci USA 73:2496

106. Pero RW, Miller DG, Lipkin M, Markowitz M, Gupta S, Winawer SJ, Euker W, Good R (1983) J Natl Cancer Inst 70:867

107. Peto R, Parish SE, Gray RG (1985) IARC Sci Publ 58:97

108. Peto R, Roe FJC, Lee PN, LevyL, Clack J (1975) Br J Cancer 32:411

109. Pitot HC (1977) Am J Pathol 87:444

110. Porta EA, Joun NS, Nitta RT (1980) Mech Ageing Dev 13:1

111. Raj HG, Venkistasubramanian TA (1974) Environ Physiol Biochem 4:181

112. Rao KN, Shinozuka H, Kunz HW, Gill TJ (1984) Int J Cancer 34:113

113. Razin A, Cedar H (1984) Int Rev Cytol 92:159

114. Riggs AD, Jones PA (1983) Adv Cancer Res 40:1

115. Ross MH, Bras G (1965) J Nutr 87:245

116. Ross MH, Bras G (1971) J Natl Cancer Inst 47:1095

117. Ross MH, Lustbader ED, Bras G (1983) J Natl Cancer Inst 71:947

118. Sacher GA (1977) In: Handbook of the Biology of Aging, CE Finch & L Hayflick, Eds, Van Nostrand Reinhold Co, New York, 582

119. Schofield JD, Davies I (1978) In: Textbook of Geriatric Medicine and Gerontology. JC Broklehurst, Ed, Churchill Livingstone, New York, 37

120. Schroeder HA, Mitchener M (1971) J Nutr 101:1531

121. Schwartz AG, Moore CJ (1977) Exp Cell Res 109:448

122. Segall PE, Timiras PS (1976) Mech Ageing Dev 5:109

123. Slinchak SM (1968) In: Multiple Malignant Tumors, Zdorov'ya, Kiev

124. Strehler BL (1962) In: Time, Cells and Ageing. Acad Press, New York

125. Stukonis MK (1979) Cancer Cumulative Risk - Based on the Three Volumes of Cancer Incidence in Five Continents. IARC Int Techn Rep No 79/004, IARC, Lyon

126. Tannenbaum A, Silverstone H (1953) Adv Cancer Res 1:451

127. Tomatis L (1985) Cancer Lett 26:5

128. Turkevich NM, Kunitsa LK (1964) In: Abstr Sympos Tumors and Organism Petrozavodsk, 67

129. Turkevich NM, Vasnetsova SS, Gutnik NS, Matveichuk JD, Samundjan EM (1982) In: Neuroendocrine System and Experimental Cancer of Mammary Gland. Naukova Dumka, Kiev

130. Vanyushin BF, Zinkovskaya GG, Berdyshev GD (1980) Molecul Biol 14:857

131. Walford RL, Naeiem F, Hall KY, Tam CF, Gatti RA, Medici MA (1983) In: Immunoregulation, N Fabris, E Garaci, J Hadden & Metchison NA, Eds, Plenum Press, New York, 399

132. Wattenberg LW (1985) Cancer Res 45:1

133. Weinberg RA (1983) Sci Amer 249:126

134. Weinstein IB, Gattoni-Celli S, Kirschmeier P, Lambert M, Hsiao W, Backer J, Jeffrey A (1984) In: Cancer Cells. 1. The Transformed Phenotype. AJ Levine, GF Vande Woude, WC Topp, JD Watson, Cold Spring Harbor Lab., 229

135. Zollars PR, Farley WJ, Cogan PS (1983) Fed Proc 421:1042

© 1987 Elsevier Science Publishers B.V. (Biomedical Division)
Concepts and theories in carcinogenesis. A.P. Maskens et al. eds.

CHRONIC STRESS AS A COFACTOR IN CARCINOGENESIS

P. EBBESEN

The Institute of Cancer Research, The Danish Cancer Society, Radiumstationen, DK-8000 Aarhus C, Denmark.

INTRODUCTION

In the last 300 years it has been useful to approach issues of disease in ways which assume a separateness of mind and body functions. This was a necessary step in the evolution of science to eliminate the influence of mysticism. The limitations inherent in such a division of labour have become more apparent in recent years due to rapid advances in immunology and brain research. Of particular interest is the emerging field of psychoneuroimmunology (1,12).

BASIC CONCEPTS

In this presentation adversive stimuli will be called stressors. Here we are dealing with the external factors, such as, death of spouse, divorce, moving, hazards etc.

The stress response is another basic concept. A condition or response of an individual exposed to a certain stressor will vary greatly. Take as an example type A behaviour patterns which in humans involves the tense, over-worked person with deficient deactivation after exposure to a stressor.

Finally, stress can also be considered as the incongruent interaction between the environment and the invidual. In this case, no external event and no psychological structure is a priori harmful. The stressor and the coping mechanisms are both significant. When the interaction between environment and individual is incongruent, the basis for illness, poor prognosis, and poor responsiveness to treatment is present.

More about the stress responses: first of all, stress responses occur both at the psychological and the social level, and stress responses are not disease-specific. Physiologically, there can be changes in hormonal, immunological, and neuroregulatory reactions (1). Psychologically, there are the subjective phenomena of anger and despair. Sociologically, stress responses can include antisocial behaviour.

Complicating the attempt to link stress with cancer, is that some say the level of a certain hormone may have little significance unless it is known how the level of several other hormones is affected. Another point of interest is that certain types of stressors can lead to increased resistance to some diseases and decreased resistance to others (2). In addition, the relationship between acute stress response and long term disease outcome is very little studied.

ANIMAL STUDIES

Animal experiments in nearly all cases have dealt with short-term stressors and monitoring of stress responses for a short period. One might not expect such an approach to give much evidence for or against the effect of stressor on cancer initiation or development.

The literature is confusing but the reviews of Fox (10) and Ader (1) show that stressors can hasten the appearance of spontaneous tumors and speed up the growth of implanted tumors. Most convincing are the studies demonstrating that stressors can hasten the onset of viral cancer in animals. Also in this respect, it is of interest to note that the pronounced influence on virally induced cancer can be obtained with such diverse forms of stressors as noise, unpredictability in mouse handling, and psychosocial conditions.

A growing animal literature shows that when coping can only take the form of giving up, as no other way of influencing the adverse or dangerous situation exists, the animal is prone to disease or death (2).

In short: there are some examples of a modest effect on cancer development of short-lasting stressors, however, chronic or repeated application of stressors might have more pronounced effects, and such experiments might be more relevant to the human situation.

Riley's group in Seattle did some of the very few studies on chronic stress situations. Among other results was the finding of a higher incidence of mammary tumors in mice maintained housed under conditions of daily stress as compared to mice kept in more stable, sheltered environment (14).

Our own experiments are still in progress. Basically, we use chronic psychosocial stress in DBA/2, BALB/c and CBA mice. From the moment of weaning, the animals are grouped either one mouse a box, or 3 or 9 mice a box for life. With 9 mice and to a lesser extent with 3 mice a box we find that males grouped with males develop a hunched posture, low weight, anemia, amyloid in spleen, kidney, and liver, and a reduced life span (6-9)(Fig.1, Table 1). Females are unaffected by the grouping stress. It is important to notice that the adverse effect on the males was independent of whether or not the animals were biting each other.

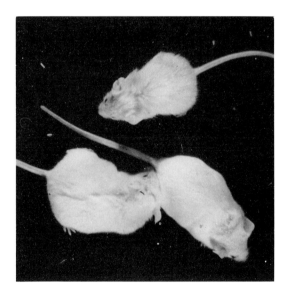

Fig. 1. 3 male BALB/c mice, all 12 months old. The smallest is from a cage with 9 males, the middle-sized from a box with 3, and the healthiest-looking was kept in isolation.

When challenged with murine sarcoma virus, the stressed males were the least resistant (Table 1).

Work is in progress to determine the rank of each male kept 3 or 9 a box and to compare the clinical picture and resistance to cancer induction with rank. It is our expectation that low rank in a small group with a stable hierarchy is associated with better health, than is the case for male mice that are living 9 a box. In the latter chaos situation where no hierarchy can be upheld. All are equally miserable.

TABLE 1

CHRONIC CROWDING STRESS RESULTING IN AMYLOIDOSIS AND SHORTENED LIFE SPAN

	Stress response (life span, amyloidosis)	Growth of murine sarcoma virus induced tumor
Male		
Male alone	0	+
Male with males	+	++
One male with females	0	+
Several males and several females	+	++
Castrated males	(+)	not done
Females		
Isolated	0	
Females with females	0	
Females with males	0	
Castrated	0	

HUMAN CANCER AND STRESS

Research on stress and the causation of cancer in humans is difficult to access. Most investigators did not consider the time lag between initiation of tumor growth and recognition of tumor presence. Furthermore, there is no evidence of a dose-effect relationship, and there is always the danger of retrospective studies that the disease itself is responsible for deviations from data of healthy controls.

A famous prospective study by Thomas (17) where 1130 former Johns Hopkins medical students were followed over 30 years indicated that conflicts in childhood were correlated to cancer incidence later in life. The same year (1979) Shekele (16) reported that a prospective study could correlate depression and incidence of cancer. Shegal (1974) found no increase in cancer incidence of concentration camp survivors, although they had enhanced indidence of cardiovascular disease. Bereavement, however, has consistently been associated with enhanced risk of several diseases, including cancer (4,13,17).

It is noticeable that a recent study of cancer patients in advanced stage of the disease found survival unrelated to psychosocial factors previously determined as predictive of longevity in the general population (5).

FINAL DISCUSSION

Stressors and stress responses seem to influence cancer development in certain instances. To what extent it is cancer initiation or progression is largely unknown. Certain histological types of cancer, e.g. lymphoid tumors and virus induced tumors, are probably more easily influenced than other tumor types.

There is a pressing need to establish good experimental models and to promote prospective human studies. This is an area where preventive measures can be envisioned, and thus an area of concern for ECP.

ACKNOWLEDGEMENTS

This presentation has drawn extensively on a 1984-report prepared by John Schneider, Ph. D., for the Danish Cancer Society.

REFERENCES

1. Ader V. (1981) In: Psychoneuroimmunology. Academic Press.

2. Ader V, Cohen N. (1975) Psychosocial Medicine 37:330-340

3. Ader V. (1976) In: Modern Trends in Psychosocial Medicine. Ed. OW Hill. Butterworth, London, pp. 21-41

4. Bastrop RW, Lazarus L, Luckhurst E. (1977) Lancet I:834-836

5. Cassileth BR, Lusk EJ, Miller DS, Brown LL, Miller C. (1985) New Engl J Med 312:1551-1555

6. Ebbesen P, Rask-Nielsen R. (1967) JNCI 39:917-932

7. Ebbesen P. (1968) J Expt Med 127:387-396

8. Ebbesen P (1972) Acta Path Microbiol Scand Sect B 80:149-159

9. Ebbesen P, Faber T, Fuursted K. (1982) Exp Geront 17:425-428

10. Fox BH. (1983) J Psychosocial Oncol 1:17-32

12. Locke S. (1983) The Mind and the Immune System. An annotated bibliography

13. Parkes CM. (1981) In: Acute Grief. Ed. P Margolis. Columbia Univ Press NY

14. Riley V. (1975) Science 189:465-467

16. Shekele RB, Raynor WJ, Ostfeld AM, Garron DC, Bielianskans Liv

SC, Maliza C, Paul O.   (1981) Psychosomatic Medicine 43:117-125

17.   Schneider JM.   (1984)   In: Stress, Loss, and Grief.   University Park Press, Baltimore, Maryland

18.   Thomas CB,   Dusynski   KR,   Shaffer   JV.   (1979)   Psychosomatic Medicine 41:281-302

© 1987 Elsevier Science Publishers B.V. (Biomedical Division)
Concepts and theories in carcinogenesis. A.P. Maskens et al. eds.

PREVENTION OF VIRUS-ASSOCIATED HUMAN MALIGNANCIES: AN EPIDEMIOLOGICAL VIEW

G. de THE

Faculty of Medicine A. Carrel, Lyon, France.

SUMMARY

Virus-associated cancers prevalent in the developing countries of the intertropical zone, provide a unique opportunity and challenge to consider primary or secondary prevention. Among the four groups of viruses and associated cancers, two represent major international health problems, namely human papilloma viruses (HPV) related cervical cancers and Hepatitis B virus (HBV) associated hepatocellular carcinoma, while two represent research models, namely Epstein-Barr virus (EBV) related Burkitt's lymphoma (BL) and nasopharyngeal carcinoma (NPC) and retrovirus associated proliferations and immuno-deficiencies. Sub-viral vaccines are either already in use for HBV, or experimentally ready for EBV, but assessment of their values in preventing human tumors raises a number of financial and technical difficulties. Early detection through viral markers is at hand for both EBV-related NPC, and HPV-related cervical carcinoma.

Beside virus-oriented interventions, one should consider other co-factors which are known to play a key role in the development of these virus-associated cancers. Among those, foods contaminated either with Aflatoxin B1 in Africa (primary liver cell carcinoma), or with nitrosamines in Asia (nasopharyngeal carcinoma). Last, but not least, one will have to consider individual genetic susceptibility or resistance to viruses or environmental carcinogens, to establish beyond prevention, predictive medicine.

INTRODUCTION

That viruses are causally related to certain malignancies in most animal species and recently to some human cancers has slowly emerged since the pionneering observations of Ellerman and Bang (6) at the dawn of this century. Since cancers are not

TABLE 1
VIRUS AND HUMAN MALIGNANCIES

	RETROVIRUSES	HERPESVIRUSES	HEPADNAVIRUSES	PAPILLOMAVIRUSES
	HTLV/1,II LAV/HTLV-III	EBV HSV-2	HBV	HPV16,18,33,x ?
Genome	Diploid RNA 10^6	DNA 10^8	DNA 10^3	DNA 10^3
	CANCER ASSOCIATED VIRUSES DO NOT HAVE "ONC" BUT TRANSFORMING GENES			
Cell-virus relationship	TAT genes integrat. DNA provirus	transf. genes latent episomal	gene rearrangement integration	transf. gene integration
Assoc. Diseases Mortality/y Morbidity/y	HTLV-I: leuk/lymph. neurological diseases LAV/HTLV-III: AIDS epidemics: 20/30,000 ? EBV or Papill. Ass.Tm.	EBV: polyclonal lymphoproliferations – Burkitt's lymph. – Nasopharyngeal ca. 90,000/y	Primary Liver Ca. 260,000/y Chronic Hepatitis 500,000/y	Genital Ca. Cervix: 460,000/y Vulva-Penis-ENT ?
Epidemiological characteristics	HTLV-I: Endemics SW Japan, Caraib Central Africa LAV/HTLV-III: Epidemic Eq. Africa, USA, Europe	Ubiquitous/world Early age infection	Endemic Eq. Africa South East Asia early age infection	Ubiquitous age effect ?
Cofactors	probably genetic ?	genetic: BL-c-myc environ: BL-malaria NPC: food habits	genetic ? environ: aflatoxin B1	genetic ? environ: HSV-2
Prevention	vaccine ? early detection	vaccine ? early detection: NPC	vaccination being implemented	vaccine ? early detection viral markers/ cytology

contagious, it appeared insane to many researchers that infectious agents could be related to non contagious diseases. This remained the case until Ludwig Gross (9) showed that a common retrovirus in mice could be etiologically related to T cell leukemias, provided that it infects susceptible individuals very early in life. It was further shown that viruses with oncogenic potential usually require a long delay between infection and development of the associated malignancies. These viruses do not replicate in transformed cells, hence the lack of contagiousness of the viral associated tumors.

The main question in the framework of this meeting is to assess the role of viruses within the widely accepted multistep carcinogenic process, operating both at the cellular and organism level. Members of four different families of viruses are involved, namely retroviruses, herpesviruses, hepadnaviruses and papillomaviruses. No "final common way" appears to exist for the different viruses to transform a normal cell into a tumorous one. Rather, as it is the case for other environmental carcinogens, viruses appear to act in different ways and means at various steps of the multistage carcinogenesis process, either in initiating or promoting abnormal growth.

That viruses do not represent the final common way of carcinogenesis does not undermine their critical importance in fundamental as well as in applied cancer research. Furthermore, oncogenic viruses opened a new avenue for controlling certain human malignancies such as genital cancers, liver cell carcinoma and nasopharyngeal carcinoma present in Western Countries and representing major public health problem in developing countries. We shall first present the role of viruses in a number of human cancers, then discuss the possible means to intervene to prevent the clinical emergence of tumors.

COMPARATIVE CHARACTERISTICS OF ONCOGENIC VIRUSES AND ASSOCIATED TUMORS

Table 1 compares the basic characteristics of the four different types of viruses having oncogenic properties in humans, as well as their impact on cancer morbidity, mortality.

Retroviruses which are associated to a number of spontaneous tumors in many animal species and to certain T cell malignancies in humans, usually behave as chronic or latent carcinogenic agents. They exceptionally represent acute transforming agents and in this case contain extra genes of cellular origin named "onc" genes which account for their immediate oncogenic potential. In contrast, slow or chronic retroviruses which do not contain such "onc" genes, exhibit transforming potential through their LTR (long terminal repeat) sequences, acting as CIS-promotors, or through TAT genes (trans-activating transcription) which can activate cellular onc genes situated at distance from the site of integration of the pro-virus.

The prototype of oncogenic herpesviruses in humans is the B lymphotropic EBV, which does not contain onc genes, nor requires integration to express a continuous mitogenic activity , leading to polyclonal expansion of target B lymphocytes. Molecular mechanism of cellular immortalization by EBV is not yet fully understood, but implies sequential steps of transcription and translation, involving at least two EBNA (Epstein-Barr nuclear antigens) genes, initiating and maintaining the transformed state (12). One further EBV gene codes for a cell-surface antigen: the lymphocyte defined membrane antigen (LYDMA) recognized by the immune system, as target for specialized cytotoxic T cells. The pathogenesis of Burkitt's lymphoma appears to imply an early and massive EBV infection in African infants who develop the disease 5 to 9 years after (5). The initiating EBV-related event leads to an expanding B lymphoproliferation, favored by specific immunosuppression of the cytotoxic T cells induced by holo or endemic malaria, as shown by Moss et al. (15). The final step is genetic, involving c-myc activation caused by chromosomal translocations 8:14, 8:22, 8:2 (13).

In nasopharyngeal carcinoma pathogenesis, the EBV oncogenic potential is probably expressed as a late event in the multistep carcinogenic process. This is because NPC develops mostly, if not only, in individuals suffering from a specific reactivation of EBV in nasopharyngeal mucosa (20). Such a reactivation, preceeding tumor development, is possibly linked to environmental factors.

Nitrosamines (11,19,16) could be associated with NPC development. Are nitrosamines or other carcinogens acting independently from the EBV or do they reactivate EBV latency in a specific way leading to tumor development? This remains unanswered. Their known tissue tropism for the epithelial cells of the nasal cavities and upper respiratory tract is to be noted. Up to the present time, no strong genetic factor has been demonstrated for NPC although HLA related genes might represent a risk marker (17,3).

Cellular transformation by hepadnavirus, such as the HBV (which does not appear to contain onc nor transforming genes), may be due to highly specific integration of the viral DNA, close to certain cellular onc type sequences controlling cellular division (18). Co-factors involved in the development of primary liver carcinoma (PLC) are related to food consumption contaminated by Aflatoxin B1 (14). Genetic resistance or susceptibility to HBV and/or to Aflatoxin B_1 may play a role, but no data are available. PLC is responsible for approximately 260,000 deaths a year in Intertropical Africa and South East Asian regions.

The most frequent cancer of viral origin is without contest cervical carcinoma responsible for more than 500,000 new cases annually around the world. Three papilloma viruses (HPV type 16, 18 and 33) among the 45 different types known today are closely associated with this tumor (8), being integrated in the tumorous cells. Whether they contain transforming genes is yet unknown, but no cellular onc sequence is detectable in their small genomes. As in the case of primary liver carcinoma, integration of papillomavirus is a prerequisite and appears to represent by itself a major risk factor for cellular transformation. Other co-factors appear necessary for the development of genital tumors and these might involve environmental and behavioural factors, such as cigarette smoking or genital herpes HSV-2 infection, acting as an initiating factor (21). Genetic factors probably control individual susceptibility or resistance to either viral or chemical co-factors.

PREVENTIVE AVENUES FOR VIRUS-ASSOCIATED TUMORS

Thus, viruses appear as priviledged oncogenic agents, acting each one on their own account, involving different ways and means on the yet to discover fundamental mechanism of oncogenesis. But the most critical question in the framework of the present symposium, is to evaluate the various avenues for CANCER PREVENTION opened by such a viral association. The first question coming to public health oriented minds is to assess the magnitude of the expected impact. A yearly 750 to 900,000 new cases of cancer around the world are associated with one of the above described viruses. If one assumes that such virus-associated malignancies, predominating in the crowded developing countries of the intertropical zone, represent 30 to 45% of incident cancer cases around the world, and estimates that 80% of those could be avoided through antiviral measures, then the impact could be as dramatic as if tobacco-related malignancies could be eliminated.

Three different types of intervention could be envisaged: primary cancer prevention by anti-viral vaccines; secondary prevention by early tumor detection using viral markers; intervention against environmental co-factors. Such interventions will be indeed most efficient on genetically susceptible individuals.

ANTIVIRAL VACCINES

Antiviral vaccines represent the royal avenue of prevention for the technically oriented occidental world. First generation of sub-viral vaccines against hepatitis B virus (HBV) is in use since more than a decade in selected groups in the northern and southern hemispheres (1). Subviral EBV vaccine has been found efficient in an experimental model (7), but has not yet been assessed in humans. Genetically engineered second generation sub-viral vaccines are being developed for HBV and are considered for EBV. Sub-viral vaccine for the human retroviruses is in stage of basic research where the difficulties due to high rate of mutation in the env gene region slow down the progress. Because of the AIDS epidemics and the number of persons at risk both in the industrialized and the developing countries, retrovirus vaccines represent a major research priority. Vaccine development for papillomaviruses is also of great public health importance, but may be hampered by the fact that three antigenically unrelated viruses are involved in genital carcinomas and that humoral immunity against papilloma viruses does not prevent new infection, mainly controlled by avaibility of virions to susceptible basal cells in mucosae.

Two main difficulties arise when considering vaccination against human oncogenic viruses. The first relates to the immunological control of experimental viral infections leading to tumor development in animals. Cell mediated immunity involving specific cytotoxic T-cells and other T-cell subpopulations appear critical to stop the spread of cell-associated viral infections, as observed with herpes and papillomaviruses. Similarly, for retroviral and HBV infections, cell-mediated immune (CMI) mechanisms are determinant for the outcome of these infections. Subviral vaccines, usually made of surface glycoproteins induce a poor CMI response, not as efficient as the natural infection does. Furthermore, the existing and successful animal and human herpes vaccines (Marek disease (2) or varicella-zoster) represent live, attenuated viruses, able to replicate in the host. Such a replicatión is usually associated with a strong cell mediated immune response, which provides active protection against clinical viral diseases. The development of human varicella-zoster virus vaccine indicates that public health authorities are not totally opposed to introducing new viral vaccines of the classical types. With regard to EBV, there is a possibility that the glycoprotein subviral vaccine might induce a poor cell-mediated immunity, unable to prevent the development of BL and NPC. The possibility of using the non-transforming P3HR1 K strains of EBV, as a possible source of attenuated live vaccine should be considered.

The second drawback of viral vaccines with regard to virus-associated human cancer relates to the cost of such vaccines and the financial inability for the concerned countries or continents to consider mass vaccination at the present time. Genetically engineered sub-viral vaccines may represent a major step toward lowering their price. The dilemma between high technology, health needs and lack of resources of the developing world, raises a new challenge for industrial countries and international governmental or non-governmental health organizations.

EARLY DETECTION THROUGH VIRAL MARKERS

Secondary prevention, through early detection of virus-associated tumors, using viral markers, can represent a major step for controlling certain cancers. At present, two situations fall in this category, which could have a major impact in large populations. The first example is that of nasopharyngeal carcinoma: large population surveys in South China, using IgA antibodies to VCA, as immuno-virological marker, permitted to detect NPC at an early stage of clinical development, where specific radiotherapy could lead to excellent survival rate (20).

Three years serological and clinical follow-up of 1,138 normal Chinese individuals having IgA/VCA antibodies in Zangwu county of the Guangxi Autonomous Region of South China, showed that individuals who lost their IgA antibodies did not develop NPC, that individuals who increased their IgA/VCA antibody titer by two dilutions or more, over two years, carried a 20% chance to develop the disease and that individuals who maintained an intermediate titer had 1.3% chance to develop the disease (4). Thus, a very minor fraction of the population (0.1 % of the population aged 35 y or more) carries a major risk for developing NPC and the possibility to carry out antiviral drugs or immuno-therapy trials in the group at highest risk, i.e. increasing their IgA/VCA titers, should be sought.

The second example refers to HPV-associated cervical neoplasias. Dysplasia where HPV-16, 18 or 33 can be detected, should be considered as high risk pre-cancerous lesions and should be treated as such. Such a detection is actually achieved by dot blot analysis, in which DNA extracted from exfoliated cells of the cervix is annealed to complementary viral RNA, to detect the presence of integrated HPV in such cells. This test is carried out in specialized research laboratories and should be incorporated in the near future in the routine cytological cervical smears, whenever severe dysplasias or flat condylomata are clinically observed (see Freese).

INTERVENTION AGAINST CO-FACTORS

Virus-associated cancers, like any other malignancy, result from a multistep process and the question arises whether intervention against co-factors other than viruses could help in controlling these tumors. We saw that anti-viral vaccines have their own problem and that even when available cannot be used widely, mainly because of their prohibitive cost for the countries concerned. The HBV vaccines represent a typical example. Approximately one billion 500 million persons in Asia and Africa are exposed to severe diseases caused by HBV, but only a very small minority can benefit from existing HBV vaccine. The presence of Aflatoxin B1 in daily consumed food represents a critical co-factor in PLC genesis. To my knowledge, no serious intervention to improve storage of crops favoring the growth of Aspergillus flavius has been implemented. No doubt that any change of habits implies a long, laborious and often deceiving process, but in the end represents the cheapest and a most efficient way to improve health. It is difficult to assess the proportion of PLC which could be prevented in this way, but Peers et al. (personal communication) have shown in Swaziland that Aflatoxin consumption emerges as the most critical determinant of geographical variation of PLC.

In nasopharyngeal carcinoma, besides EBV, other co-factors are associated with certain ethnic life styles, where food habits appear to play a key role (10). The presence of nitrosamines in preserved foods, daily consumed as described above, in South China and in North Africa (16), opens a new opportunity for assessing the possibility of modifying, possibly through minor changes, the mode of preparation of such preserves, eliminating highest exposure to nitrosamines. The wide variations observed in nitrosamine contents between dried fish preparation in South China and Greenland and between Touklia and Harissa preparation in Tunisia (16), suggest that modification in the preparation of such foods might lead to important effect on NPC incidence.

In the case of genital cancers, there is no doubt that beside the human papilloma viruses, other co-factors associated with hygiene play a critical role. The intervention of chemical carcinogens associated with bacterial, fongic infections of the genital tract, may be important. Reinforcing hygiene by education may have a major impact in developing countries, where genital cancers prevail. In the industrialized countries, one should look for genetic factors controlling susceptibility or resistance to either viruses or co-factors associated with a given tumor.

Predictive medicine, a notion promoted by J. Ruffié and J. Dausset, is based on characterizing genetic risk factors to develop certain diseases, as well as genetic markers of resistance or susceptibility to environmental agents (biological or chemical). Such an approach will need long term prospective studies on large populations, but represents a new and very promising field for decreasing the unbearable cost of medical care in the western world.

REFERENCES

1. Blumberg BS (1984) In: Virus-Associated Cancers in Africa. Williams A, O'Conor G, de Thé G, et al (eds), IARC Scientific Publications 63, Lyon,pp 243-263

2. Calnek BW (1982) Develop Biol Stand 52: 401-405

3. Chan SH, Day NE, Kunaratnam N, et al (1983) Int J Cancer 32: 171-176

4. de-Thé G, Zeng Y (1986) In: "The Epstein-Barr Virus. Recent Advances". Epstein MA, Achong B (eds), William Heinemann Medical Books, London, pp 236-249

5. de-Thé G, Geser A, Day NE, et al (1978) Nature 274: 756-761

6. Ellermann Y, Bang O (1908) Centralbl f Bakt Abt 1 (Orig) 46: 595-609

7. Epstein MA, Morgan AJ, Finerty S, et al (1985) Nature 318: 287-289

8. Gissman L, Boshart M, Durst M, et al (1984) J Invest Dermat 83: 26-28

9. Gross L (1951) Proc Soc Exp Biol Med 78: 27-32

10. Hubert A, de-Thé G, Nasopharyngeal carcinoma: an anthropological approach to environmental factors, (Submitted)

11. Huang DP, Gough TA, Ho JHC (1978) In: Nasopharyngeal Carcinoma: Etiology and Control, de-Thé G, Ito Y, Davis W (eds), IARC Scientific Publications, Lyon, 20: 309-314

12. Kieff E, Hennessy K, Fennewald S, et al (1985) In: Burkitt's Lymphoma: A Human Cancer Model. Lenoir G, O'Conor G, Olweny CLM (eds), IARC Scientific Publications 60, Lyon, pp 323-339

13. Leder P (1985) In: Burkitt's Lymphoma: A Human Cancer Model. Lenoir G, O'Conor G, Olweny CLM (eds), IARC Scientific Publications 60, Lyon, pp 341-357

14. Linsell CA, Peers FG, (1977) In: Origins of Human Cancer. Hiatt HH, Watson JD, Winsten JA (eds), Cold Spring Harbor Conferences on Cell Proliferation, Cold Spring Harbor Laboratory, vol. 4: 549-557

15. Moss DJ, Burrows SR, Castelino DJ, et al (1983) Int J Cancer 31: 727

16. Poirier S, Ohshima H, Bourgade MC, et al Volatile nitrosamine levels in common foods from Tunisia, South China and Greenland, high risk areas for nasopharyngeal carcinoma. (Submitted)

17. Simons MJ, Wee GB, Day NE et al (1974) Int J Cancer 13: 122-134

18. Tiollais P, Pourcel C, Dejean A (1985) Nature 317: 489-495

19. Yu MC, Ho JHC, Lai SH et al (1986) Cancer Res 46: 956-961

20. Zeng Y, de-Thé G (1985) In: Epstein-Barr Virus and Associated Diseases, Levine PH, Ablashi DV, Pearson GR et al (eds), Martinus Nijhoff Publishing, Boston, Dordrecht, Lancaster, pp 151-163

21. Zür Hausen H (1982) Lancet ii: 1370-1372

INDEX OF AUTHORS